"I'm a medical journalist, consumer, mother of four grown children, and now a grandmother, and all of these roles color my point of view. I've always hated people telling me what to do, so I've written a book in which no one tells you what to do, either. Instead, I provide you with the information you need to make your own decisions . . . I also explain medical options in detail, including both their risks and benefits."

—Diana Korte,
from the Introduction

More praise for *Every Woman's Body*

"*Every Woman's Body* is exceptionally interesting, accurate, comprehensive, unbiased, and positive. It is the only book I know that covers both sides of the controversial issues, like abortion, and lets the reader choose. It is an excellent sourcebook for all women and health professionals alike."
—Lucy R. Waletzky, M.D.
Co-founder and Co-director,
Medical Illness Counseling Center,
Chevy Chase, Maryland

"Diana Korte's book is a valuable tool for women who are trying to take control of their own health."

—Sara Paretsky

EVERY WOMAN'S BODY

EVERYTHING YOU NEED TO KNOW TO MAKE INFORMED CHOICES ABOUT YOUR HEALTH

DIANA KORTE

FAWCETT COLUMBINE · NEW YORK

A Fawcett Columbine Book
Published by Ballantine Books

Copyright © 1994 by Diana Korte
Illustrations Copyright © 1994 by Dana Burns-Pizer

All rights reserved under International and
Pan-American Copyright Conventions. Published in the
United States by Ballantine Books, a division of Random House,
Inc., New York, and simultaneously in Canada by
Random House of Canada Limited, Toronto.

Grateful acknowledgment is made to *Ms.* Magazine
for permission to reprint
an excerpt from "Bodily Harm — Help for Women
Trapped in the Binge-Purge Cycle," by Pamela Eren.
Copyright © 1985 by *Ms.* Magazine.
Reprinted by permission.

Library of Congress Catalog Card Number: 94-94047

ISBN: 0-345-38652-3

Cover design by Kathleen Lynch

Text design by Holly Johnson

Manufactured in the United States of America

First Edition: July 1994

10 9 8 7 6 5 4 3 2

To Juliana, who helped me with this book more than anyone else, and who is the finest daughter a mother could have. May she and my daughters-in-law — Deborah, Jillian, and Kuniyo — always know that they have choices. Here are these four women, left to right.

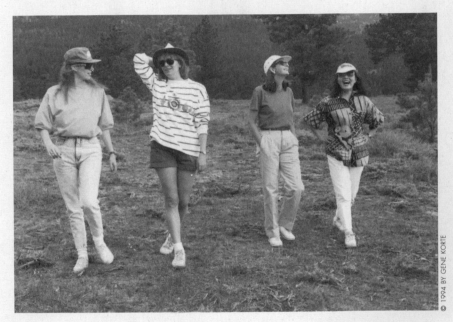

Contents

ACKNOWLEDGMENTS

I thank Gene, of course. He makes everything possible and, besides, he was a good blind date. I include our four kids here because their rearing taught me about consumer health care. And now that they're older, they help me in other ways as well.

Juliana spent many an hour in libraries, while coping with her worries that she either did have or soon would have at least one of the maladies mentioned in this book. Neil kept the house running smoothly in the early years of the project, while occasionally surviving the dusty levels of a library for the cause. Aren with his peerless research skills and investigative tendencies spent much time in libraries for me as well. Drew and Kuniyo and Aren and Jillian continued my consumer health education by bringing my wonderful grandchildren, Akio and Hope, into the world. A special thanks, of course, to all three daughters-in-law — Deborah, Jillian, and Kuniyo — for their editorial comments, wit, and affection.

I thank the following colleagues: Pam Novotny for reading manuscript pages early on, Genevieve Paulson for helping me see the path, Karen Pryor for her good advice, Judy Sanders for her constant friendship, and Lucy Waletzky for her insights. I'm indebted to Lynn Seligman, matchmaker for this project, and to Ballantine's Joëlle Delbourgo, who, in asking me to write this book, became its godmother. Appreciation goes to all the other

Ballantine helpers, known and unknown, including my many editors—
"Book Doctor" Nellie Sabin, Sherri Rifkin, Lynn Rosen, Nancy van Itallie,
and Jane Bess Wooten—illustrator Dana Burns-Pizer and this project's
managing editor, Stephen McNabb.

And where would this project be without IBM, the company that
carefully transported my files through two international moves? Part of this
book was written while living in Europe and discovering the wider world
of other health care systems, not just our own. I am grateful, too, to Fran
Carpentier at *Parade* magazine who insisted on double-checked sources
years ago and Tom Wicker, formerly of *The New York Times,* for telling me
to search for the hidden story. Special thanks go to primo medical reviewer,
Bob Rountree, a physician who not only does his homework, but who also
has "heart."

I thank the women whose stories I've told, including the letter-writers
to my co-authored book, *A Good Birth, A Safe Birth.* Appreciation also goes
to those whose comments were originally published elsewhere in the following newspapers and magazines: *Boulder Daily Camera, Esquire, Isthmus of
Madison, Medical Self-Care, Mothering, Ms., People's Doctor,* and the *Washington
University* Magazine. Also, a thank you to the newsletters of these organizations: American Anorexia/Bulimia Association, Anorexia Nervosa & Related Eating Disorders, Inc., Endometriosis Association, International
Cesarean Awareness Network, and the National Women's Health Network.

I'm indebted to all of the women who wrote the books that preceded
mine, who described the politics of women's health care so thoroughly that
I didn't need to. They allowed me the freedom to say to you, the reader:
We don't have to be mad about our health care treatment anymore. We just
have to make it our own. Thanks, too, to the thousands of dedicated
researchers throughout the world who, with little recognition, regularly
publish important information in obscure journals.

Much of the information that includes numbers or percentages came
from the United States government, often the National Center for Health
Statistics (NCHS), along with the Centers for Disease Control and Prevention and the National Institutes of Health, among others. I am especially
indebted to researchers at the NCHS, in particular Paul Placek, for his help
with childbirth data, his advice and guidance on accessing and evaluating
government information, and his suggestions for finding other resources.
I am grateful, too, to Selma Taffel, William Pratt and William Mosher,
Robert Hartford, Mary Moien, Sam Notzon, Bob Pokras, Stephanie Ven-
tura, Ron Wilson, and others at NCHS for their many hours of help.

Among the other organizations and their public information officers to
whom I say thanks are the American Public Health Association, the American College of Obstetricians and Gynecologists, and the American Medical

Association. These are the three organizations, among many, that I've contacted the most.

In addition, I'm grateful to the following for many forms of past and present assistance and have listed them alphabetically: the anonymous medical reviewers who didn't always agree with me, Trisha Bosak, L. Joseph Butterfield, the late Janet Chusmir, Jean and Andy Greensfelder, Molly Griesen, La Leche League International, John Meyer, midwives everywhere, Roberta Scaer, and all those I may have unintentionally overlooked.

I've used libraries in many states and countries, but the two I have used the most are the University of Colorado's Norlin Library in Boulder and the Boulder Public Library. Thank you to David Fagerstrom and his staff at the CU library. At the Boulder Public Library, I'm grateful to Carla Gustafson-Reardon and her colleagues. And in particular, my appreciation goes to the women in the Reference Room who, with nary a complaint, answered hundreds of questions for me — Beth Armstrong, Barbara Buchman, Jane Perlmutter, Lynn Reed, Connie Walker, and Judy Waller.

And a final tip of the hat to naysayers and all those who made me more careful than I might otherwise have been by their criticisms.

EVERY WOMAN'S BODY

INTRODUCTION

The body changes from one decade to another and from one life-style to another, just as it changes when you are ill. There is no single "Lifetime Plan" that will suit all your needs over time, and there is no one medical treatment that will always be right for all women. At different stages in your life, you may find that you need to change what you eat, choose a different method of birth control, or embrace a little-known alternative health care option. No one path is best for everyone. Only you will know what's best and normal for you. That's why it's important for everyone to be aware of the choices available in health care today.

I'm not a health care professional. I'm a medical journalist, consumer, mother of four grown children, and now a grandmother, and all of these roles color my point of view. I've always hated people telling me what to do, so I've written a book in which no one tells you what to do, either. Instead, I provide you with the information you need to make your own decisions. Whenever possible, I describe ways in which you can doctor yourself—for example, preventive measures you can take or home remedies you can try. In addition, I also explain medical options in detail, including both their risks and benefits.

The women's health groups that I participated in for years taught me that women know best about women's health issues. I also learned that the information resources you need to make most health care choices are available. In this book I've compiled enough material to enable you to make informed choices about many aspects of your health, no matter what your age or life-style might be.

Most women get health information from the media, not just from doctors, friends, and family. However, most newspaper, TV, and radio reporters get much of their information from only a few medical journals. That's why you'll notice my information is often different. I used as wide an array of sources as I could, including not only information from the medical establishment, but also the results of up-to-date international research published in more than 400 medical journals, hundreds of books, and dozens of magazines, newspapers, and newsletters. I also drew on correspondence and conversations with women, health care providers, and researchers in twenty countries. You'll find hundreds of women's personal stories in this book — women explaining in their own words what did or didn't work for them. These quotes all came directly from conversations with women or from printed sources.

Many comprehensive health care books are written by traditional doctors in a "this is what you're going to get" tone. Then there are books, often written by consumers, which, although helpful, lean toward doctor-bashing. Either group may have books that make readers feel sick because the implied messages are that your body is your enemy, not your friend, and that it's impossible to do all the "right" things for good health.

Blaming someone — you or the doctor — is not the issue. I think it's time for a new-generation women's health book, one that offers you choices in a nonjudgmental way and empowers you so that you can build on the life-style you've already chosen and find your own ongoing passage to good health.

This book has four major sections. Part I is aimed at helping you stay healthy. It includes descriptions of the female body and how it functions, as well as information on the kinds of everyday life-style choices that affect our immune system and, more than we sometimes realize, determine whether we're well or sick. There's also a discussion of doctors, hospitals, and common medical tests and how to get what you want from all three. Finally, this section describes the health needs of women who are often overlooked: poor and disabled women, caregivers, and women who are or have been abused.

Part II, the largest part of the book, is an alphabetical guide in which you'll find descriptions of 39 health issues that were chosen either because they mostly affect women (pregnancy, birth control, osteoporosis) or they affect women differently than men (AIDS, cancer, heart disease). I approached all the research and data with one basic question: "How does this affect women?"

Over a lifetime no one of us avoids illness, even if only the occasional cold or flu, because a preventive life-style is not enough to keep us healthy all of the time. If you are faced with making decisions about any of the issues in Part II, each entry will give you an overview of what you need to know, including a rundown of the options available. Whenever a subject is controversial, I present the facts and let you make up your own mind. Examples are why doctors love the birth-control pill . . . and women often leave it; Alzheimer's and the aluminum connection; and why some women get depressed after a cesarean and some don't.

Part III is a Resource Directory that lists nearly 400 organizations that will give you information about different topics. Many provide referrals to local groups or health care providers; some offer publications and other materials; dozens maintain hot lines for support and immediate help.

If you want more information, Part IV lists my recommendations for further reading. It's been my experience with other projects that some of you will want to not only know where I got my information, but also where you can go for more. For you, Recommended Reading lists books and articles I've compiled.

The source notes partly answer the question that you ought to be asking me about this material, namely, What is your information based on? Like all authors, I select some sources and reject others. I owe it to you, however, to display my list. And for those of you who want the rest of the answer, see page 625 for information on how to obtain a complete set of the source notes (about 500 manuscript pages).

If you're on a quest for more information, be aware that you can find medical journal articles at most state university or medical school libraries, both of which usually are open to the public. You may also want to use the computerized search systems that they have, in particular Medline, one of several such data bases I used extensively for this book. Your local library will have most of the magazine and newspaper articles. (If you want to hire someone else to do your homework on a particular topic, see "Research Services" on page 593 in the Resource Directory.)

If there's something you especially like, or if you have other comments, please let me know. Use the "Here's What I Think" questionnaire at the back of the book.

A Note on Gender: Because the enrollment of women in medical schools has increased fourfold in the last twenty years, and women are already the majority in some health care specialties, I've used female pronouns when referring to medical providers throughout this book.

One last comment. Take only what works for you from this book and ignore the rest.

PART I

YOUR PASSAGE TO GOOD HEALTH

CHAPTER 1

YOUR BODY AND ITS SYSTEMS

Our bodies are composed of systems that work together. If we understand how these systems function and incorporate the steps that keep them functioning at their best, we are more likely to live with vitality. Here are brief descriptions of the eight major body systems.

THE IMMUNE SYSTEM

The immune system is our defense against invaders such as viruses and bacteria. The first barriers against these substances include skin, nose hairs, and mucus in the nose and throat. The second barrier is composed of cells that clean away the detritus (unlike red blood cells, which carry food and oxygen). If unwelcome microscopic objects overcome the first two barriers, they are met by a third barrier, the antibodies. These substances are produced by the body to fight serious invaders — for example, the human immunodeficiency virus (HIV) that causes Acquired Immune Deficiency Syndrome (AIDS).

The mastermind of the immune system is the *thymus gland*, located

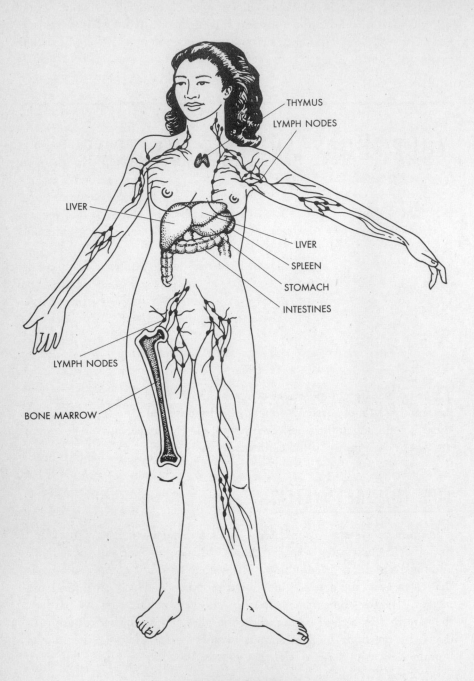

THYMUS

LYMPH NODES

LIVER

LIVER

SPLEEN

STOMACH

INTESTINES

LYMPH NODES

BONE MARROW

IMMUNE SYSTEM

behind the breast bone. When functioning correctly, the thymus gland knows what belongs in the body and what does not. When the thymus and other parts of the immune system are not functioning correctly, however, it's possible for someone to develop one of the 40 or so *autoimmune diseases* (for example, allergies, lupus, or rheumatoid arthritis) in which the body's own antibodies attack other cells, causing a "civil war."

Many different parts of the body make valuable contributions to the immune system, including bone marrow (the factory for blood cells), the lymph nodes, the liver, spleen, stomach, and intestines. When our immune system is functioning at its best, all three layers of its defense mechanism work together to keep us from succumbing to a variety of ailments. Sometimes body invaders (flu and cold viruses, for example) overwhelm the immune systems of even the healthiest people. In addition, our genetic inheritance can make our bodies susceptible to ailments, such as migraine headaches, allergies, or arthritis.

But for most of us, the biggest influence on the health of our immune system is not our ancestors or killer viruses, but our everyday life-style habits — loosely defined as some combination of what we eat and drink, how active we keep our bodies, and how much we enjoy life. You'll see references throughout the book about the effect of certain practices (for example, smoking or eating a vitamin-rich diet) that can either suppress or boost the immune system, that is, literally decrease or increase the number of our white blood cells — our second barrier of immune defense. (See "How to Stay Healthy" on page 25 for specific information on how to keep your immune system up to par.)

It's believed by some researchers that women have superior immune systems, the result of a double dose of immune-regulating genes that are necessary for pregnancy. Statistics show that baby girls are more likely to survive the first year of life and that in the United States, women live an average of seven years longer than men. However, the flip side of our allegedly superior immune system is that sometimes it may work too well. Women are, in fact, more likely than men to have one of the autoimmune diseases.

THE ENDOCRINE SYSTEM

The endocrine system is a collection of interworking glands that produce hundreds of hormones, substances that travel via the bloodstream to targeted cells that these chemical messengers regulate. (Other glands, like sweat glands, mammary glands, and tear glands move secretions out of the body, rather than send regulatory messages.) Although the precise mechanism of each gland and its secretions is not known, it is known that these chemical messengers function best when we're in good health and that the endocrine system can be adversely affected by illness, stress, or age.

The following glands comprise the endocrine system:

• The *pituitary gland*, located deep in the brain, regulates the other glands in the endocrine system and also controls many body processes including growth, urine production, and skin darkening. The pituitary produces several secretions that affect uterine contractions during childbirth as well as breast milk and its production. Although women are accused of being naturally more weepy, women may cry more emotional tears, researchers say, because their bodies have twice as much *prolactin*, a pituitary hormone associated with producing fluid, including milk in the mammary glands. (Prior to puberty, girls and boys have similar prolactin levels and cry about the same amount.) The pituitary also produces the hormone *oxytocin*, which triggers orgasm, the start of labor, and the release of milk from the breast. When the pituitary malfunctions, it may cause infertility in some women by releasing inappropriate amounts of follicle stimulating hormone (FSH) and/or lutinizing hormone (LH), both of which are necessary for reproduction.

• The two triangular-shaped *adrenal glands* sit on top of the kidneys. These glands produce several hormones and secretions, including adrenaline, or epinephrine, and noradrenaline, that help us cope with emergency situations. Adrenaline speeds up respiration and raises our blood pressure, and noradrenaline causes the blood to move more quickly through the body. Other adrenal secretions include hormones such as estrogen, progesterone, and cortisone.

• The *pancreas* helps our bodies maintain blood sugar levels and metabolize carbohydrates by producing and releasing insulin. One of the results of a malfunctioning pancreas is diabetes mellitus, a disorder in which the pancreas does not produce enough insulin, resulting in abnormal blood sugar levels.

• The *thyroid gland* produces the thyroid hormone that affects the heart and metabolic rate. The thyroid is the easiest of the glands to examine because it's located below the Adam's apple in the neck and can be felt from the outside. Women are five times more likely to have thyroid disorders than men. A woman who is *hypothyroid* has low levels of certain hormones produced by the thyroid gland. She feels constantly cold, drowsy, and slow-moving. She may also have a heavy menstrual flow, constipation,

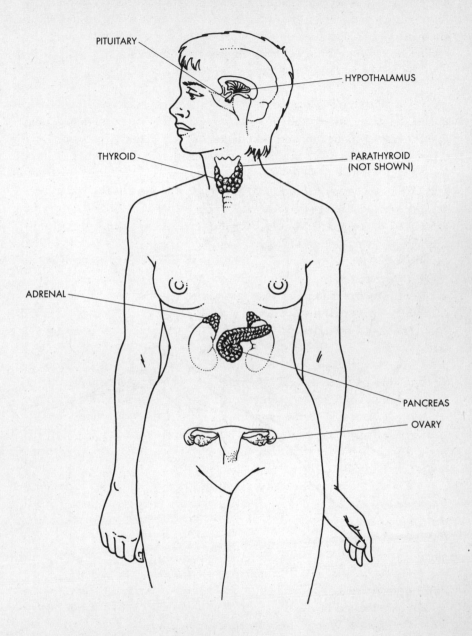

PITUITARY

HYPOTHALAMUS

THYROID

PARATHYROID
(NOT SHOWN)

ADRENAL

PANCREAS

OVARY

ENDOCRINE SYSTEM

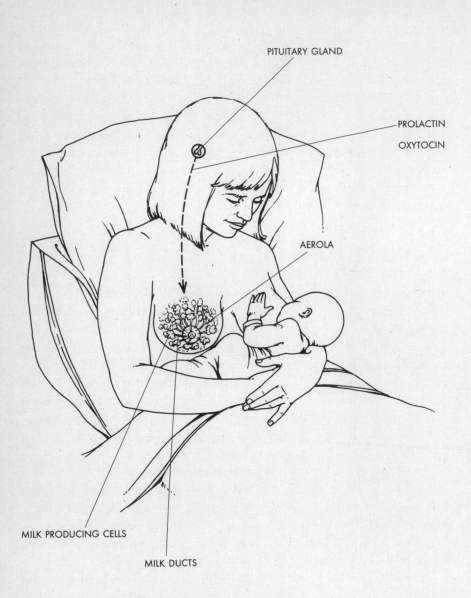

PITUITARY GLAND

PROLACTIN

OXYTOCIN

AEROLA

MILK PRODUCING CELLS

MILK DUCTS

BREASTFEEDING

and muscle and joint aches. Conversely, a woman who is *hyperthyroid* is jumpy, and she may lose weight and have eye problems.

• The four *parathyroid glands*, tiny glands adjacent to the thyroid gland, produce a hormone that affects the metabolism of calcium, phosphorus, and vitamin D. This in turn affects muscle and nerve function as well as bone strength. (One of the drugs used for osteoporosis is a synthetic form of one of the secretions of the parathyroid glands.)

• The *hypothalamus*, attached to the pituitary gland, secretes many hormones that regulate the pituitary and the release of adrenaline from the adrenal gland. The hypothalamus also regulates body temperature and appetite, affects sexual development, and influences how we react to anger or fear. Two examples of appetite disturbances that may be associated with a malfunctioning hypothalamus are anorexia (eating too little) and obesity (sometimes caused by eating too much).

THE MUSCULOSKELETAL SYSTEM

Bones, muscles, joints, ligaments, and tendons work together to hold up our bodies and allow them to move. Our bones, which make up the skeleton, build their strongest mass in our teens and 20s. That's why these are the years when it's important to have a high-calcium diet. Bones naturally begin to lose some of that mass starting in the mid-30s in women as well as in men, but in women the loss may accelerate when the ovaries no longer produce estrogen, which helps maintain bone mass. Significant loss of bone density is called osteoporosis, a condition characterized by brittle bones. However, most women who exercise regularly at all ages halt the bone loss. (See "Osteoporosis" on page 431.)

A *ligament* is a band of tough tissue that connects one bone to another or holds an organ in place; a *joint* is the place where two bones are joined; and a *tendon* is inelastic tissue that connects a muscle to a bone or some other structure. When we move our bodies inappropriately, whether exercising too long or lifting objects that are too heavy, we can pull ligaments, muscles, or tendons, causing pain and impaired movement.

A *muscle* is the only body tissue, whether located in your heart or in your arm, that moves by contracting itself. Each of the 600 named muscles in our bodies is made up of interlocking fibers and each muscle has its own role to play. Some muscles have to be consciously moved, like those in our arms and legs. Others, like the heart or the powerful muscles in the wall of the uterus that move a baby down the birth canal, move involuntarily.

BONES

MUSCLES

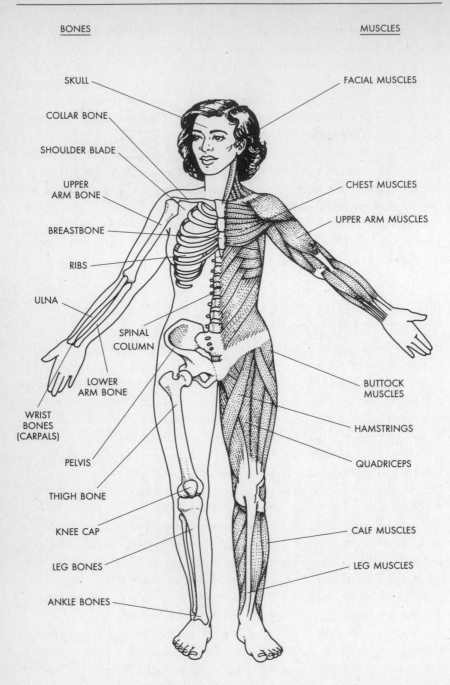

SKULL

FACIAL MUSCLES

COLLAR BONE

SHOULDER BLADE

CHEST MUSCLES

UPPER
ARM BONE

UPPER ARM MUSCLES

BREASTBONE

RIBS

ULNA

SPINAL
COLUMN

LOWER
ARM BONE

BUTTOCK
MUSCLES

WRIST
BONES
(CARPALS)

HAMSTRINGS

PELVIS

QUADRICEPS

THIGH BONE

KNEE CAP

CALF MUSCLES

LEG BONES

LEG MUSCLES

ANKLE BONES

MUSCULOSKELETAL SYSTEM

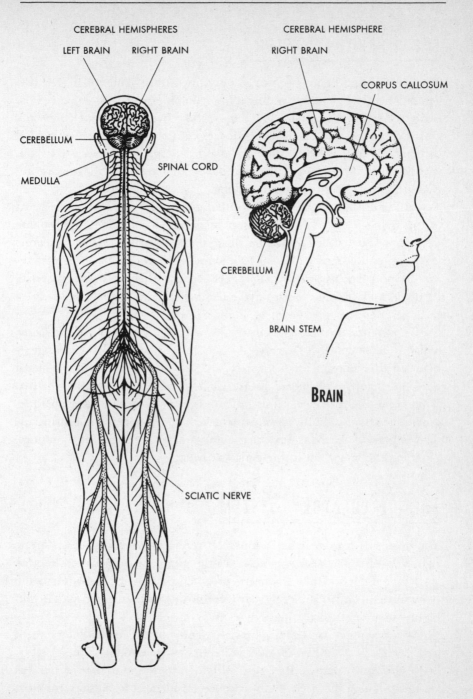

CEREBRAL HEMISPHERES

LEFT BRAIN   RIGHT BRAIN

CEREBELLUM

MEDULLA

SPINAL CORD

SCIATIC NERVE

NERVOUS SYSTEM

CEREBRAL HEMISPHERE

RIGHT BRAIN

CORPUS CALLOSUM

CEREBELLUM

BRAIN STEM

BRAIN

THE NERVOUS SYSTEM

The three-pound brain is protected by ¼-inch-thick skull bones. The two cerebral hemispheres (left and right brains) comprise nearly 90 percent of brain tissue; they control thought, senses, and movement and are connected by the *corpus callosum*. The *cerebellum*, located at the back of the head behind the ears, controls balance and muscle coordination. The *brain stem*, which is about three inches long, is the link between the brain and the spinal cord; it also controls heartbeat and breathing.

The brain and spinal cord comprise the *central nervous system*. A large part of the brain's job is to receive sensory information and initiate appropriate responses. Often called the master gland, the brain releases many secretions including endorphins and enkephalins, mood-altering substances that resemble morphine. We may feel the effect of these when we laugh, give birth, let down milk, have an orgasm, take recreational drugs, or exercise vigorously (a phenomenon known as "runner's high").

The central nervous system works with the *peripheral nervous system*, which is made up of all the nerves — bundles of fibers — that carry signals between the central nervous system and the rest of the body. When a person develops Alzheimer's disease, millions of nerve endings in the two brain hemispheres tangle, causing the loss of memory and other malfunctions. There is also the *autonomic nervous system*, which operates automatically, digesting food in the stomach, moving wastes through the intestines, pumping the lungs, and contracting the heart.

THE CIRCULATORY SYSTEM

The heart is a four-chambered muscular pump that receives blood on its right side through the *veins*, sends it to the lungs for oxygenation, returns it back to the left side of the heart, and then propels it back out into the body through *arteries* and eventually into the *capillaries*, microscopically thin blood vessels entwined with body cells.

Blood supplies cells with a constant supply of oxygen and nutrients; it also carries away carbon dioxide and other waste products. In a healthy body, circulatory pathways are clear, although they tend to narrow some as we age. But if our life-style habits or genetic tendencies lead us toward heart disease, then these pathways can become clogged. Nutritious food and regular exercise are two ways to help keep the pathways clear.

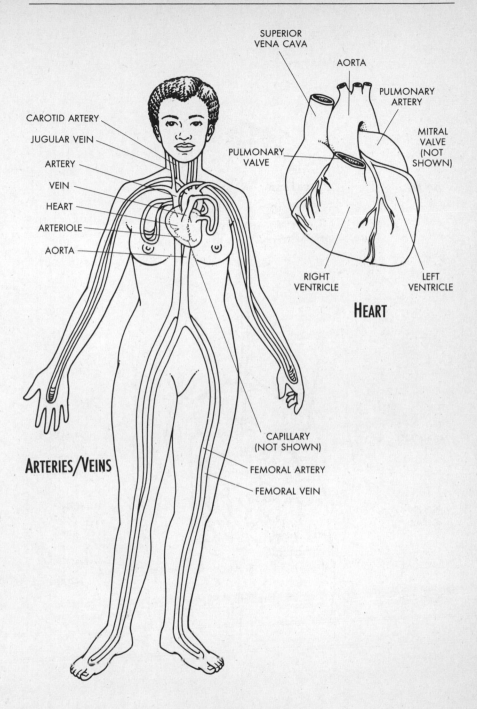

SUPERIOR
VENA CAVA

AORTA

PULMONARY
ARTERY

MITRAL
VALVE
(NOT
SHOWN)

PULMONARY
VALVE

CAROTID ARTERY

JUGULAR VEIN

ARTERY

VEIN

HEART

ARTERIOLE

AORTA

RIGHT
VENTRICLE

LEFT
VENTRICLE

HEART

CAPILLARY
(NOT SHOWN)

FEMORAL ARTERY

FEMORAL VEIN

ARTERIES/VEINS

CIRCULATORY SYSTEM

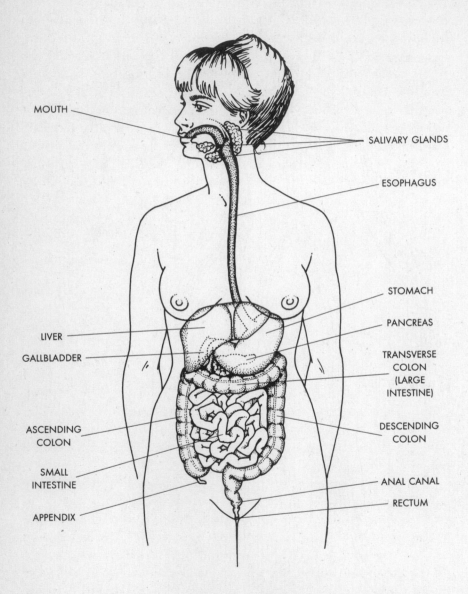

MOUTH

SALIVARY GLANDS

ESOPHAGUS

STOMACH

PANCREAS

LIVER

GALLBLADDER

TRANSVERSE
COLON
(LARGE
INTESTINE)

ASCENDING
COLON

DESCENDING
COLON

SMALL
INTESTINE

ANAL CANAL

RECTUM

APPENDIX

DIGESTIVE SYSTEM

THE DIGESTIVE SYSTEM

Digestion begins in the mouth with an enzyme present in saliva. When food is swallowed, it passes down through the esophagus into the stomach, where it is broken down and mixed with strong acids and enzymes. Next, this well-mixed food enters the small intestine, where more enzymes are added, along with bile from the gall bladder.

Digestion is completed in the small intestine with help from the liver, pancreas, and the kidneys. Eventually, the digested food becomes small enough to pass into the bloodstream as molecules. The large intestine, which includes the colon, absorbs water and retrieves certain chemicals from the remaining material, finally converting what's left into feces that move out through the rectum. The entire digestive system from mouth to anus is called the *alimentary canal* and is 30 feet in length.

THE RESPIRATORY SYSTEM

Air passes into and out of the lungs through a series of ever smaller and thinner tubes, entering through the nose or mouth and proceeding through the bronchi and the bronchioles until it enters the *alveoli*, tiny air sacs within the lungs. The network of alveoli covers 600 square feet; oxygen in the air passes through these thin walls into the bloodstream and is exchanged for the carbon dioxide we exhale.

Air is inhaled and exhaled according to the movement of the *diaphragm*, a sheet of muscle that separates the abdomen from the chest. People who exercise regularly improve the ability of their lungs to move air in and out. That's why with conditioning we can climb more stairs or walk more blocks without huffing and puffing. When alveoli become flabby and stretched — as with habitual cigarette or marijuana smoking — emphysema and other diseases that result in shortness of breath can occur. Healthy pregnant women, on the other hand, eventually experience difficulty in breathing, especially while lying down, because the growing baby puts pressure on the diaphragm.

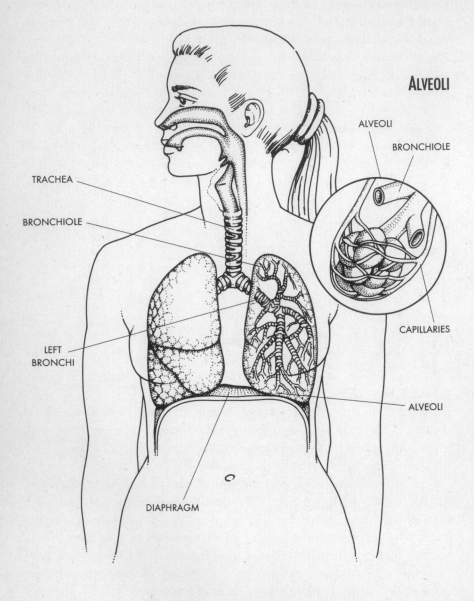

ALVEOLI

ALVEOLI

BRONCHIOLE

TRACHEA

BRONCHIOLE

CAPILLARIES

LEFT
BRONCHI

ALVEOLI

DIAPHRAGM

RESPIRATORY SYSTEM

THE REPRODUCTIVE SYSTEM

Unlike men, who have only one sexual function (intercourse), women have three: intercourse, menstruation/pregnancy/childbirth, and breastfeeding —all of which are influenced by the same network of body parts, hormones and glands. Our reproductive system busies itself from month to month with a menstrual cycle that begins at puberty and ends with menopause. (See illustration on menstruation on page 406.)

Even if we aren't reproducing, we experience hormonal changes according to the progress of our cycle from week to week. And if we are reproducing, our bodies undergo tremendous changes as our children grow within us. (See illustration of conception on page 162.) Most of the female reproductive organs are inside the pelvic cavity, including the *vagina* (which

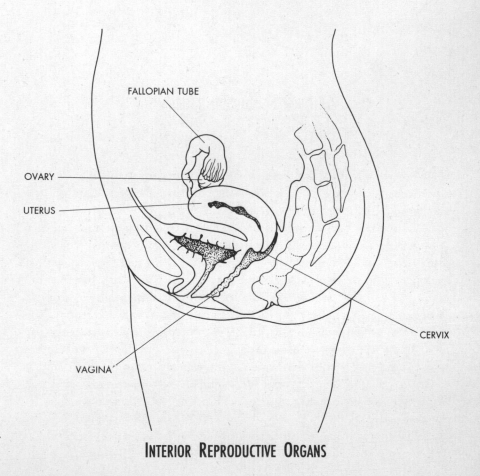

FALLOPIAN TUBE

OVARY

UTERUS

CERVIX

VAGINA

INTERIOR REPRODUCTIVE ORGANS

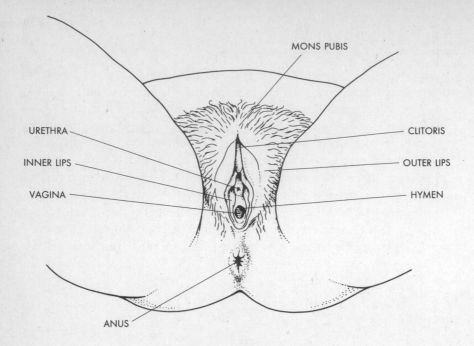

MONS PUBIS

URETHRA

CLITORIS

INNER LIPS

OUTER LIPS

VAGINA

HYMEN

ANUS

EXTERIOR REPRODUCTIVE ORGANS

is also the birth canal), the *uterus* (also called the womb), the *fallopian tubes*, and the *ovaries*. The two ovaries take turns releasing an egg each month, and they produce estrogen and progesterone as well.

Although our entire bodies can respond to sexual stimuli, the area around our genitals, as well as our breasts and nipples, are what we usually think of as our sex organs. The most sensitive is the clitoris, located near the opening to the vagina. It has as many nerve endings as a man's entire penis. No wonder the clitoris is the focus of sexual pleasure for women! Other external organs are the *mons pubis*, a pad of fatty tissue in front of the pubic bone which is covered with hair, the outer lips *(labia majora)* and the inner lips *(labia minora)*. Below the clitoris is the opening of the urethra where urine comes out. The hymen is the slender fold of membrane that covers the vaginal opening until it's stretched by tampons, sex, or some form of exercise. (See Recommended Reading for "Your Body and Its Systems" on page 603.)

Now that you know a little about how our bodies work, let's look at how to keep them in good shape.

CHAPTER 2

HOW TO STAY HEALTHY

The key to staying healthy and avoiding or reducing the impact of many illnesses is life-style. An ounce of prevention is truly worth many pounds of cure. Our day-to-day habits can either enhance or inhibit our immune system, which is the body's first line of defense in preventing disease. They affect our vitality—our energy and power to endure—more than any other factor. As many women with chronic disease will tell you, it is much more difficult to get back to good health than it is to maintain it when the immune system is strong.

Being sensible about your genetic inheritance also enhances your health. People in your family may be susceptible to certain health problems. For example, some people can probably live on ice cream, burgers, and fries right into their 90s, while that same diet could kill someone else at 50. If you're aware, you do not necessarily have to get the diseases of your ancestors. If a parent or sibling was diagnosed with a certain disease while still relatively young—at age 40 or so for many cancers and heart disease, or ages 50 to 60 for Alzheimer's—then you may have a *genetic tendency*. When these diseases start at later ages, they are not usually considered to be hereditary. That's why it's important to know what "runs" in the family and at what age, and then take appropriate preventive steps.

All of us indulge in some unhealthy habits at least occasionally. That's normal. Healthy daily habits on average, however, will improve our odds. Although nothing can guarantee a disease-free life, a healthy life-style helps reduce our risk (or lessen the impact) of many illnesses, including cancer, heart disease, and other chronic ailments. Most important, our life-style habits regarding food, recreational drugs, exercise, friends and lovers, emotions and stress, skin, eyes, and teeth are largely within our control.

FOOD

What we eat and drink — and don't eat and drink — has a profound effect on our vitality. Women need certain foods, vitamins, and minerals in abundance, especially to make the passage from illness to good health.

What foods you need depends partly on your age, your body constitution, your genetic inheritance (as in an inability to digest gluten in wheat products, for instance), and what demands are currently being made of your body either by you (smoking or drugs of any kind) or by outside forces (for example, environmental pollutants). It's important for each of us to know about food and to learn about it from a variety of sources. But beware of "prime time" as a source. Food advertised on TV tends toward too much sugar, salt, and fat.

Body weight is a major issue for many women. Most women go on weight-loss diets, and when they do, they generally follow regimens that add and subtract different foods. What can be said universally is that everyone goes off these diets sooner or later, and most women don't end up weighing appreciably less than they did before (though some clearly do). Since dieting is not a lot of fun and can be stressful to the body, particularly when essential nutrients are omitted, women who eat sensibly day in and day out, maintaining a reasonable weight, are healthier than women who repeatedly go on weight-loss diets.

The closest you can come to a perfect diet is the trust-your-body diet, the one that babies are born with and men more than women are likely to follow. The key to this diet is listening to your own body. Your body's needs change over time, and each of us has a biochemical individuality. We all don't have the same nutritional requirements, just as some of us need seven hours of sleep at night and others eight or nine. The more in tune you are with your body, the more you will eat absolutely the right things, provided you have access to them. Sometimes you eat for pleasure and fun, sometimes for strength. There is no one diet that fits everybody all of the time.

Some feel better eating meat regularly, others feel better when they eat meat infrequently or not at all. Some are allergic to dairy products, wheat, or citrus, and need to get the nutrients each of those supply from other foods. If you trust your body, you'll learn to eat when you're hungry and eventually you'll feel at home with moderation.

Following are 11 different diets geared toward specific needs you may have. At some time in any woman's life one or more of the brief diets listed below will probably apply.* They don't promise weight loss; rather, they are focused on the food and supplements you may be deficient in because of a life-style choice, age, or a medical condition. (For dietary suggestions for specific problems, see "Premenstrual Syndrome" on page 408, for "Dysmenorrhea (Cramps)" on page 411, and for "Osteoporosis" on page 431. If you want to find a nutritionist, see Morales on page 604 in Recommended Reading.)

Most of these diets recommend vitamin or mineral supplements. Although clearly the best source of vitamins is food, an estimated one half of U.S. women regularly use supplements. The use of vitamin and mineral supplements is controversial, unregulated by the FDA, and arguments both for and against often lack overwhelming evidence. All vitamin and mineral suggestions in the following diets, however, are backed up by published research. (See "Food" on page 604 in the Recommended Reading for books, in particular those marked with an asterisk, that suggest specific supplemental dosages.)

Two of these diets use the word organic. One issue is the question of what an organic label means. Until a federal 1990 law is put into action, there is no nationwide, uniform interpretation of *organic*, although some states have standards. *Organic* generally means that the food is produced free of hormones and antibiotics or chemical pesticides, herbicides, or fertilizers. Until uniform labeling is enforced, when you're buying food labeled organic, ask the seller to describe the product's pedigree (where and how it was raised or grown).

Another dispute is whether organic food is healthier for you than nonorganic food. Many people think it is. A Louis Harris poll in 1989 showed that about half of us have eaten food labeled organic, and we do it because we believe there are health benefits. However, like the issue of vitamin and mineral supplements, arguments for and against often lack overwhelming evidence. Some people rest easier knowing they are eating food that was produced without chemicals, while others do not think chemicals are worth worrying about.

In at least one case, many researchers believe organic is definitely better

---

*I am indebted to Nan Kathryn Fuchs, author of *The Nutrition Detective* (Jeremy Tarcher Publishing, 1985), for the idea of providing special diets for certain common conditions.

for you. Liver, more than other cuts of meat, may store toxins, so choose organic liver only.

THE ANTI–BREAST CANCER, HEALTHY HEART DIET

Japanese women who still eat the traditional low-fat diet have one-fifth the breast cancer rate of American women. However, Japanese women who eat the Western-style diet have no such advantage. Whether the link between diet and cancer can be proved without a doubt (research is definitely mixed), the following suggestions are considered prudent for an anticancer diet (particularly — studies show — for cancers of the colon, rectum, cervix, endometrium, and lung). Other studies show that adopting these guidelines may improve your heart's health and general condition. (See "Cancer" on page 231 for more life-style recommendations.)

• Eat five servings of vegetables and fruit each day. Focus on vegetables and fruit with color — dark green (such as spinach and chard), orange and yellow (such as cantaloupes, carrots, and winter squash). Make friends with cruciferous vegetables — broccoli, Brussels sprouts, cabbage, rutabagas, turnips — a couple of times a week. Start increasing them in your diet gradually to avoid intestinal gas. (Notable offenders are beans, Brussels sprouts, raisins, apple juice, and prune juice.)

Less than 10 percent of us in the United States eat a total of five servings a day of vegetables and fruit, so most of us will have to gradually work our way toward this goal. A typical serving size is one medium fruit, ¾ cup of 100 percent fruit or vegetable juice, ½ cup cooked or raw vegetables or fruit, one cup of raw leafy vegetables, or ¼ cup dried fruit. (See "Beano" on page 580 under "Food" in the Resource Directory for a food enzyme product that prevents gas from whole grains, soy and other beans, and many vegetables like cabbage and broccoli.) It's essential to include in your anticancer diet vitamins C, A, E, the B vitamin complex (folic acid in particular, to reduce your risk for cervical cancer), and the minerals selenium, calcium, and magnesium. If you get enough vegetables and fruit, you'll be well on your way.

• Eat 20 to 35 grams of fiber per day. (The average American in 1991 ate 11 grams of fiber each day.) Fiber is found only in whole grains, fruit (whole fruit, not usually juice), vegetables, nuts, and legumes, especially dried peas and beans. Read package labels and find cereal (crunchy cereal is not necessarily high in fiber) that you like that has at least five grams of fiber per serving. Add bran to your diet. Oat and rice bran are associated with improved heart health, and wheat bran may reduce the incidence of breast cancer. Remember, as with the cruciferous vegetables mentioned above, introduce high-fiber foods gradually to avoid flatulence.

Eat fresh fruit with the skin on, and choose stone-ground whole-wheat and other whole-grain products. Many products have their fiber content listed on the package. Generally speaking, the less processed a plant food is, the more fiber it has. A fast food that provides more fiber than most selections is a bean burrito (to reduce the fat content, skip the cheese).

• Eat a serving of fish two times per week. Among the best are salmon, tuna, mackerel, herring, sardines, and halibut. To avoid contaminated fish, do not cook and eat fish that has a strong odor. If it smells bad, it is.

• Add soybean products, such as tofu, soy milk, and soy yogurt, because of their tendency to reduce your breast cancer risk.

• Avoid excessive alcohol and don't smoke.

• Choose fish or poultry (white meat) over red meat because of their lower fat content.

• Avoid fats and oils. Be aware that much Chinese food and many fast-food sandwiches (including those made with chicken or fish) are prepared with high amounts of both.

• Limit your use of salt-cured, smoked, and nitrite-preserved food.

• Try to reduce fats to 30 percent or even less of your *total* diet (not necessarily each bite you eat).

How to Find Fat in Your Food

Some fat is essential to our health. Although polyunsaturated fats (safflower, corn, sesame, soy, sunflower, olive, canola, and many fish oils) are better than those fats that are saturated (dairy and other animal products, and coconut and palm oil), generally speaking fat is fat.

To achieve a diet that derives 30 percent (or less) of its calories from fat, eat about 50 to 60 grams of fat per day. Eat less fat if you want to lose weight. (Men can get away with 80 grams or even more because of their larger — on average — size.) Some researchers believe a fat intake of 10 percent or lower can unplug heart arteries.

Finding fat in your food has just become easier. By May 1994, food product labels are required to include the number of grams of fat, fiber, and salt (sodium) along with calories and other information. Certain advertising labels will finally have uniform definitions, too. "Low fat" means no more than three grams of fat per serving, for example, and "less" and "reduced" apply to products that have at least 25 percent of the fat removed.

Avoid food that has more than five grams of fat per serving. Substitute picante sauce or mustard for mayonnaise, and choose oil-free salad dressings. (Most salad dressings have five grams of fat per tablespoon — and typical salad bar salads may have more fat than fast-food burgers and fries.) Drink skim milk or eat nonfat yogurt (if you're not sensitive to dairy products) and avoid most cheeses. Eat a serving of meat no bigger than the palm of your hand, and stay away from fried foods. Cut the fat in recipes by at least one third, and season foods with herbs and spices instead of butter or margarine.

If you want to compute the actual percentage of fat in any one product, multiply grams of fat per serving (found on the package label) by nine (which is the number of calories per gram of fat). Then divide your result by the total number of calories. With practice, it's easy to roughly figure which foods are acceptable and which are not. A cup of whole milk has 150 calories and eight grams of fat. This means whole milk is 48 percent fat. A quick rule of thumb: If the product has about 300 calories, it should have 10 grams or less of fat.

If you do your "fat math," you may discover, like most other Americans, that your diet is higher in fat than you thought it was. But once you know what your fat intake is and where it comes from, you can look at your eating habits over a week's time and see what you are willing to adjust. Over time, fat math will become automatic. (See "Fat Counters" on page 605 of Recommended Reading for helpful books. Also see "Food" on page 580 of the Resource Directory for more information about anticancer foods.)

THE ANTI-ADDITIVE, ANTI-PRESERVATIVE DIET

Chemicals (about 9,000 of them) are used to alter the smell, taste, color, and texture of our foods. Although these are labeled safe by the U.S. government, some of these chemicals can cause a variety of unpleasant side effects. If you're sensitive to certain additives or preservatives, you may need to do some detective work to find out all the ways in which they are used. Some say if these chemicals are not a problem for you, don't worry about them. Others say it makes sense to avoid potentially troublesome additives, since the likelihood of your being affected increases with the amount of the chemical you ingest.

Following are three commonly used food chemicals that have potentially severe side effects:

• The additive *NutraSweet* (or *aspartame*) is the most commonly consumed artificial sweetener. Despite the fact that it turns up everywhere, its safety continues to be questioned. Although your experience may be different, research shows that many users gain weight using this product because it can trigger hunger. (Similarly, it's suspected that fake fat products reinforce the taste for fat.) Other symptoms that have been implicated with aspartame use are headaches (including migraines), dizziness, swelling of the larynx (upper part of the windpipe), severe rash (including hives), swelling, itching, memory loss, blurred vision, seizures, hyperactivity, insomnia, fatigue, menstrual disorders, and behavioral disorders (more often in women and children than in men).

Avoid or limit the use of "sugar-free" products when NutraSweet or aspartame is listed in the ingredients. People with the inherited disease phenylketonuria, or PKU, should avoid NutraSweet altogether. Artificially sweetened items include soft drinks, desserts, and yogurt, as well as products aimed toward your children, such as Kool-Aid, Jell-O, chewing gum, and children's vitamins.

• The preservative *sulfite* prevents the browning of potatoes, the wilting of lettuce, and the souring of beer and wine. The FDA estimates that at least one million Americans — many of whom have a history of asthma — are sensitive to sulfite. Toxic side effects usually begin within five to 20 minutes and start with tingling and flushing, followed by any of the following: headache, vomiting, wheezing, a feeling of heat, hives, dizziness, cramps and/or explosive diarrhea, unconsciousness, and occasionally, death. Manufacturers are required to list sulfite when it's used, but if you are eating in a restaurant or you are at a wedding reception or a conference dinner, you won't be able to read the labels.

For those who are sensitive to sulfites, which includes many people with asthma, avoid those products that are legally treated with sulfite, but are not necessarily labeled as such, including mushrooms, cider, U.S. produced beer (50 chemicals are permitted), and shellfish (shrimp, scallops, clams, crab, lobster, and the like).

Also avoid those products that are required by law to show sulfite on the label. It is also listed as sulfur (or sulphur) or sulfur dioxide, potassium or sodium metabisulfite, potassium or sodium bisulfite, or calcium or sodium sulfite, or sulphite. Affected products include dried fruit (unless product is labeled "unsulfured"); potatoes, including chips and mashed, baked, and boiled varieties (but not fresh, due to 1990 FDA ban); guacamole; prescription drugs; and some canned vegetables and juices. Most wine has sulfites added, but even so-called organic wine may have minuscule amounts of sulfites that are created by the fermenting process itself.

Chicken, eggs, meat, and cheese are not generally treated with sulfite, so if you know you're sulfite-sensitive, choose these when eating in an unfamiliar restaurant.

Select nonpackaged, nonprocessed foods in their natural state to reduce your overall exposure, and if you're a wine or beer drinker, find brands that use the least amount of preservatives. For instance, some beers produced at small, local companies do not use preservatives.

• The additive *monosodium glutamate* (MSG) is frequently used as a flavor enhancer in Asian food and in packaged products, where it is listed on the label as hydrolyzed vegetable protein. In people who are sensitive, MSG can cause symptoms within 30 minutes, although they usually are not as severe as the reactions to sulfite. These symptoms include chest pain, facial tightness, a sensation of heat over the neck and shoulders, abdominal cramps, and headaches. (See "Additives, Preservatives, and Other Food Chemicals" on page 550 in the Resource Directory.)

THE BIRTH-CONTROL PILL DIET

Birth-control pills change the way your body absorbs specific vitamins and minerals. Some researchers say that if you compensate for this in your diet, you'll reduce your risk for side effects. Others say that Pill users don't need extra vitamins. If you try this diet, see how you feel. You be the judge.

• You'll need extra B_6 (found in whole grains, brewer's yeast, and vitamin supplements), B_{12} (found in vitamin supplements, lean meat, fish, and liver), and biotin (found in brewer's yeast, egg yolks, liver, and brown rice), another B vitamin.
• Be sure you especially get enough of the B vitamin folic acid, which is found in green leafy vegetables, liver, and brewer's yeast.
• You'll need extra vitamin C, which is found in citrus, garden peppers, many fruits and vegetables, and vitamin supplements.
• You'll also need vitamin E, which is found in raw nuts and seeds and vegetable oils, as well as vitamin supplements.

THE MENOPAUSE DIET

Some body changes that occur at menopause are associated in part with eating habits. By being careful about what you eat and what you don't eat, you can avoid or reduce certain symptoms.

• Reduce both the frequency and intensity of hot flashes (transient feelings of heat), a common menopausal symptom, by avoiding the following known triggers: excessive amounts of sugar, animal fats, highly processed foods, chocolate, and hot drinks.
• Avoid large amounts of caffeine and alcohol as well as the consumption of large amounts of food at one time. These excesses can raise your body temperature and, consequently, trigger more flashes. Moderation is the key.
• Make sure you are eating whole grains, cold-pressed vegetable oils, legumes, nuts and seeds, fish, and liver to strengthen your body so it is up to par and able to regulate the hormonal shifts during this time with the most ease.

• Eat soybean products, such as tofu, soy milk, and soy yogurt regularly because soy reduces hot flashes in some women due to an estrogen-like ingredient.

• Drink lots of water and try herbal teas or supplements that include ginseng, dong quai, and black cohosh to reduce hot flashes.

• Consider a multivitamin/mineral preparation. Some health care providers suggest that you take supplements of vitamin E, vitamin C, and bioflavonoids to help strengthen your body's temperature-regulating mechanisms; B complex to avoid moodiness; and calcium-magnesium supplements (1500 mgs. of calcium daily after menopause begins significantly slows bone loss) to keep your bones strong as your estrogen levels drop. (See "The Menopause Diet" on page 605 in Recommended Reading for more about specific dosages.)

The Over-The-Counter and Prescription Drug Diet

Many drugs, especially if taken over a long period of time, can affect how the body absorbs certain vitamins and minerals, which may lead to undesirable side effects. (See "Prescription and Over-the-Counter Drugs" on page 592 in Recommended Reading for a list of books that describe many commonly used drugs and their side effects.) Three valuable drugs commonly used by millions of women are:

• *Aspirin*, the world's most used medicine, can irritate the stomach lining; cause nausea, vomiting, internal hemorrhage, ringing or buzzing in the ears; block the absorption of vitamin C and the B vitamin folic acid, and occasionally cause allergic reactions. Take vitamin C while you're using aspirin and consider a less toxic painkiller, especially for children, who are more susceptible to side effects than are adults. If you are advised to take aspirin for an extended period of time for any reason, be sure to discuss with your physician the pros and cons for you.

• *Antibiotics* can slow down protein synthesis and destroy helpful bacteria in the colon. Their use can lead to yeast infections, diarrhea, and other intestinal problems. While you are on antibiotics, eat yogurt, which contains live cultures. Among these are L. *Acidophilus,* B. *Bifidus,* S. *Thermophilus,* and L. *Bulgaricus.* Afterwards, take *lactobacillus acidophilus* powder to help restore helpful bacteria.

• *Cortisone* (also known as prednisone) is used for many chronic autoimmune diseases, such as arthritis, lupus, and severe allergies. It inhibits the absorption of calcium, and long-term use can lead to osteoporosis. Counteract this by getting enough calcium and magnesium (along with regular exercise), vitamin B complex, and vitamin C.

THE PREGNANCY DIET

The best way to grow a healthy baby without depleting your body is to eat quality foods wisely during pregnancy, and better yet, for some months beforehand. Plan to take a folic acid supplement *before* you conceive, for example, as an insurance policy against eating an inadequate amount of this vitamin. (It's found in fortified cereals, dark green leafy vegetables, brewer's yeast, whole grain breads, and beans.) It must be in your system at conception and during the first month of pregnancy to help avoid the birth defect, neural tube defect. (See "Neural Tube Defects" on page 454.) Folic acid is, of course, necessary throughout pregnancy.

The ideal diet is a combination of foods to add and substances to avoid. The current recommended weight gain is about 25 to 35 pounds for women whose prepregnancy weight was in the normal range. (See "The Pregnancy Diet" on page 605 in Recommended Reading and "How to Avoid Birth Defects" on page 453 for additional safer-pregnancy suggestions.)

• Add protein in greater amounts than you probably usually consume. Some researchers suggest 75–100 grams per day. The National Academy of Sciences recommends that vitamin-mineral supplements should not be taken routinely although they do recommend supplements of iron and the B vitamin folic acid for all pregnant women. Other experts suggest a full-range multivitamin and mineral supplement, including iron, folic acid, B$_6$, and calcium-magnesium.

• Avoid *all* recreational drugs, including alcohol, nicotine (in cigarettes), cocaine, and marijuana, as no amount has been determined by research to be safe. (See "Pregnancy and Recreational Drugs" on page 451.)

• Avoid *all* prescribed and over-the-counter drugs. If your physician recommends that you use any drug, make sure you understand why it's both necessary and safe. Follow the steps in "Do Your Homework about Prescription Drugs" on page 74. Be aware of safe substitutes. Daily aspirin use (aspirin is the most used drug during pregnancy), for example, has been suggested to treat high blood pressure during pregnancy. However, calcium has been shown to reduce high blood pressure in pregnant women as well.

• Avoid large amounts of caffeine (more than three cups of coffee daily or 300 milligrams of caffeine), which occurs naturally in coffee, tea, and chocolate, but is also added to soft drinks and over-the-counter drugs.

• Choose fresh foods whenever available and avoid foods that use additives and preservatives.

• Avoid products sweetened with NutraSweet (aspartame), as it's possible — though rare — for some babies to be affected by this additive in utero.

THE SKIN DIET

Skin blemishes, acne, rashes, poor skin tone (including a washed-out appearance), and wrinkles are all affected by what we eat. To help your skin stay healthy:

• Eat whole grains, fresh fruits, vegetables, eggs, and cold-pressed vegetable oils.

• Be sure you get enough beta-carotene (vitamin A) and vitamin C.

• Avoid fats (including fried foods), refined foods, caffeine, alcohol, smoking, and chocolate.

• Don't smoke. Some research suggests that smoking accelerates the appearance of facial wrinkles by as many as seven years.

THE SMOKER'S (AND PASSIVE SMOKER'S) DIET

When tobacco burns, about 4,000 chemical compounds are produced. Since smoking cigarettes affects all the cells of the body, it's important to replace the nutrients that smoking destroys. That's true whether you're the smoker or you breathe other people's smoke. A 1990 U.S. government survey indicated that smokers are not likely to eat adequate vegetables, fruits, and grains, nor are they likely to take vitamin-mineral supplements. If that description fits you, and cigarettes will remain in your daily diet, you can still help your body.

• You need extra vitamin C. Each cigarette destroys 25 milligrams and each pack uses up 500 milligrams. A glass of orange juice typically has 60 milligrams of vitamin C, so supplements are likely your best option.

• Choose a high-vegetable diet (for beta-carotene, which converts to vitamin A in your liver, and vitamin C, as well as fiber), including deep-orange, red, and dark-green vegetables, especially carrots, sweet potatoes, broccoli, spinach, and peppers.

• Get plenty of vitamins E, folic acid, and B_{12} and the mineral selenium to help protect your lung tissue.

• Avoid food additives, high-fat foods, and excessive alcohol.

THE SOCIAL DRINKER'S DIET

You don't have to be an alcoholic for alcohol to cause some damage. You can minimize that possible damage by replacing the nutrients alcohol destroys.

• Whenever you consume alcohol, add some vitamins B_1, B_{12}, and folic acid to your diet.
• Add magnesium, which is found in dark-green vegetables, but may be more readily available in supplements (along with calcium).

THE STRESS DIET

When your emotional stress is of the unhealthy variety, or your body is run down from environmental stresses (like smog, carbon monoxide from vehicular exhaust, or the chemical fumes inside air-tight buildings), your immune system may suffer, leaving you feeling run-down and vulnerable to a variety of ailments.

• Be sure you eat lots of fresh vegetables, legumes, whole grains, and fish.
• Consider taking a vitamin B complex supplement and vitamin C.
• Avoid sugar, caffeine, alcohol, white flour, excess fats, and junk food (often the first choice for people who are feeling stressed).

THE VEGETARIAN DIET

Most of the world eats vegetarian or near vegetarian, and an estimated 12 million or more Americans do, too. Vegans are strict vegetarians who eat no animal products whatsoever. Most U.S. vegetarians, however, eat eggs and dairy products. As a group, vegetarians have less heart disease, obesity, diabetes, rheumatoid arthritis, and osteoporosis than meat eaters.

Although protein balancing (serving vegetarian food that combines a full range of amino acids) was once thought to be necessary, newer information shows that it is not. An essential addition to the vegetarian diet, however, is vitamin B_{12}. This vitamin is only found in animal foods, such as meat, dairy products, and eggs or in fortified foods, such as certain breakfast cereals, breads, and specific brands of nutritional yeast. It is also absolutely necessary for nursing mothers who are vegetarian to take B_{12} supplements because body stores are not enough. (See "The Vegetarian Diet" on page 605 in Recommended Reading and "Vegetarian" on page 580 in the Resource Directory.)

RECREATIONAL DRUGS

Alcohol, tobacco, marijuana, cocaine, and anabolic steroids, among other substances, are part of many women's life-styles, whether rarely or regularly, often beginning in the early teens. Their effects on women are sometimes different than their effects on men. (See "Pregnancy and Recreational Drugs" on page 451 for the effects these drugs have on unborn children.) Following is a description of these drugs, listed in order of their use by U.S. women, along with their consequences and suggestions for users.

ALCOHOL

Women, perhaps especially those less than 50 years old, get drunk twice as fast as men because their stomachs do not digest alcohol as well, with the result that the alcohol enters the bloodstream quickly, and they feel the toxic effects sooner. Alcohol-related problems — alcoholism, hypertension, obesity, anemia, liver damage, gastrointestinal bleeding, and death from alcohol toxicity — all may occur sooner and often more severely in women than in men.

Toxic effects of alcohol are one or more of the following: nausea, dizziness, lack of coordination, slurred speech, trembling, headaches, sweating, nervousness, mental confusion, and poor judgment. Too much alcohol is also associated with ulcers; diabetes; cancers of the breast, cervix, throat, mouth, and rectum; infertility; menstrual cramps and menstrual cycle irregularities; birth defects; miscarriages; early menopause; osteoporosis; pneumonia; suicide attempts; and inability to have an orgasm (a parallel side effect in men is the inability to maintain an erection).

In addition, some people have mild to severe reactions to the chemicals used to enhance, stabilize, and preserve U.S. alcoholic beverages.

Alcoholism is repeated drinking that causes trouble in the drinker's personal, professional, or family life and is more likely to be chronic in women past the age of 35. One third of alcoholics are women, but the number is growing because new female drinkers outnumber new male drinkers, beginning with the college-aged. Drinking that becomes a prob lem is more common among women who are lonely, those who use other addicting drugs, the unemployed, the divorced, the sexually abused, those living with alcoholic men, and perhaps those who are lesbians. (See "Alcohol" on page 605 in Recommended Reading for more information about women and alcohol. See also "Alcohol" on page 552 in the Resource Directory for helpful organizations.)

TOBACCO

Less than half (23 percent) as many U.S. women smoke as drink alcohol (55 percent). The women most likely to smoke are older than 35, unemployed, less educated, poor, and, if pregnant, unmarried. Smokers are also three times more likely to drink alcohol, especially beer. In general, more men than women smoke and men smoke more cigarettes than women, although most all smokers average nearly a pack (20 cigarettes) a day.

Toxic effects of smoking (including clove cigarettes) are cancers of all kinds (risk increases with intake): bladder, cervix, esophagus, kidney, larynx and oral cavity, lungs, pancreas, and stomach. Smoking, particularly as a teenager, may be a risk factor for breast cancer, and smoking is a suspect for colon cancer as well. In addition, there's a doubled risk of heart attack for women who smoke, even as few as one to four cigarettes daily (the risk of heart attack increases to tenfold when smoking is combined with use of the Pill).

Other toxic effects are: destruction of vitamin C (which can cause bruising and bleeding gums), ulcers, migraine headaches, chronic bronchitis (women are more susceptible than men), emphysema (lung damage), asthma (recurrent attacks of breathlessness), decreased fertility, early menopause, premature wrinkles, and increased risk for cataracts (clouding of lens of eyes), ectopic pregnancy, and perhaps osteoporosis (particularly after menopause even while using estrogen replacement therapy).

Sidestream (also known as passive or secondhand) smoking causes many of the same toxic side effects (including heart disease, lung cancer, and other respiratory diseases) not only for humans but perhaps for pets as well. In addition, smoke can cause headaches and allergies of all kinds, as well as increased incidence of asthma, pneumonia, and other infections in children.

MARIJUANA

Many people still believe that marijuana, a smokable mixture from the hemp plant, is good for you, or at least not bad for you. However, that's not the case, particularly for regular users and for the fetuses of pregnant women. It's estimated that about one third of young U.S. women have used marijuana, and most who still do also smoke cigarettes, drink alcohol, and have a high intake of caffeine.

Toxic effects of marijuana, which contains more than 400 chemicals, are confusion, mood swings, and lung and bronchial tube damage. Damage to the respiratory system may show up sooner than it does in cigarette smokers because marijuana contains 50 percent more cancer-causing materials than tobacco, and the tar content is greater. Other effects of marijuana use are premenstrual sugar craving and binging, headaches, fatigue, disturbance in hormone production and disruption in menstrual cycle; and decrease in short-term memory (possibly permanent), especially with daily use, difficulty in organizing thoughts, and may precipitate schizophrenia (a psychotic illness).

COCAINE

One in five U.S. women has used cocaine in some form at least once, government estimates claim, and most cocaine users also use marijuana and alcohol. Cocaine's appeal is its intense effect of euphoria, sometimes with heightened sexual passion. This sexual effect, however, occurs only in early use, and then only for some people. Regular use causes sexual depression (impotence in men). Typically, an intense high is followed by a crash of unpredictable effects that lasts from eight to 50 hours. This is often followed by one to five days of near normal functioning, followed by profound depression, anxiety, boredom, irritability, and violent behavior.

Toxic effects of cocaine were first reported 100 years ago and include: damage to nasal passages and sinuses (including chronic sniffling and/or nosebleeds, along with decreased sense of smell); damage to the brain, which can be permanent; migraine-like headaches; seizures and/or heart attacks (caused by spasms in blood vessels) that are sometimes fatal, as well as long-term effects to the heart, resulting in rapid beating, which may not show up until years later after cocaine use has stopped.

ANABOLIC STEROIDS

These are synthetic versions of the male hormone testosterone, and when used appropriately under close medical supervision have legitimate medical uses (such as Danazol for the treatment of endometriosis). It's the unregulated use of anabolic steroids that is the problem. They enhance muscle delineation and growth, improve speed, and give the user a sense of invincibility while often causing aggression. Although these drugs have reportedly been used most often by male athletes, women athletes and body-builders have reported using them, too.

Toxic effects of anabolic steroids include: deeper voice, depression and/or violent anger; clitoris enlargement, facial hairiness, male pattern baldness, breast reduction, liver damage, elevated cholesterol levels, insomnia, fatigue, and menstrual irregularities, all of which may be reversible.

Long-term, known side effects of steroids may result in psychiatric disturbances and drug addiction, including substance craving and withdrawal symptoms.

SUGGESTIONS FOR USERS OF RECREATIONAL DRUGS

Pay attention to your genetic predisposition and your history. The woman most likely to have an ongoing problem with substance abuse may have a childhood history of sexual, physical, or emotional abuse, may have parents or grandparents who were dependent on alcohol or other substances, or may be someone who is emotionally very fragile. The woman most likely to smoke has one or both parents who also smoked.

Recognize the difference between reasonable use of a drug and a drug problem. Some researchers believe that one or two drinks per day is a safe and moderate amount, except of course when you're pregnant. Many others believe that amount can inhibit the immune system and lead to a variety of ailments and accelerated aging. Our bodies all vary in their capacity for toxic overload, and be aware that alcohol hits women hardest in the two weeks before their period begins. If you're having unpleasant side effects (headaches and depression, for example) with one or two drinks per day, then this is probably not a safe and moderate amount for you.

Because of potentially dangerous drug interactions, avoid using alcohol when you're taking drugs, such as aspirin or prescription drugs, including Valium, Librium, Miltown, Thorazine, phenobarbital, Darvon, Demerol, and antihistamines. (A mix of cocaine and alcohol is particularly lethal.) Be aware that alcohol use can increase your need for certain nutrients (see "The Social Drinker's Diet" on page 36).

There is no known safe amount of daily cigarette smoking. Even a single cigarette per day can change your body chemistry (see "The Smoker's [and Passive Smoker's] Diet" on page 35 for suggestions on how to counteract some of the unhealthy effects of smoking). But what about low-tar, low-nicotine cigarettes? Theoretically, they reduce your risk, but in reality they don't, especially for women. Most people who smoke these cigarettes end up smoking more in total and inhaling more deeply, so that they end up with the same amount of tar and nicotine.

Be realistic about stopping substance use altogether, and plan for success. It's one thing to stop using a substance you've barely begun. It's quite another to stop a well-entrenched habit, especially if that habit involves more than one recreational drug. Fewer than 10 percent of women alcoholics are successful at stopping altogether for as long as four years, and the most likely to succeed are milder alcoholics without serious family histories of drinking problems.

As for smoking, 90 percent of all quitters stop cold turkey. Also, people who are not depressed (particularly severely) are more successful, as are quitters who make new nonsmoking friends to reinforce their new non-smoking life-style. If you want to quit smoking, don't wait for your physician to suggest it, as studies show that's not likely to happen, especially if you're still in your 20s or 30s. (See "Tobacco" on page 605 in Recommended Reading for information on how to quit smoking.)

Some women smoke to lose weight, so it's no surprise that women are usually concerned about putting on pounds if they quit smoking. Not all exsmokers gain weight, but for those who do, a typical gain is about five pounds (although a few gain as much as 30 pounds). It's mostly due to an adjustment in metabolism, and some experts suggest that an additional mile walk per day will usually readjust your metabolism. If you do choose to quit, health benefits start immediately, no matter what your age.

Some experts say that the treatment program of choice for cocaine abuse has three parts: detoxification, personal counseling, and community support groups. Although this is apparently the most effective approach, the dropout rate is still often 50 percent or more. Acupuncture, the stimulation of points on the body using tiny needles, helps some people stay off of cocaine by affecting their brain chemistry. (See "Acupuncture" on page 82.) Despite individual cures, treatment specialists agree no one really knows how to cure drug addiction in everyone. The general rule of safety for any addictive drug is once-a-week use is better than once-a-day use, once-a-month use is better than once-a-week, and so on.

EXERCISE

Regular exercise, according to numerous studies, has many benefits. It can:

• *Boost your immune system,* add years to your lifetime, increase your sense of well-being, and enhance your self-esteem.
• *Reduce your feelings of stress* and mild or severe depression and fatigue, while reducing your risk for heart disease because it lowers your cholesterol (not so, however, if you smoke), the level of fat in your blood, and blood pressure (two alcoholic drinks per day erase the blood pressure benefit, however) particularly when combined with weight loss. It also reduces your risk for endometriosis (a disease in which patches of the uterine lining, or *endometrium,* show up in other places in the pelvic cavity), arthritis (joint inflammation), and adult-onset diabetes mellitus.
• *Decrease your risk for cancer of the breast,* uterus, ovary, cervix, vagina, and colon. Long-term studies have shown a reduced incidence of these particu-

lar cancers in women who exercise on a regular basis — and the more years the better. The influence of exercise on other cancers is unknown.

• *Help you to lose weight* (research indicates 45 minutes of exercise five times per week is best for this).

• *Minimize cramps and premenstrual syndrome* (PMS) symptoms (including headaches, bloating, breast tenderness, and weight gain), reduce your monthly menstrual flow by as much as 20 percent, and lessen common discomforts during pregnancy, like morning sickness (see "Exercise and Pregnancy" on page 450).

• *Improve your overall fitness and breathing capacity,* alertness and decision-making ability, your skin coloring due to improved circulation and, as a cosmetic plus, minimize bags under the eyes and reduce the risk and/or severity of varicose veins.

• *Make your bones denser and stronger* (calcium intake alone is not adequate) thereby reducing the risk for osteoporosis and bone fractures.

If there ever was a magic pill for many people, exercise is it. Although most researchers agree that moderate exercise is healthful, they often disagree about what constitutes regular exercise, and how much is enough. Comprehensive research reported in 1989, however, suggests that a little goes a long way — *if* the exercise is regular, such as 30 minutes of walking (brisk is best) three days per week. (The U.S. Centers for Disease Control and Prevention's definition of sedentary is fewer than three 20-minute sessions of somewhat vigorous physical activity per week.) How you measure what's enough for you depends, in part, on what you want to accomplish. If you want to become a marathoner, you will, of course, do more than walk three times a week.

Many advocates of one or another form of exercise, whether jogging, swimming, or aerobic dancing, swear by what they do and believe it is best for all. It's not. Some women love the organization of a class, others despise it. Some will walk for miles in the country, but hate walking even a block in the city. Know yourself. Change from one form of exercise to another when you lose interest.

Investigate exercise helpers, such as videos, audio cassettes, and TV programs. Whatever exercise you choose, be sure to take care of your feet and knees and they'll help take care of the rest of your body. Get shoes with lots of padding and plenty of toe space, which may mean you'll need a larger size. If your knees bother you after exercising, consider wearing high-top shoes if your knees normally turn in. (See "Exercise" on page 604 in Recommended Reading.)

Walking is the exercise that most people do, and it's also the safest (although it's wise to avoid streets with heavy traffic because of noxious fumes and carbon monoxide). You won't be injured unless you fall off a curb, and you don't have to have a certain body type to do it safely. Walking is also the choice with the most staying power. (You might quit tennis because of elbow pain, or you'll quit jogging because of leg cramps.)

Walking is as effective as any other form of exercise, including running. You'll begin to reduce tension, anxiety, and blood pressure on the first day if you walk as little as one mile briskly (or three miles at any pace). To start a walking exercise program, you don't have to take lessons, go to a special place like a health club (though more and more walkers go to shopping malls in the winter), or get new clothes. All you need is a good pair of shoes.

No one is too old to start exercising regularly. Some women begin in their 70s or later. A group of frail 90-year-olds increased their muscle strength, size, and mobility in just eight weeks with weight-training three times a week.

Those women who do go to health clubs usually want to use free weights (which are especially beneficial for building bone mass), body-sculpting machines (such as Nautilus), or they want an organized class where someone else does the thinking and they just have to follow a routine.

If you're considering a health club, ask about the qualifications of the instructors, although there is no uniform certification process. Instructors with lots of experience and dance or kinesiology (the study of human muscular movements) background, for instance, are usually savvy about avoiding injuries. (The safest aerobics taught today is low impact. It's just as effective as high-impact jumping and is not fraught with potential injuries.) Good instructors not only know exercises, but also understand anatomy and how the muscles work. Beware of instructors who only pay attention to themselves in the mirror and not to you.

Try different instructors to find the one you like best, because if you don't, you'll discover lots of reasons not to go. If you're not interested in using the locker room, arrange your schedule so that you don't need it. If you don't want to use weight rooms along with men, find a club that has women-only facilities. Some clubs cater to large people. Find out if there is a trial membership period, and inspect the club during the time you would use it. Is it overcrowded? Does it have facilities you wouldn't use (saunas and hot tubs) that raise the price? Will the club refund your money if you move away or are injured? Ask the Better Business Bureau how the club handles complaints.

Some women feel worse each and every time they exercise. (And, no, it can't all be explained away by saying these women are out of shape. Bodies respond differently. Some women, including athletes, have exercise-induced asthma, for instance.) If you have this problem, look for ways to build exercise into your daily life. When you walk to the car or climb the steps, be aware and do it consciously. Park your car a little farther than you need to from the store or your job. Sing—in the shower, the car, the church choir. It will improve your heart-lung functioning, and it may also help keep your voice youthful, avoiding the hoarse, wavering tones associated with old age.

While you exercise, play music, whether that means listening to a tape while walking or playing energetic music during a demanding workout. Consider yoga. It's a peaceful series of postures that increase your circulation, improve your breathing, and help limber and stretch your body. (See "Yoga" on page 59.)

FRIENDS AND FAMILY

People came into this world for eons in interdependent tribes held together by location and genetics. Our ancestors stayed with each other not only because of a shared need for food and shelter, but also for the physical need for companionship, which is still true today.

Everyone needs friends, but women with special needs for support networks are: caregivers to the old and sick; single moms; women experiencing grief, whether from widowhood, divorce, a partner's loss of a job or a move to a new city following a partner's transfer; and women who have recently had operations. The women who make friends with the most ease, researchers say, may be single women without children who never married. They learn early how to keep other people in their lives.

You can expand your network and keep it active by paying attention to friend-making and friend-nurturing the same way you pay attention to other health habits. Evaluate the effect on your life any change in your social network might make. Find someone with whom you can share your feelings and/or whom you can see at least once a week. If you have a mate, work on making that tie the best it can be. Try to work in a congenial atmosphere. Your co-workers can enhance or inhibit your health, and your allies at work are your first line of defense in fighting stress. For many women, office conversations have taken the place of over-the-fence chats with neighbors.

Select your support network based on your particular needs. You have different friends for different needs. If your parent just died, you'd probably turn to your partner or your siblings. If you just received a professional award, you might turn first to a colleague who understands your career goals. And if you want to appreciate a walk on a warm spring day, your dog might be the perfect companion. Cats, dogs, and other animals provide companionship, especially if you stroke their fur and talk to them. Studies indicate those actions may lower your blood pressure and reduce stress.

Don't feel bad if you like your friends a lot more than you like your relatives. Some people choose not to see some or all of their relatives. That may be a good health decision, since being around people who make us feel bad can literally make us sick. Other wise moves include contacting a self-help group whether for a disease or condition that you have or for one someone you are caring for has. Help someone else; volunteer your time.

Feeding your hermit is what you're doing when you're alone and enjoying it. Solitary time can feed your soul as well as improve your health. Loneliness is when you don't have as much intimate contact with people as you need. Continued for a long time it leads to depression, unhappiness, alcoholism in those who are susceptible, loss of morale, and a twofold increase in death from heart disease. Some research indicates that for many of us loneliness may be more devastating to our health than smoking. (See "Friends and Family" on page 606 in Recommended Reading for more information about our need for social ties.)

SEX

Movies, TV, magazines, newspapers, popular songs, and books teach us more about sex than we ever realize. According to the cultural messages, women who are having sex are young, attractive, single, childless, healthy, possessors of large breasts, "ready, willing, and able," and, oh, by the way, they never need to think about birth control. The reality is that women who enjoy sex do think of birth control if they're having sex with a man, are of any age and appearance, and may be married or single, with or without children.

Sexuality is a natural expression of being human. Like other appetites, some women have more interest in sex than others. And some have more sexual partners. (In a comprehensive 1989 survey, on average, women reported having had three sexual partners since age 18.) But regardless of how much you are interested, wanted sex empowers whereas unwanted sex depletes. Wanted sex, no matter whom you do it with, improves your circulation, keeps your vagina healthy, and releases tension. A woman's sexual capacity varies, but it usually increases after she has had a baby, which causes her pelvic blood network to enlarge, resulting in an increased capacity for orgasmic sensation.

History doesn't record much about what women say about sex, but many women today report sex gets better as one grows older — if there's an opportunity and there are no mental or physical complaints. As women age, they experience more orgasms, especially after age forty, and many women experience an increase in sexual desire after menopause due to an increase in the male hormone, androgen.

Throughout our lives, our interest in sex waxes and wanes, often depending on our life circumstances at the moment. Some sexual turning points can be pregnancy (see "Sex During Pregnancy" on page 451), the early years of raising young children, or the loss of a mate. Some women choose to sublimate their sexual energy into a career or expressions of creativity. A sexually active woman may want to consider what enhances and empowers her sexual pleasure, and what inhibits it. (See "Sex" on page 606 in Recommended Reading for more information about women's experience of sex.)

ENHANCING SEXUAL PLEASURE

To enjoy sex, it helps to feel good about your physical body and have body confidence. Do what you enjoy, experience your version of pleasure, and ignore the rest. Women are sexually extraordinarily adaptable and can experience pleasure with or without stimulation of the clitoris, G spot, vagina, or other "magic" places. Be well rested, avoid unhealthy stress, and take vacations (they're known to stimulate sexual desire). If you work at a job you like, you're in luck. Women who enjoy their work report more sexual satisfaction. When you're avoiding pregnancy and want to avoid anxiety as well, use a form of birth control in which you have confidence, and use it all the time.

Be with a partner who matters to you. If women care more deeply about their sexual partners, on average, than men do, it's not just because of early training or cultural norms. It's physical. The hormone oxytocin flows in our bodies more than it does in men. And research shows that this "good feeling" hormone stimulates caregiving tendencies. It becomes a trigger for bonding, whether with a mate or with an infant. That's true during orgasm (resulting in a sense of well-being and pleasure), during labor (stimulating contractions) and breastfeeding (pleasurably releasing milk from the breasts).

Exercise your pelvic floor muscles. All forms of muscular exercise improve our pubococcygeus (PC) muscle, the master muscle of support in the pelvis, but the Kegel pelvic-floor exercises are the best. Childbirth is almost universally blamed for damage to the PC muscle, but some researchers believe this is true only in the case of muscles that were already weak at the time. Ordinarily, a strong PC muscle is not weakened in birth unless there is unusual trauma or many children. A strong PC muscle may result in more feeling in the vagina, more orgasms, and enhanced vaginal lubrication. It also may reduce or sometimes eliminate a number of other problems that result from weak muscles in the pelvis, including menstrual cramps; urine leaking from laughing, sneezing or coughing; and early symptoms of uterine prolapse (a fallen uterus). Elderly women who have leaked urine for years to the point of having to wear pads have learned to do Kegels with very favorable results: improvement for nearly all and total cure for many, often avoiding surgery.

KEGEL EXERCISES

To do Kegels, isolate the PC muscle by sitting on the toilet, start to urinate, then stop. The muscle you feel when you start and stop urinating is the PC muscle. You can feel it also when you put two fingers into your vagina and contract and release the muscle. If you're not sure which is the right muscle, find a health care provider who uses either her fingers or a perineometer (a muscle tester than can be inserted into your vagina to measure the strength of the PC muscle) to help you.

Now that you have found your PC muscle, you're ready to exercise. Quick squeezes are called flicks (contract and release your PC muscle to the beat of your heart or the rhythm of music), longer ones are called holds (contract for 10 seconds, squeeze once rapidly, then release for 10 seconds).

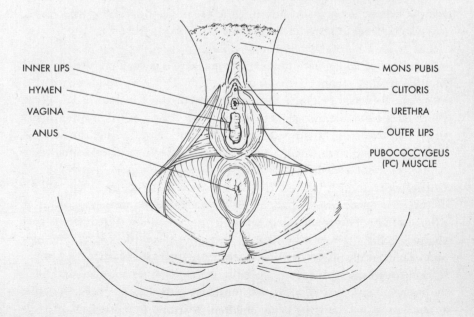

INNER LIPS

HYMEN

VAGINA

ANUS

MONS PUBIS

CLITORIS

URETHRA

OUTER LIPS

PUBOCOCCYGEUS
(PC) MUSCLE

BODY PARTS FOR KEGEL EXERCISE

Estimates vary on how often and how many of these exercises you need to do, but you will be the best judge for you. You should feel results in about three weeks; if you don't, consider increasing the exercises. It's recommended by some experts that you do flicks and holds for a total of 15 minutes every day, or a total of 50 to 100.

In some cultures daughters learn this simple exercise from their mothers just as they learn how to take care of the rest of their bodies. But in Western cultures, mother-daughter sexual instruction has been taboo. Some doctors are not familiar with these exercises either, so don't assume that they can help you with them.

THINGS THAT INHIBIT SEXUAL PLEASURE

Many women enjoy sex less when they don't feel good about their bodies. Insecurity about the way you look can affect any woman at some time in her life, but those who have had cancer or disfiguring operations or have just had a baby are especially susceptible to feeling physically inadequate. Stress, fatigue, illness, and feeling low can also interfere with sexual pleasure. Some infections and conditions can reduce or eliminate sexual desire and pleasure, either because of pain (for example, due to an ovarian cyst) or itching (from, say, a yeast infection), or both. Too much alcohol reduces interest in sex and increases the likelihood that a woman will not experience orgasm, although the use of alcohol often precedes sex for many women. Occasionally, uterine fibroids interfere with orgasms as well.

Drugs, including barbiturates; tranquilizers like Valium, Ativan, and Xanax; Depo-Provera, a birth control injection; Provera, used for excessive menopausal bleeding; DES, the Pill (although the freedom from worry about birth control may make this sexually enhancing as well), and progesterone, all may possibly impede sexual pleasure. Episiotomy, the surgical cut to widen the birth canal during childbirth, may result in painful intercourse, at least for awhile.

Oophorectomy (removal of ovaries) and hysterectomy (removal of uterus) have mixed results. For some women, sexual pleasure increases after a hysterectomy because it solves a problem that had interfered with sexual pleasure before. However, for other women, pleasure decreases. The biggest killer of sexual desire is an oophorectomy, because it castrates a woman by removing her ovaries (see "Oophorectomies, Hysterectomies, and Sex" on page 362). Some women who have had oophorectomies will experience a return of sexual desire by taking a drug combination of estrogen, progestin, and testosterone (androgen).

This may all sound bleak, but other women have had these problems and have found ways around them, so don't feel that your current problem, whatever it may be, will be a life sentence. If you're not enjoying sex as much as you'd like, here are some things you can try:

• *Remember that you are sexually unique.* You may normally want more or less sexual activity than your partner, and your normal response to sexual stimuli may be more or less like other women's.

• *Find time for sex and know that you deserve its pleasure.*

• *Discover your particular sexual pleasures* and let your lover know how to provide pleasure to you.

• *Avoid all sexual overtures that you don't want.* You'll not only feel more in control of your life, but you will experience sex as a pleasure — not a punishment.

• *Avoid any drug that you know inhibits your sexual desire.*

• *Learn to retrain your body's sexual responses,* if necessary. (See Wigfall-Williams on page 617 in Recommended Reading for suggestions on sexual retraining.)

• *Change your diet* if ovarian cysts or uterine fibroids interfere with your sexual pleasure. (See "Ovarian Cysts" on page 437 and "Uterine Fibroids" on page 522 for dietary recommendations.)

EMOTIONS

Emotional ills can be as debilitating to the immune system as cancer cells, drugs, and the AIDS virus. That's why it's just as important to maintain good emotional health habits as it is to eat well and to exercise. The ingredients of women's and men's emotional health are very similar, but women usually know more about emotions because biologically we're childbearers and culturally we are permitted to express feelings. Love is the essence of life, and women usually are the ones who understand this and provide the glue in a family. But on the flip side, women are susceptible to three normal emotions that can become negative when taken to extremes. We all would do well to recognize and manage them before they become problematic.

DEPRESSION

Some consider depression the common cold of emotional ills, with all of us at least having the blahs — a mild form of depression — from time to time. Some of the reasons for depression are not mental but physical: a genetic predisposition, deficiencies of specific vitamins — in particular the

B vitamins — (see Werbach on page 606 of Recommended Reading) a drug side effect, or a lack of sun in the winter, called seasonal affective disorder, or SAD. SAD is often treated successfully with exposure to more light. (See "Seasonal Affective Disorder" on page 606 in Recommended Reading.) Other reasons for depression can be frustration, changes in our lives, or what some call spiritual crises. Depression may also accompany a chronic ailment or serious illness.

Many think our bouts of mild depression can be used to teach us about ourselves and should be welcomed, not dreaded. Some researchers recommend exercise as the best all-around cure for mild depression, because it releases mood-altering chemicals in the body. (And as depression can be "catching," you would do well to avoid depressing people.) However, severe depression — when symptoms are so intense that a person is unable to function at work or at home — often requires both counseling and drug treatment. For best results, if you seek treatment for depression, find someone who will take a thorough history from you to avoid misdiagnosis.

GUILT

Although it's an uncomfortable feeling, guilt is a plus if it's used for self-correction. It's a minus if it is a constant companion in your life. Constantly feeling guilty is like driving down the street while looking in the rearview mirror. You can't see where you're going, and you're likely to mess up what's ahead. As women, and especially as mothers, we may be programmed to blame ourselves for everyone else's problems, but for our good health, we must begin to question that script.

WORRY

Some women worry all the time, and think it's virtuous. Many spend hours a day fearing the what-ifs of the future. Like guilt, worry is helpful if it's used to look out for real danger. Otherwise, worry doesn't seem to be helpful. It can escalate to phobias, interfere with living, and cause indecision and procrastination. (See "Worry" on page 607 in Recommended Reading and "Emotional Health" on page 577 in the Resource Directory for organizations which are helpful with a variety of emotional problems.)

ACCENTUATING THE POSITIVE

To avoid the downside of depression, guilt, and worry, try to cope effectively with what life hands you — no more, and no less. It may take hard work and much time to develop this learned response, but it is possible to do so. Your resilience influences how well you handle crises of all kinds. Coping well contributes to feeling healthy and in control; helplessness and hopelessness suppress the immune system. Be positive, be an optimist.

Expect the best to happen. Imagine good things in your life. If this doesn't come naturally, then pretend. As a result, you may adjust to an illness better than others, cope better with problems in general, and will certainly be more pleasant to be around. Most people pick their optimistic or pessimistic style early in life and stick with it, but if you want to change from being a pessimist to being an optimist, it's possible with lots of practice.

Take responsibility for what happens to you. We all experience setbacks that are beyond our control, but embracing our problems is empowering. Do what you have to do to feel you have control over your life. When you feel more control over life events, even when other more "realistic" people say it's impossible, your health will be enhanced. If you feel better at the beach or in the mountains or in the midst of an urban crowd, arrange your life so that you can be in those places at least some of the time. If certain pieces of furniture or other objects, like books or photographs, make you feel good, keep those in a prominent place in your life. Avoid overlooking the contentment you enjoy now in the search for "perfect" happiness.

HOW TO FIND A THERAPIST

If you are finding that a problem is becoming all-consuming, and you need more help than what you can get from friends and family, self-help groups, clergy, or books, you may benefit from some form of therapy. Whether or not therapy helps you depends in part upon finding a therapist who suits you, so keep the following guidelines in mind:

• *Think about what your problem is and put it into words.* If you can't sleep at night or are afraid to drive, say that. If you were just divorced, despise your job, or feel depressed, say that. Or if you're in the midst of a messy relationship with no one to turn to, say that. No matter how vague the problem seems to you when you put it into words, you'll waste your time (and money) and that of the therapist if you don't have some idea of what part of your life needs attention.

• *Give some thought to what kind of therapy is most likely to help you* (though what seems to matter more is how much you like the person, regardless of her training). There are more therapists now than ever before and many therapies are available, but here are two of the most common. *Psychotherapy,* which usually takes six months to five years, focuses on understanding your unconscious feelings and developing insights. *Brief therapy*, which usually takes 10 to 12 weeks (but can be as brief as one session), focuses on how you can solve a specific conscious problem. Most people stop therapy in less than six months, and research shows that the short approach is usually as effective as the long, particularly for people who have a clear idea of what their problem is and who want to solve it quickly.

• *Check your insurance plan.* The coverage you have may vary depending on the type of therapist you choose. Clinical social workers have at least a master's degree, plus at least two years of clinical experience. Clinical psychologists have either a master's degree or doctorate in the study of human behavior with at least two years of supervised experience. Psychiatrists are medical doctors who, in addition to medical school training, have four years of specialty training in mental disorders; they are the only therapists who can prescribe drugs. Psychoanalysts are psychiatrists or psychologists with specific training in the theories and techniques of Sigmund Freud and his followers.

• *Shop around.* First, gather some names. If you are African American or Latina, for example, and want an African American or Latina therapist, narrow your focus. Ask your friends about their experiences with therapy. Call the mental health department of your local health department and ask if they make referrals. Yellow Pages are a resource, if only to narrow your search. Don't let lack of funds stand in your way. If you do not have cash or insurance to pay for a therapist, call your local United Way, health department, or family and children's organization to find out what services they offer.

• *Talk with therapists on the phone to narrow your search.* If you don't like the therapist on the phone, you're not likely to enjoy her in person either. You can tell whoever answers the phone who you are and that you have some questions of a personal nature for the therapist. Ask if there is a fee for this phone conversation. Ask what time would be convenient for you to call back or whether the person would prefer to call you later. When you are speaking to the therapist, among the questions you may ask are:

> *Have you successfully treated other women with a problem like mine?*
> *About how long will the treatment take?* (Be aware that this may be hard to determine before an in-person interview.)
> *Do you think you can help me?* (If this person doesn't sound optimistic about your success, look elsewhere until you find someone who does. Plan for success, not failure.)
> *What do you expect of me?*
> *How long is a therapy session?*

What happens if I am late?
How much do you charge?
Can you accept direct payment from my insurance?

• *Make a get-acquainted appointment first.* See how the first session goes before committing yourself to a therapist. Clarify why you're there and have the therapist explain your rights as a person seeking help as well as what the therapist sees as her job. The hallmark of a helpful therapist is that she understands you. Some believe that people leave therapists more because they feel misunderstood than for any other reason. Although both sexes can be helpful, women psychiatrists in particular give patients more time and may pay more attention to preventive health.

The therapist should not be prejudiced against you because you are a woman, a member of a minority, lesbian, divorced, battered or otherwise abused, a user of recreational drugs, a believer or nonbeliever in God, nor for any other reason. This person should help you see your strengths, not just your problems. A therapist with a negative attitude will slow your recovery. Don't waste your time thinking that the therapist will overcome any initial personal bias by working with you. That's not likely, nor is it time well spent. (See "Finding A Therapist" on page 607 in Recommended Reading.)

WOMEN AND HYPOCHONDRIA

Sometimes women, including those who seek therapy, are thought to be hypochondriacs (people who imagine illnesses). Traditionally, many men have thought that women are sentimental and weak, often full of imaginary ills. Despite evidence to the contrary, this belief in women's inherent weakness is alive and well today.

Women typically are more interested in health matters than men. They often take prevention more seriously, ask more questions, and will go sooner to doctors or therapists with a problem. Those actions may sound to you like taking responsibility, but to many others it's considered problematic behavior. Since men don't go to doctors or therapists as quickly, their ailments are often taken more seriously. According to many studies, men complaining of headaches and depression, for instance, are given more time by health care providers than are women with similar maladies.

In addition, women have a host of ills that are difficult to diagnose or treat. Men don't get endometriosis, for example — a disease that has a wide range of symptoms, some of which can be rather vague. Sometimes women have to go to several doctors before they find one who can really help. This search for the cure doesn't prove that we're hypochondriacs. Rather, it says that the successful treatment of some ailments may require more effort on our part.

A true hypochondriac lives in terror of disease and is preoccupied with bodily symptoms and functions for no reason. Some women, indeed, have vague feelings of illness or discomfort, a kind of "cosmic flu," that can't be identified — just as some men do. And some women enjoy poor health — just as some men do. But society's perception of those women and men may be quite different.

If you are troubled by a health problem, trust your instincts and keep seeking help until you are given a diagnosis that makes sense. Because women are sometimes considered malingerers, you may encounter skepticism, and you may have to be more diligent than you would like. Remind yourself, if necessary, that you do have a problem, and that finding the right help is not necessarily a popularity contest.

STRESS

Stress is the spice of life. Sometimes it gives you indigestion and sometimes it adds zest. Good stress adds incentive, mobilizes us for action, and gives us a measure of excitement. When their lives become too calm some people fall ill as easily as others get sick when their lives become too hectic. It's the negative stress over a long period of time that inhibits our immune system.

The women most likely to feel positive stress — and are healthier for it — are those who have multiple roles in life. They are happily married and/or have families at home, have strong mutual support networks, and are employed. Even though women are more likely to have the most stressful jobs in the workplace and increasing numbers of women moonlight with a second job, work is still a positive experience for many women. On the other hand, the women most likely to feel negative stress are those who are poor, are single parents, have a chronic illness, live with chronic pain, or care for someone who does (see "Chronic Pain" on page 607 in Recommended Reading.)

Symptoms of negative stress include headaches, acting in a rude and curt manner toward the people around you, excessive drinking, ulcers, depression, leaving work undone, and failure to hear what other people say. Negative stress can raise your blood pressure, increase your heart rate, and cause pain, for example, in the lower back, not explained by any organic or systemic dysfunction, or in the face, as in temporomandibular joint, or TMJ, syndrome (see "Temporomandibular Joint Syndrome" on page 502).

Following are suggestions for relieving negative stress and promoting relaxation, though no one strategy is best for everyone. (See "Stress" on page 607 in Recommended Reading.)

• *Use creativity.* When you can't be creative in your relationships or on the job, be creative in other parts of your life. (See "Creativity" on page 607 in Recommended Reading.)

• *Listen to your body.* You may be relaxing, but not enough for you. You may be eating well, but not well enough for *you.* (See "The Stress Diet" on page 36.)

• *Do whatever is calming for you.* If seeing a police car in your rearview mirror makes you anxious, breathe slowly (one of the quickest ways to reduce stress), turn on classical music (usually soothing), and don't drive over the speed limit. Relax your shoulders, and feel the tension lessen. Whether you're doing the dishes, stuck in a traffic jam, or sitting at a day-long meeting, take a few moments to consciously relax.

• *Get enough rest.* Most people sleep seven to eight hours daily. Women, however, are more likely than men to report sleeping fewer than six hours at night. This is especially true of mothers of young children. Too little sleep interferes with your creativity and sense of well-being, and it may make you susceptible to fatigue and illness. (See "Fatigue" on page 344.)

• *Get enough exercise.* Exercise releases tension quickly and reduces anxiety.

• *Laugh a lot.* Find and nurture friends who are funny. Laughter that leaves us weak for the moment is beneficial and healing: it enhances our immune system, reduces blood pressure, eases muscle tension, and improves breathing and the nervous system. It also can increase your creativity on the job or at home, can reduce pain and inflammation, aids sleep and digestion, and some say it offers a natural alternative to drug-induced highs.

• *Change your stressful environment.* That may or may not be easy. If it would involve a job change, think through what you would have to do. It may reduce your stress just to figure out what the steps would be. Cut out irritating noise and listen to soothing music instead. That can slow your heartbeat, making it easier to relax.

• *Change your perspective.* Much stress occurs when your mind irrationally worries your body that some awful thing is going to happen. Stress can also occur when you put everyone else's needs before your own.

• *Choose moderation.* Too much of almost anything — sunlight, exercise, high-fiber foods, junk food, work, even leisure — will suppress your immune system.

• *Limit your exposure to environmental hazards that stress your body.* Examples are: toxic chemicals on the job, in the home, or in the outside environment, air pollution, and enclosed buildings with poor air circulation.

• *Have a good cry.* You may rid your body of potentially harmful stress chemicals.

• *Talk out your problem with someone you trust.* Unwanted stress can make you feel like a pressure cooker. Talking about your worries lets off steam.

• *Try a massage, or take a hot bath.* Either one increases blood flow and helps relax muscles. (See "Massage" on page 607 in Recommended Reading.)

Other ways of minimizing the negative stress in your life include the ancient practices of therapeutic touch, acupressure, yoga, and meditation.

THERAPEUTIC TOUCH

Therapeutic touch is the no-touch version of the laying on of hands. This ancient technique was rediscovered in the 1970s by Dolores Krieger, a nurse. It's used to relieve pain and promote relaxation. Research has shown that it increases levels of certain helpful chemicals in the blood, and it may speed the healing of ulcers and bone fractures.

Therapeutic touch can be performed by someone well versed in this therapy, or it can be done with practice by someone following directions. You can find a practitioner in the Yellow Pages of your phone book in some cities, or try calling your local hospital (some nurses perform this therapy on request) or nursing school and ask for a referral.

Here's how therapeutic touch is done. The therapist takes a moment to feel peaceful. Then, palms out, she places her hands two to four inches away from your skin while you're standing, sitting, or lying down. She may do this all over your body, or she may focus on specific parts of your body. Sometimes she may make rapid up-and-down wiping motions. It might feel warm in some body parts after the therapist has done this, and many people feel relaxed. It's not clear why therapeutic touch may cause warming and relaxation, but it's believed this effect is the result of a manipulation of a suspected energy field around a person's body. (See "Therapeutic Touch" on page 607 in Recommended Reading.)

ACUPRESSURE

Acupressure is self-administered, needleless acupuncture. It's the pressing of certain points on the body that has a beneficial effect at the painful site and on certain ailments. Acupressure stimulates circulation and aids in relaxation. It can also give relief from headaches, motion sickness, tension,

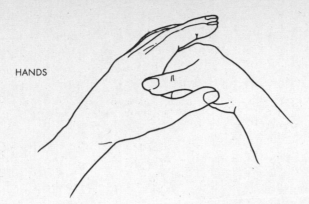

HANDS

Squeeze the point where the thumb and index finger of the other hand meet. Hold for 15 seconds. Switch hands and repeat.

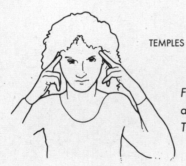

TEMPLES

Find the depression between your hairline and the outer edge of your eyebrows. Then press.

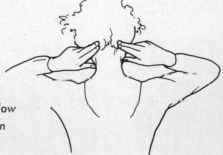

BACK OF HEAD

Massage the back of the neck just below the base of the skull about one inch on either side of the spine.

ACUPRESSURE HEADACHE RELIEF

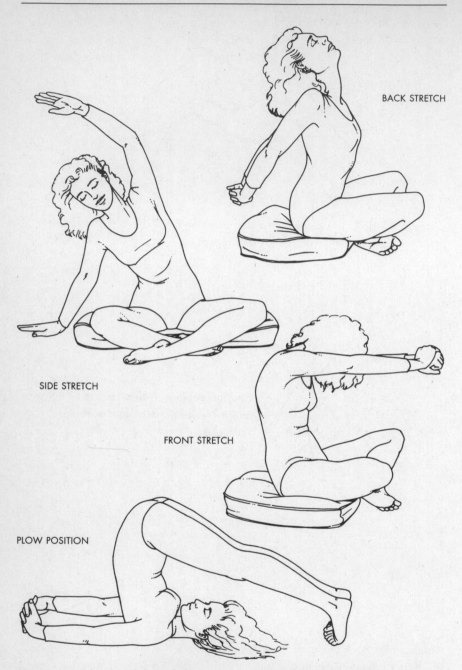

BACK STRETCH

SIDE STRETCH

FRONT STRETCH

PLOW POSITION

Start on your back with legs in front of you. With palms down, lift legs over your head.

YOGA

constipation, and fatigue, and can be helpful in premenstrual syndrome, morning sickness in pregnancy, labor, birth, breastfeeding, menopausal symptoms, and tension. (See "Acupressure" on page 607 in Recommended Reading.)

YOGA

Yoga is a system of postures that strengthen and stretch. Yoga tones and increases the suppleness of both the spine and the rest of the body. Deep breathing oxygenates the blood and invigorates the brain and nervous system, and deep relaxation and meditation ease tension and stress. Yoga is also helpful for people who have had injuries or who have chronic pain. It can relieve asthma by improving breathing capacity, helps prevent uterine prolapse and urine incontinence, and provides general well-being for the whole body. (See "Yoga" on page 608 in Recommended Reading.)

MEDITATION

Meditation is a quiet state that brings relaxation along with lowered metabolism, heart rate, breathing rate, and blood pressure, as well as slower brain waves and, for many, a decrease in pain. It literally slows down the body.

One common guide for relaxation involves this sequence: Sit or lie down quietly in a comfortable position. Close your eyes. Relax your muscles. Breathe slowly and naturally. As you breathe out, feel yourself beginning to relax. Feel the tension leave your body. Imagine that you're doing this in a calm and relaxing place — at the beach or at the foot of a mountain. Don't worry about how you're doing. Continue for 10 to 20 minutes. Do this once or twice a day and your concentration will improve over time with practice. (See "Meditation" on page 608 in Recommended Reading.)

SKIN HEALTH

Sunlight is intoxicating, may brighten your mood, and is essential for life. It can give your body needed vitamin D, perhaps even reduce your blood pressure and soothe your stomach. But adequate amounts of beneficial sun can be obtained in 15 minutes, before burning or tanning occurs. Too much sun can be harmful, even deadly. Following are suggestions for maintaining healthy skin while delaying the onset of wrinkles and reducing your risk for skin cancer and cataracts.

• *Protect your skin from direct sunlight as much as possible.* Wear a hat or sun visor, long-sleeved shirts, and long pants. Protect your eyes by wearing sunglasses that block ultraviolet light. Consider wearing a wet-suit if you're going to spend hours in the water while white-water rafting, surfing, or snorkeling.

• *Wear sunscreen every day* to reduce your risk of sunburn and skin aging, particularly if you live in a high-altitude area or near a beach. Protect infants and children also. Most of us get 80 percent of our total lifetime sun exposure by age 21. And despite many parents' belief that a child with a tan is a healthy child, one bad sunburn in childhood can lead to skin cancer in adulthood. As the ozone layer (that part of the atmosphere that blocks out many dangerous ultraviolet rays) decreases, you'll burn sooner and—though it won't entirely prevent sun damage—adequate sunscreen will be more important than ever. An added benefit of lip balm to reduce the number of flare-ups of painful cold sores (or herpes blisters) around the lips is its sunscreen.

Many experts recommend that you use a product with a sun protection factor (SPF) of at least 15, which theoretically allows you to stay in the sun 15 times longer than if you had no protection. (For most people, that's 15 minutes.) If you use SPF 15, supposedly you could be in the sun for three hours and 45 minutes before burning (or SPF 15 multiplied by 15 minutes). That only holds true, though, when the product is *liberally* applied. Generally one ounce is needed to cover one adult body. Keep the sunscreen creams away from your eyes because of possible allergic reactions.

Unfortunately, no sunscreen product offers protection from all harmful ultraviolet rays—that means no product offers full protection from skin cancer or photoaging. Most products on the market now are only effective against ultraviolet B (UVB) light and not ultraviolet A (UVA) rays, which until recently were considered benign. (The SPF system measures only UVB radiation protection.)

It makes sense then to avoid long periods in the sun, even with liberal use of sunscreen, and then to use the higher number SPF products as much as possible. In the future, look for products that protect you from both kinds of UV rays. But remember that no product will ever be 100 percent effective, so you still need to use common sense about how long you stay out in the sun. Be aware, too, that some drugs, like antibiotics, the Pill, or anti-inflammatory agents may make your skin more sun sensitive. And too much sun can be a trigger for lupus (see "Lupus" on page 391).

• *Eat a healthy diet.* Since your skin reflects what you do (and don't) eat, eat well. (See "The Skin Diet" on page 35 and "Skin Health" on page 608 in Recommended Reading.)

• *Have your skin checked periodically by a dermatologist* if you already have had skin cancer (there is a 50 percent chance of reoccurrence within five years), if you have a family history of skin cancer, if you live in areas of high altitude or mostly sunny days, if you smoke, or if you have new, unusual skin eruptions.

• *Avoid tanning booths.* Their lamps produce light that is more harmful than natural sunlight. Overexposure in tanning salons may also burn the corneas of your eyes and cause cataracts. If you *must* tan (although tanning of any kind always damages the skin), a tan from the sun is safer than one from a tanning salon. The safest tan, however, comes from the more than 35 self-tanning products on the market.

• *Avoid smoking.* It will accelerate wrinkling, sometimes by as much as ten years, due to the effect of nicotine on the surface of your blood vessels, and it increases your risk for skin cancer.

• *Exercise regularly.* This increases the circulation to your skin and helps keep it healthy.

Don't believe cosmetic companies' claims for wrinkle-reversal products. They're not true. Cosmetic manufacturers can claim almost anything because the Food and Drug Administration (FDA), the policing agency for false product claims, is usually too busy keeping up with other products and drugs. However, the FDA does keep track of complaints about cosmetics. (See "Skin Health" on page 596 in the Resource Directory if you have a problem with a cosmetic or skincare product.)

One miracle product you may have heard about is Retin-A. This prescription-only derivative of vitamin A has been approved by the FDA for the treatment of acne and sometimes skin cancer. It's also used now as an antiwrinkle cream, because it may make the face smoother and pinker while erasing fine wrinkles. It's also effective in making so-called liver spots or dark patches of skin caused by sun damage lighter. That's the good news.

The bad news is that changes, which may be only subtle, take months to appear and will fade quickly if you use this expensive drug for only a few months. Retin-A use requires daily sunscreen protection and the avoidance of sun exposure because of the skin's increased sensitivity. Retin-A nearly always causes some short-term reaction, including skin peeling, cracking, stinging, and red, scaly patches. This product has not been in use long enough for researchers to know if it has long-term side effects.

DENTAL HEALTH

The care of teeth is the same for women and men with the exception that pregnancy affects the gums, and women are more likely to have temporomandibular joint, or TMJ, syndrome (see "Temporomandibular Joint Syndrome" on page 502). Many women's gums bleed easily during pregnancy. Along with regular dental hygiene, many women have found that taking vitamin C, especially when combined with calcium and magnesium, reduces the bleeding and tenderness. (See "The Pregnancy Diet" on page 34.)

FILLINGS

Amalgam fillings are the 100 million fillings, known as silver fillings, that dentists use every year to restore decayed teeth. The concern of some dentists is that they are 50 percent mercury, and mercury is toxic. Researchers agree that mercury can indeed make its way into the body, but there's no agreement on what that means. In Sweden dentists cannot put amalgam fillings into the teeth of pregnant women, but here in the United States, the National Institutes of Health in 1991 said no confirmed effects on a fetus have been reported and the American Dental Association says these fillings are safe for all. They point out that if these fillings were causing problems, the number of complaints would be overwhelming. More recently, the U.S. Public Health Service agreed with this statement, but also allowed that long-term health problems can't be ruled out because of insufficient research.

Signs of mercury toxicity are: irritability, depression, anxiety, and insomnia. To complicate matters, however, mercury can also depress the immune system, which can result in a flare-up of a number of diseases. If you're interested in investigating whether or not you have mercury in your body, you can obtain a blood test. Substitutes for amalgam fillings are usually made with gold, ceramics, or plastic and are usually more expensive than amalgam. (See "Dental Health" on page 608 in Recommended Reading for more information and page 574 in the Resource Directory for a toll-free number to obtain the names of dentists who offer mercury-free dental fillings.)

DENTAL X-RAYS

Dentists routinely x-ray teeth because in some combination they believe that the information obtained is essential, or consumers want it, or it also helps pay the overhead. Dental x-rays are not perfectly safe, because no form of this radiation is perfectly safe, nor are all x-ray machines properly calibrated to give you the least amount of radiation. Many states, but not all, have mandatory inspections of dental x-ray machines every three years.

But doesn't the use of dental x-rays outweigh the risks? That depends on why you're having the x-rays. For instance, have you wondered what would happen if you didn't have the routine "bite-wing" x-rays to determine if you have hidden cavities? In most cases, nothing would happen. That's because, when there's no visible sign of tooth decay, only one in 10 x-rays will turn up such hidden decay. So what happens if you don't get the x-rays and all the while you have had a cavity? Eventually that cavity will be visible, and you and your dentist will proceed with the appropriate treatment — perhaps not as quickly as you might have with an x-ray, but well before the tooth is in serious trouble. The effect of all radiation adds up, and the less you are exposed, the less risk there is to your body.

Your children are more susceptible to the radiation of dental x-rays than you are because the younger people are, the more susceptible they are to tissue damage. (See "X-Rays" on page 608 in Recommended Reading and on page 599 in the Resource Directory.)

Eye Health

The care of eyes is the same for women and men though women are more likely to use certain drugs that may affect the eyes. The Pill, for instance, makes the wearing of contact lenses uncomfortable or impossible in some women, because of a change in the curvature of the cornea.

About 50 percent of people in the United States wear glasses, with 20 percent of that group also using contact lenses. Women, especially younger women, are more likely to use contacts than any other group. These lenses are available in hard or soft, daily or extended wear, bifocal, colored (the preferred colors are shades of blue), permanent or disposable. However, not all of these lens options nor the solutions to clean these products are equally safe.

All contact lenses need to be kept scrupulously clean, following each product's directions for cleaning, wetting, soaking, and lubricating. That means no homemade cleaning solutions to reduce costs. When contact lenses are not handled as directed, users are more likely to get eye infections. If you are allergic to a particular lens care product or your eyes burn when you put in your contact lens, try switching to a lens-cleaning product that does not use any preservative, especially thimerosal.

Be careful about the use of extended-wear lenses (which can be left in for two weeks or so before cleaning) or disposable contact lenses (which can be left in one week and then thrown away). They may be more convenient than lenses that are removed daily, but many eye experts say that keeping a contact on the cornea for prolonged periods increases many times over your risk for red eyes, corneal abrasions (cuts on the surface of the eye), corneal ulcers, and allergic eye symptoms, especially in those who are prone to allergies anyway. More seriously, contacts that are left on for days increase your risk for serious infections, some of which cause severe vision loss and require corneal transplants.

To keep your eyes healthy, wear sunglasses that protect eyes from ultraviolet (UV) light. (Not all sunglasses filter UV, so select carefully.) Have a special UV-screening coating added to your contacts or eyeglasses. Cutting down on your exposure to UV rays reduces your risk for the formation of cataracts (thin layers of cells that become opaque and blur or block vision). Eat a diet rich in vitamin A to reduce incidences of burning, itching, and conjunctivitis in your eyes. Include the B vitamins to reduce eye twitching and clouding of the cornea, and add vitamin C to prevent cataracts and glaucoma (a disease that damages the optic nerve).

CHAPTER 3

How to Get Better Health Care by Taking Responsibility for What Happens to You

Everyone has occasional aches and pains that are normal and ordinary. However, when discomforts or illnesses interfere with our pleasure in living, or our bodies are passing through stages that are foreign to us, acceptance and enjoyment of the way things are may not be enough for us anymore. It may be time to gather information, alter our behaviors appropriately, and determine the right health care providers with whom to work on a given problem.

Making health care choices is not always easy because the same solutions don't work for everyone. Also, contradictions in reported research results add to the confusion. In addition, we may have to overcome a reluctance to choose new options, especially if family and friends won't easily support unfamiliar choices or when our current health care provider is skeptical.

Following are a dozen suggestions to help you make health decisions that are in your own best interests.

AVOID ''PEDESTAL POWER''

You are in charge of your own health. Doctors and other health care providers do not determine your health. *You* do (though you don't have total control, either). By assuming that doctors control your health, you give them "pedestal power" — you've put them on a pedestal. When pedestal power is strong, you're either elevating doctors in your mind or trying to knock them down with as much force as possible. Stand on level ground with doctors. Ideally, your doctor should be a well-informed ally, not a demigod. Doctors give you the best information they have, but you heal yourself, sometimes with the aid of others, including doctors. It's *your* body that recovers from a cold or the flu, and it's *your* body that regenerates bone when you've had a break.

BRING A FRIEND

Take a friend with you to the hospital or to your doctor's office. Research shows that people heal faster, enjoy labor more, and leave the hospital sooner when they have lots of love and support from friends. Also, discussions at office visits are clearer when you have brought someone to make sure you don't miss any information. This is especially true when you're upset, sick, or unsure of yourself. In this case, two heads are indeed better than one. Ideally, the person you have with you is someone who cares about you and with whom you feel comfortable. Many hospitals and health care providers welcome this helper because she often reduces the workload of hospital nurses, and she can be a clarifying presence in a doctor's office. (See "Bring a Friend" on page 608 in Recommended Reading.)

BE YOUR OWN HEALTH DETECTIVE

Many conditions and diseases are not simple to diagnose. Our own observations and thoughtfulness about symptoms can be as important as the comments of our health care providers. One woman became her own health detective after she developed asthma in her 50s. None of the tests her allergist gave her answered the question, Why?, and the only appropriate treatment seemed to be drugs.

Since she was a scientist, she decided to keep a diary of her symptoms daily, nearly by the hour. She took that diary to her physician, and after he read it, he recognized that her daily symptoms were those of a particular allergy to red cedar that he had never seen outside of a logging camp. After questioning her further, the physician discovered that her new home was built from red cedar, and red cedar logs were burned in the fireplace, as well as stored by the furnace ducts in the basement spreading essence of red cedar every time the furnace came on. The allergist wouldn't have known to ask her questions about red cedar if this woman hadn't shown him her symptom diary. You don't have to be a scientist, however, to be a careful observer of your symptoms. (See "Health Detective" on page 608 in Recommended Reading.)

KNOW THE ODDS ARE IN YOUR FAVOR

Don't assume that if others get an ailment, you'll get it, too. It's easy to get the impression from media coverage of health that *you* will get breast cancer, *you* will have hip fractures and osteoporosis, and *you* will have a miserable menopause. The truth is that most women don't develop any kind of cancer, most women don't have hip fractures or osteoporosis, and most women don't find menopause miserable. Most of the time, most of us beat the odds.

RECOGNIZE PERSONAL BIASES — YOURS AND THEIRS

Everyone has biases, those tendencies or preferences that color the way we receive and give information. People of different points of view, in good faith, can look at the same information and come up with opposing opinions.

If you think you're not biased, think of this: If I said there are hundreds of studies that prove the superiority of breast milk over synthetic milk, would you breastfeed your infant for more than a few weeks? If I wrote that Chinese herbs work as well for some women as estrogen replacement therapy for menopausal hot flashes, would you find an acupuncturist who uses Chinese medicine or an herbalist? If I told you that there is a fabulous contraceptive that helps prevent AIDS, sexually transmitted diseases (STDs), and pregnancy, all without side effects (the condom), would you use it?

You know the answers to these questions, not me. If you recognize and accept your personal beliefs as your health care silent partner, your decision making may be easier.

Your everyday life-style choices are also part of your personal beliefs. Maybe you smoke or eat lots of junk food. Maybe you detest smoke, and think junk food is poison. Are you judgmental about other people's habits? Are you defensive about your own? Whatever your choices are, recognize them as your own, make sure you're well informed, be realistic about and plan for their consequences, and — if you wish to hold onto them — enjoy them as much as you can.

Health care providers have personal biases, just like everyone else. If you and your doctor have totally opposing viewpoints on a question of choice — for example, those dental x-rays we discussed in Chapter 2 — recognize that the doctor is entitled to her viewpoint, and you are entitled to yours. Look for health care providers who can tolerate other points of view — or better yet — share your views.

KEEP THE ROLE OF ATTITUDE IN PERSPECTIVE

If you've tried to avoid a cold or the flu through will power and you got the bug anyway, or you tried visualization and optimism and you're still stuck with a chronic condition like ulcers, allergies, or a more serious disease, or you tried for a natural childbirth and ended up with a cesarean, join the crowd. You've got lots of company. Chronic fatigue syndrome, cystitis, infertility, and many other diseases and conditions are sometimes said to be due to a state of mind. However, the mind-body connection is not clear, nor is it simple.

Since earliest times people have believed that our minds and hearts can affect our bodies. Today, some researchers describe the cancer-prone personality (masochistic, sexually inhibited, depressed, generally hostile), and they can give you details about who's likely to get a heart attack (someone who distrusts others and is in a hurry). What if you have had cancer or a heart attack? Was your self-esteem and/or state of health improved by knowing those descriptions? Or did they add a form of tyranny and a greater burden to your healing process?

Even though others may blame you for your illness, you cannot flunk the mind-body connection. Be aware that clinicians who call themselves holistic (treating the whole person, not just the particular ailment), whether they are traditional doctors or alternative healers, often seem the most insistent that your emotions have caused your illness. Who gets what disease when is in fact due to a combination of genetic triggers, environment (that includes bacteria, viruses, chemical pollutants, inappropriate diet), other unknown factors, and the mind-body connection in an as yet unexplained ratio.

If you have had one of the many diseases or conditions with mind-body profiles attached to them, here are some suggestions about what to do when you discover the psychological profile. Take from the descriptions only what is helpful to you. Ignore the rest. You know yourself best. For example, let's say you get migraine headaches. Women who get migraines are often considered oversensitive and perfectionists and their headaches are often ascribed to stress or crankiness. If it seems there is a connection between your migraines and stress, then by all means see if alleviating the stress eases your headaches. However, if stress doesn't seem to be a trigger for you, you can keep looking for another cause — say, a food allergy — or, at least for the time being, you can decide that your migraines are part of your life, and you'll cope with them.

Be sure to run to the nearest exit — if you're mobile — if someone says they are telling you about your shortcomings "for your own good." If the description is something you've read, dismiss any characteristics that don't apply, which may be all of them. When you hear it from others, you can say, "I know you mean well, but I don't believe it. If I want information, I'll ask for it. If I don't ask, please don't volunteer it."

Suggest to those who want to help you what they could do for you. You might say: "I know that you're telling me this because you want to help me, but I don't find this description helpful. Instead, let me tell you what would be helpful to me in a practical way." And then tell them. Change your health care provider if that's the person who is giving you a negative message. If this person is insistent that you have psychological problems in addition to your physical problems, and this doesn't ring true to you, you are not being aided by this person. In order for doctors and others to help you heal, you need to feel mutual trust and believe that they are helpful, not humiliatingly demeaning, or persistently wrong.

Studies show that our mind's best ally in overcoming illness is the belief that we — not someone else — will steer the course if not to complete recovery at least to a conviction that we did our best. And if we die as the result of a disease, it's because we're mortal — not because we have a bad attitude. (See "Attitude" on page 609 in Recommended Reading.)

BE YOUR OWN EXPERT

Choose an experienced health care provider, but be your own expert and use what works for you. Doctors almost always have more background information on a particular topic than you do, and they surely have seen many health trends come and go, which gives them a valuable perspective. But undisputed guidelines for standard care hardly ever exist, which is a large part of the reason why Dr. A suggests one remedy and Dr. B recommends something else.

Besides, no one is looking out for you in particular. That's your job. You're the one who knows you, your biases, goals, and limitations. You don't have to accept without question what one person tells you. Gather as much information as you can, and make your own well-informed choices. Although making choices is no guarantee that you'll have complete control over your health, you can still have the satisfaction of weighing the known risks against benefits. You can investigate claims, whether in traditional medicine or alternative treatments, and decide for yourself if the product or procedure is appropriate for you. Pay attention to your own body and experiences when making choices.

In spite of the media's common portrayal of health information as black and white, in the everyday world, health choices are gray. For example, an interpretation of a mammogram may accurately diagnose whether or not you have a cancerous lump in your breast. On the other hand, mammogram interpretations also can miss an existing tumor or falsely indicate that you have cancer when you do not. Other tests and procedures can also produce questionable or false results. The more information you gather, the more accurate a picture of the situation you'll have.

Be aware that most medical research in this country studies white males, although this gender (and sometimes racial) gap began to change in 1990 with the creation of an Office of Women's Health Research and Development at the National Institutes of Health. (See "Women's Health Research" on page 598 in the Resource Directory.) But for now, sometimes it's just a guess whether recommendations for men are good (or bad) advice for women. Even when research is only about women, recommendations can be contradictory. As an example, opinions about estrogen replacement therapy (ERT), a drug used by women during and after menopause, range from troublesome to troublefree — depending on which research is featured. To use or not to use ERT is only one of many health care decisions that you will make over time. (See "Estrogen Replacement Therapy" on page 337 for a discussion of the troublesome/troublefree issues.)

You can improve the outcome of any choice you make by working with and building trust with a health care provider who has lots of knowledge about and experience with what you want. That means if you need a hysterectomy, open-heart surgery, or a cesarean, find a surgeon who has performed the operation hundreds of times. If you want to avoid an episiotomy (the surgical widening of the birth canal), find a midwife or a doctor who knows the techniques that will help you avoid this. And if you want to consider alternative healing methods for cancer, find an alternative healer, not a traditional oncologist.

DON'T BE SEDUCED BY MEDICAL TECHNOLOGY

According to the American Medical Association, in 1987 in the United States, 19 billion tests were performed. That's an average of nearly 80 tests for every woman, man, and child! In spite of the widespread use of high-tech medicine, the U.S. Office of Technology Assessment, an advisory group to Congress, has found that only a minority of the high-tech medical procedures used in the United States have been proven beneficial.

If high-tech medicine doesn't help as many people as once thought, then why do many doctors use it and why do we love it so? Because most of us believe technology is the ultimate in thoroughness, and sometimes it delivers on that promise. High-tech, state-of-the-art products or procedures are also high in status. Further, insurance companies usually pay for them, making the use of high-tech medicine seemingly financially painless. However, this is changing. Insurance companies, in some instances, are reducing or eliminating payments for high-tech procedures.

High-tech medicine has become a mainstay for the 84 percent of U.S. doctors surveyed by the American Medical Association in 1992 who said they practice defensive medicine — the use of tests and procedures to protect physicians in case of a malpractice suit. Medicine may once have been a calling for many, but now high-tech tools and insurance coverage have made it a business for a large number — a complaint made by physicians (as witnessed by dozens of medical journal articles) and patients alike. But it isn't only physicians who may overuse medical technology. Sometimes consumers insist on having high-tech tests performed or exotic drugs prescribed despite their doctors' reluctance to do so.

Inform yourself about the effectiveness and safety of tests, procedures, or medical devices that are suggested to you in order to make the best use of technology and avoid unnecessary, potentially inaccurate high-tech medicine. Many medical procedures and tools, like research in many fields including heart disease, are necessarily works-in-progress. Usually there is no last word on the best approach to use. Physicians use their best judgment, and so should you. Although your health care provider will give you information to help you in your decision making, it's your responsibility to ask for more information, if you need it, or to do your own research.

You may come across some startling facts. For example, research indicated for decades that the less drastic lumpectomy (partial removal of the breast) combined with radiation is as effective for most breast cancers as mastectomy (complete removal of the breast). However, only now are lumpectomies being performed in increasing numbers. Many physicians didn't believe that early research warranted using the less invasive procedure. And perhaps that belief is still true. For unexplained reasons, however, research consistently shows that which operation you have depends mostly on what part of the country you live in.

Before agreeing to a high-tech test or procedure, ask yourself and your physician the following questions:

- *Will it improve my quality of life?* (If it won't, do you know why you want to use it?)
- *What exactly is involved? How long does it take? Will it hurt?*
- *What are the risks?*
- *How can I prepare for it?*
- *Is there a simpler and/or safer way to get the information?*
- *What is the usual accuracy level?* (If you opt for this test, take that into consideration when you get the results.)
- *How much does it cost?*

Know that you can stop the use of technology if you want to, although that may be difficult for you because it's clear that wherever high-tech machines and procedures are available, they are used.

Recently, doctors have come under scrutiny for making extra money by performing unnecessary procedures, ordering lab work from labs in which they have a financial stake, or charging excessively high prices for services that are available more cheaply elsewhere. Probably you'll never know if your doctor has an investment interest in your medical tests, but you can make inquiries and cost comparisons.

Avoid doctors who go strictly "by the book" and thus rely heavily on tests. Look for health care providers who have enough experience and insight to also use intuition, attentive listening, careful questioning, and judgment—all of which are characteristics of the art of medicine, rather than the science of medicine. If your health care provider doesn't communicate well with you, answer your questions, or describe the risks versus benefits of a test or procedure, find someone else who will. Be responsible for your choices. Say no to procedures and operations that you know you'll regret later, even though at the time you may be embarrassed to disagree.

Be aware that consumers tend to assume the complete accuracy of tests and procedures that are, in fact, fallible. The calibration of machines can be off, lab procedures can be performed incorrectly, and devices can be faulty. In addition, the interpretation of an accurately run test can be wrong or open to dispute. (See "Seduction of Medical Technology" on page 609 of Recommended Reading.)

BEWARE OF QUACKERY

What we call quackery depends on our point of view, as many people will call quackery whatever they don't know or understand. But if quackery is the use or promotion of unsafe and unproven treatments, then many products and procedures — some questionable, some highly accepted — are inappropriate. By this definition, electronic fetal monitors (EFMs), which are used during 75 percent of all U.S. labors, as reported by the Food and Drug Administration, can be considered a form of quackery or junk science.

International research has consistently shown that despite the promise that the added information these monitors offer, the use of these machines does not improve babies' outcomes, and in fact, is associated with increased risk because it leads to unnecessary cesareans. Despite these studies, there are no plans in the United States to discontinue using EFMs, in part because of hospital nursing shortages. (See "Electronic Fetal Monitors" on page 484 for more information.)

Don't assume other medical devices you are offered have been thoroughly tested for safety and effectiveness either. The use of silicone gel breast implants, for example, was limited by the FDA in 1992. Reports of injuries and illnesses for some women who had these implants and the revelation that thorough studies had not been performed to determine the safety of these products were the immediate cause of this ban. However, some women's problems with these implants had been reported in the medical literature for many years. (See "Cosmetic Surgery" on page 300 for more information about breast implants.) In fact, other implants, such as the mechanical heart valve, have also had troubled histories, including reports of withheld research information. The good news is that in 1993 the FDA started MEDWatch, a program to teach the adverse effects of drugs and medical devices. (See "International Implant Registry" on page 587 in the Resource Directory if you are considering an implant of any kind.)

According to the U.S. General Accounting Office, more than 90 percent of all medical devices marketed since 1976, many of which are used routinely in hospitals and doctors' offices, have *not* been reviewed for safety and effectiveness by the FDA. A 1990 law, however, requires the FDA to stop the production of medical devices that could cause death or serious negative health consequences — and if this occurs, the device manufacturers are then required to notify consumers.

DO YOUR HOMEWORK ABOUT PRESCRIPTION DRUGS

Drugs can be lifesaving, such as insulin for women with severe diabetes mellitus, or life-enhancing, such as cortisone for women with arthritis or lupus. But sometimes we're prescribed drugs that have severe or fatal side effects not reported until after years of use. Or we're given drugs that are too strong for our needs, unnecessary, ineffective, or too expensive when other drugs that are available would be more suitable. And although the FDA approves drugs for specific uses, some doctors prescribe drugs for other reasons which may or may not be supported by research.

Physicians, starting in medical school, are the target of intense campaigns by drug companies to use their products, and consumers are, too, through magazine ads. In addition, many physicians are given gifts, free airline travel, dinners, and entertainment expenses by these drug companies. Although many doctors keep up on the latest drug research and evaluate all the brands to see which is best for you, some doctors don't. Some physicians get used to prescribing the same drugs (and baby formulas for newborns) year after year. Or they get most of their information from drug ads in medical journals, 92 percent of which were either somewhat inaccurate or very misleading — sometimes dangerously so — according to a 1992 study.

To avoid errors when you're given a prescription, you can ask:

• *What are the advantages to taking this drug?* If you're requesting the drug yourself (which happens one third of the time with new drug products), make sure you understand in this conversation how the drug will be of benefit to you.
• *What would happen if I didn't take it?*
• *What are the known possible side effects?*
• *How can I counteract side effects?*
• *What happens if I take this drug along with other drugs?* (Bring along to your appointment all other drugs that you use — both prescription and over-the-counter. Although there may be information about side effects from a particular drug, it's often not known what the consequences are when two or more drugs are combined.)
• *Will this drug be affected by any condition I have (such as an allergy)?*
• *Is there an alternative to this drug?*

Before you leave the office or the hospital, make sure you understand how and when to take any drug you're given. When you take the prescription to your pharmacist, you can ask for the patient insert, a description printed by the drug company that describes side effects that have been reported. Ask the pharmacist if this drug has a known interaction with other drugs, including alcohol or over-the-counter medications you may be using.

You can also ask the pharmacist if there is a more effective, less expensive, or safer preparation. Generic drugs are cheaper copies of brand-name drugs that are no longer covered by patent laws. Some people avoid brand-name medications, thinking they are unnecessarily expensive; some people avoid generic products, fearing the manufacturers may be sacrificing quality for economy. The FDA reports that there is ordinarily little difference between the two in their effects, but sometimes there is. Since some insurance companies and health maintenance organizations (HMOs) offer financial incentives to consumers to buy generics whenever possible, ask your doctor or pharmacist which is best for you. It's probably not a good idea to switch from one type to another during the course of your treatment without consulting your doctor.

It's a pharmacist's job to keep up to date on drug preparations, although as in all fields, some do a better job than others. If you buy your prescription drugs from your physician, as 15 percent of U.S. consumers do, you can ask your physician these questions, or call a local pharmacist. (See "Prescription and Over-the-Counter Drugs" on page 609 in Recommended Reading for information about specific drugs and their side effects as well as about how to choose a pharmacist. See "Prescription and Over-the-Counter Drugs" on page 592 in the Resource Directory for information about obtaining drugs for free, if you have a low income. See also "The Over-the-Counter and Prescription Drug Diet" on page 33.)

Once you have started taking a prescription medication, pay attention to how the drug makes you feel. Older people in particular are more susceptible to drug side effects because their body organs — for example, the liver and kidneys — don't function as well as they once did. In addition, they are more likely to have diseases that affect the body's response to drugs, and older people take more drugs simultaneously, which may cause dangerous interactions.

Individual responses to medication vary enormously. When you are taking a drug for the first time, you might want to ask for fewer tablets in the initial prescription in case the drug doesn't agree with you. Ask your family to tell you if they notice any changes in your behavior, such as symptoms like depression, hostility, or memory lapses, among others. If symptoms do occur, notify your physician and discuss your options, which may be to continue with the same drug on a different dosage, to change drugs, or to alter treatment altogether. Adverse symptoms sometimes become apparent within hours, but sometimes it takes months, even years, before the toxicity level in the body builds enough to cause side effects.

BE AWARE OF YOUR DOCTOR'S MALPRACTICE FEARS

Medical malpractice is defined as injurious or unprofessional treatment or blameworthy neglect of a patient by a physician or other health care professional. What is considered "injurious" or "unprofessional" varies from year to year and place to place, but whatever is decided in court today in a malpractice suit is a powerful influence on what physicians do tomorrow with patients.

It's unusual for a doctor who has supported his diagnosis and treatment with high-tech procedures to lose in court. Malpractice litigation is most often triggered when unexpected events happen — such as unusual complications or malfunctioning or misused medical technology — or when substandard care has been provided. Every study examining medical negligence concludes there is far more negligence than suits filed. (See "Malpractice" on page 609 of Recommended Reading.)

The number of malpractice suits has increased enough that both female and male obstetricians/gynecologists, in particular, are sued at a two- to three-times greater rate than they were years ago, and today more than 75 percent have been sued at least once. Along with orthopedic surgeons and neurosurgeons, obstetrician/gynecologists pay the highest insurance premium rates. In 1950 a typical premium cost $36; in 1992 the average cost was $34,300 and individual rates have topped $200,000 per year. Since doctors pass these expenses along to patients via higher fees (contrary to popular belief, many ob/gyns earned, after expenses, twice as much money in 1990 than they did in 1980), we are all paying for them.

As real as doctors' fears of malpractice suits are, according to a report of the American College of Obstetricians and Gynecologists, more than 70 percent of all malpractice claims are settled in favor of physicians, and unjustified payments to plaintiffs are rare. But the process is time-consuming (typically five years) and tedious for all parties. Those suits won by patients usually involve severe injuries or the use of older medical technologies. Nevertheless, fear of malpractice litigation often results in defensive medicine by your doctor with more tests and procedures and — again — higher fees for you. The American Medical Association estimates that defensive medicine costs all of us $15.1 billion each year.

If a doctor is afraid to take on your care for fear of a malpractice suit — for example, if you are pregnant and labeled high risk or have a low income — she may not treat you at all. That's due in part to the erroneous belief of many doctors that the poor are more likely to sue them than are the middle class. (What is true is the uninsured are twice as likely to suffer negligent medical injuries.) Malpractice fears also may result in some uneasiness, at least initially, between you and your doctor (what former Surgeon General C. Everett Koop refers to as "exasperation on both sides of the stethoscope").

Do your part to avoid an adversarial relationship. If your doctor is afraid you might sue, she will likely practice defensive medicine — something you don't want. Families who have sued said their physicians did not listen to them, would not talk openly, were misleading, and didn't make certain consequences clear. Those involved in malpractice law know that happy patients don't sue. So choose health care providers who communicate well, who want to work with you, who encourage you to voice your opinions, and who clearly explain any diagnosis or treatment.

UNDERSTAND THE ROLE OF MEDICAL INSURANCE

Until the promised 1990s health care overhaul happens, we rely on a patchwork of private insurance, publicly subsidized services, and increasing out-of-pocket payments to pay for medical care in the United States. Some insurance companies are showing large profits, many others are losing money because of escalating health care costs, and some have already declared bankruptcy. What that means for the approximately 70 percent of you who have medical insurance is that some policyholders, including retirees who had been promised lifelong medical benefits, will now be held personally responsible for outstanding medical bills.

And though there's been much talk in the 1990s about the U.S. need for equitable medical insurance, which all other developed nations have, aside from residents of a few states (in particular Hawaii), children and women — particularly those past the age of 45 — are the least likely to have insurance.

As companies look for ways to control costs, they are taking higher monthly payroll deductions for health insurance premiums (average annual out-of-pocket medical expenses for families by 1991 were $1,362) — and nine out of 10 employers say they plan to reduce or eliminate coverage altogether. The insurance companies, too, are looking for ways to cut costs.

Fees for certain tests, procedures, and addiction programs that once were paid for by insurance companies are no longer reimbursed. Some insurance companies accept only healthy individuals, will not cover any preexisting conditions, and raise the rates if you do get sick later on. (See "Medical Insurance" on page 588 in the Resource Directory.)

Your daily life-style habits may also affect your insurance premiums. Some companies are offering cheaper insurance coverage to people who don't smoke and who join wellness programs where their weight, cholesterol, and blood pressure are monitored. Some companies won't insure people who have life-style – related illnesses, like AIDS, recreational drug abuse, or alcoholism. A few charge fees to overweight or smoking employees. And unless you live in states such as Montana or Massachusetts, you may be paying more for health insurance you have purchased yourself just because you're a woman — perhaps because women typically use medical care more than men. Call your state's insurance commission office for information about specific insurance companies.

Of all medical insurance holders today, more than 70 percent belong to a so-called managed-care program that offers comprehensive medical care for a fixed or reduced fee. This trend will continue to grow, taking the place of the once all-powerful free-choice plans. To control health care costs, some states are doing away with, and many companies are no longer offering, insurance plans that allow you to choose a health care provider or facility.

With health maintenance organizations (HMOs), which are the largest of the managed-care, prepaid, or discount-rate health plans, most of your medical expenses are covered. You don't fill out insurance forms and wait for reimbursement, you're more likely to get preventive care, and you're less likely to have an unnecessary test, hospitalization, or surgery.

On the other hand, you must ordinarily use only participating doctors and hospitals. You don't always see the same doctor for each visit, and some HMO physicians may perform too few tests to save money. Most HMOs discourage their physicians from referring patients to outside specialists because that raises costs, and some HMO physicians get a year-end bonus if they don't refer patients to specialists.

As with medical insurance, sometimes women pay more for HMO coverage than men. One HMO in the Northwest, for example, charges 28 percent more for women who are in their 40s than men of the same age. (See "Medical Insurance" on page 609 in Recommended Reading and on page 588 in the Resource Directory for more information about HMOs and other medical insurance plans.)

B y knowing these 12 rules of the road for your passage to good health, you are privy to some inside information. By incorporating these suggestions, you'll not only take responsibility for your health care, you'll avoid making hit-or-miss decisions about the people, places, and products in the health care world.

CHAPTER 4

HOW TO CHOOSE YOUR HEALTH CARE

You'll probably look for different kinds of health care for different problems, depending on your needs and personal preferences. All forms of healing therapy, whether conventional or so-called alternative, are not effective for every ailment or every person.

CONVENTIONAL MEDICINE

Conventional (also called traditional or orthodox) medicine is what's taught in most medical schools, practiced at nearly all hospitals, approved by the American Medical Association, and reimbursed by insurance companies (although increasingly the costs of some of the alternative therapies are reimbursed by some insurance companies). Those who practice conventional medicine include:

• *Medical doctors* (M.D.s). After four years of college and another four years of medical school, new M.D.s spend three or more years in specialty residencies. For example, an obstetrician/gynecologist residency is four years, pediatrics is three to four, and family practice is three years.

• *Osteopathic physicians*, or doctors of osteopathy (D.O.s). After four years of college and another four years of an osteopathic medical school, new D.O.s specialize in residencies — much like M.D.s. In addition, however, D.O.s complete a medical curriculum in manipulation, a form of manual pressure applied to joints, bones, and muscles.

• *Nurses.* All nurses from the following three programs pass the same state exam after graduating from an approved degree program. Nursing programs vary from associate (two-year), hospital diploma (three-year), to bachelor's (four-year) degree to master's and doctorate programs. In some states, nurses are able to prescribe medications in addition to their other duties.

• *Nurse Practitioners.* After state nursing certification, these nurses have an additional one to three years of training and clinical work in a specific specialty, such as pediatrics, obstetrics/gynecology, or geriatrics.

• *Physicians' Assistants.* The training of these health professionals began during the Vietnam War with well-trained medics. After a two-year certification program and exam, P.A.s usually work in medical group practices or hospitals and are able to perform physical exams, take patient histories, and prescribe medications in many states.

• *Midwives.* (See a description of midwives on page 255.)

CHIROPRACTIC MEDICINE

Chiropractic care may be viewed as an alternative to traditional medicine, but it's hardly unconventional in the United States. Chiropractors-to-be spend at least two years at the college level in a science curriculum, then another four or five years at a chiropractic college. The last year is spent studying the spine. Chiropractic involves manipulation of the spine and is most useful in neck and back problems. Chiropractors believe that spinal-nerve pressure or irritation can cause a disturbance of delicate body functions resulting in susceptibility to disease. Chiropractors may use other therapies, too, like heat, cold, water, massage, exercise, and dietary suggestions.

Research has shown chiropractic to be particularly effective in relieving lower-back pain and neurological complications, and it often can produce results quicker than conventional medical treatments. In addition to neck and back problems, some of the conditions treated successfully by chiropractic are headaches, pain or numbness in the limbs, and pain in the joints like arthritis or tendonitis.

Sometimes chiropractors, just like some M.D.s and dentists, are accused of taking too many x-rays. Whenever you're asked to have x-rays taken, be clear on their benefit. (See "X-Rays" on page 599 and "Chiroprac-tic" on page 571 in the Resource Directory.)

ALTERNATIVE MEDICINE

Alternative medicine comprises more than a dozen nonsurgical healing therapies, many of which are centuries old, that are not mainstream American medical practices (although they may be very traditional in other parts of the world).

A common complaint made by traditional medical practitioners about alternative medicine is that the therapies have not been reviewed with rigorous research in the United States. That may change with the recent establishment of the National Institutes of Health Office of Alternative Medicine. This group will be looking at homeopathy, herbal medicine, acupuncture, mind-body techniques such as visualization, nutritional treatments, and other practices.

According to a 1993 study, one third of Americans have tried at least one form of alternative therapy. People choose these treatments because they are often given nutritional counseling (a known weak spot for most traditionally trained M.D.s); they are usually given ample, individualized attention; and they were not helped by conventional medicine and chose alternative therapies as a last resort. It's not unusual for some people to combine conventional and alternative medicine to get the best of both worlds. This is especially true with those who have chronic ailments or terminal diseases.

Since the alternative healing methods are likely to be the most unfamiliar methods of health care to you, following are descriptions of two of the more popular (and some would say more credible) ones.

ACUPUNCTURE

Acupuncture is the 2,000-year-old Oriental practice of medical stimulation of specific points on the body by the insertion of tiny, solid, several-inch-long needles away from the site of the discomfort. (This is in contrast to acupressure, which uses finger pressure only.) In an initial evaluation, traditional acupuncturists usually take the pulse in 12 places, six in each wrist, along with an extensive medical history and an evaluation of the tongue. Acupuncturists who are also M.D.s often dispense with pulse diagnosis and go right to the needling of points. Some acupuncturists transmit electrical stimulation through the needles.

Reaction to acupuncture needles is very individual. Some women re-

Disposable needle pressed into
acupuncture point.

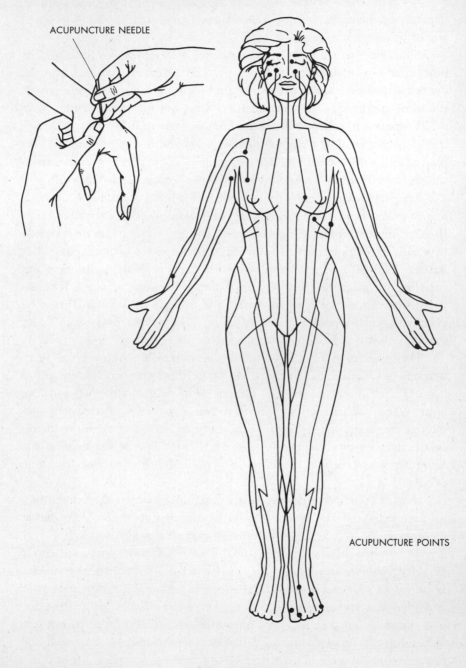

ACUPUNCTURE NEEDLE

ACUPUNCTURE POINTS

ACUPUNCTURE

port that the needles are painless, others report that they cause some discomfort. Some needles are left in for a few minutes, others for 20 to 30 minutes. The length of time, as well as the location and number of needles, depends on the acupuncturist, your response, and the condition for which you're being treated.

Although research is far from complete, acupuncture has been studied more than any other alternative therapy. The results are mixed. Like conventional medicine, acupuncture is helpful for some but not for others with the same condition, or it's helpful for a time, but not permanently.

Acupuncture seems to be most consistently helpful with pain relief, including that stemming from athletic injuries or chronic problems. It also may relieve some of the side effects, such as nausea and vomiting, from cancer chemotherapy when conventional medical methods fail to do so.

Acupuncture gives relief to some women for many conditions, including: migraine headaches; chronic fatigue syndrome; endometriosis; menstrual cramps; morning sickness in pregnancy (only if acupuncture is started very early in the pregnancy); labor pain; depression; lupus; menopausal hot flashes (especially when combined with Chinese herbs); drug craving (whether for illegal drugs or alcohol); herpes flare-ups; multiple sclerosis (particularly its neurologic symptoms); and allergies of all kinds. It may be effective against repeated (three or more) miscarriages, and may correct irregular ovulation in women who want to get pregnant.

The explanation for acupuncture's success remains controversial. Practitioners of Oriental medicine say that the needles balance *Qi* (pronounced "chee"), the body's vital energy. Others say it releases electrostimulation. Some Western researchers who have studied acupuncture say that acupuncture releases endorphins, the pain-deadening and mood-lifting body chemicals that often produce euphoria — which may be the explanation for acupuncture's success in overcoming alcohol and drug craving for some people.

If you choose acupuncture, find a practitioner who is accredited (two to three years' training) by the National Commission for the Certification of Acupuncturists (see "Acupuncture" on page 550 in the Resource Directory and on page 610 in Recommended Reading). Choose someone who is knowledgeable about Chinese herbs, since herbs often enhance treatment. Look for an acupuncturist who has successful experience in treating your condition and who also uses sterilized disposable needles (to prevent disease transmission). Ask the same questions you would of a physician (see "Choosing the People" on page 86). Many acupuncturists work with and for conventional medical doctors.

HOMEOPATHY

Homeopathy is a gentle 150-year-old treatment based on the idea that a substance that in large doses would produce a certain set of unwanted symptoms in a healthy person will, in tiny doses, cure a sick person with those same symptoms. Homeopathic remedies are prepared from mineral, plant, and animal extracts in minute doses usually in tablet form and are used to stimulate your natural immunologic defenses. The level of potency used in a remedy depends on the person's state of health and how severe the ailment is.

To practice homeopathy in the United States, a health care professional must first be a licensed medical practitioner (usually an M.D. or D.O.), must have graduated from a two- or four-year homeopathic program, and must be licensed by her individual state (state laws vary in specific requirements). Homeopathy is far more popular in England and France than it is here today. In Germany, the national health care system pays for it. Among the ailments it has successfully treated, according to more than 100 controlled European studies, are rheumatoid arthritis, fibrositis (a common "aches and pain" condition), hay fever, migraine headaches, postoperative infections, and influenza. (See "Homeopathy" on page 610 in Recommended Reading and on page 583 in the Resource Directory.)

OTHER ALTERNATIVE THERAPIES

Among the other more popular alternative therapies are: acupressure, yoga, and therapeutic touch. (See "Acupressure" on page 56, "Yoga" on page 59, and "Therapeutic Touch" on page 56.) Other popular therapies are naturopathy (healing through nutrition, herbal medicines, and "natural" practices — see "Naturopathy" on page 590 in the Resource Directory), reflexology (manipulation of the feet), rolfing (deep, sometimes painful massage to realign the body), the Alexander technique (pain relief through improved posture), and medicinal herbs. (See "Alternative Medicine" on page 609 in Recommended Reading for information about these and other alternative healing therapies.)

BIOFEEDBACK

Biofeedback is not a method of healing, although it's often associated with alternative medicine. It is a treatment technique that trains you to use your own body signals by watching and/or listening to sensitive recording devices. Biofeedback teaches you to regulate processes that are not usually under your conscious control.

With some uses of biofeedback, you'll be asked to lie down or lean back in a comfortable chair and shut your eyes, while the technician attaches to your forehead several surface electrodes coated with conducting fluid. The electrodes are connected to an electromyograph machine, which monitors muscle tension. Other biofeedback devices can be managed by yourself and are connected to various parts of the body.

With biofeedback, you will learn through a series of tones to measure your state of relaxation and then go on to control your responses. Biofeedback may be effective in controlling tension and migraine headaches, reducing pain, and lowering heart rate and blood pressure. It also has helped people correct visual disorders, reduce the distress of stomach ulcers and other digestive disorders, and manage epilepsy. Some athletes use biofeedback to improve their performance by making them aware of anxiety and tension.

If you choose biofeedback, find an accredited practitioner. (See "Biofeedback" on page 554 in the Resource Directory.)

CHOOSING THE PEOPLE

Most of the time there's more than one way to solve a health problem. An M.D., for instance, can give you a drug to relieve the pain of migraines, but an acupuncturist may be able to reduce your number of headaches without drugs. Whether she is a traditional M.D. or an alternative health care practitioner, the professional will know best and believe most in what she practices. That means most orthopedic surgeons are not likely to recommend a podiatrist for a foot problem, and many chiropractors are not likely to recommend a gynecologist for menstrual pain. For any one problem, you have more courses of action to choose from than you may realize.

You usually have to find different practitioners yourself. There is no independent health service broker, no place where you can be diagnosed and offered all options of treatment. Hospital or medical center referral services will refer you to members of their staff. Other referral services usually operate on fees received from the doctors to whom patients are referred.

Following are step-by-step suggestions for finding and working with health care providers you will like. (Sometimes your order of the steps will be different from this list, depending on your circumstances and your understanding of your ailment or condition.) Use these suggestions in addition to the guidelines from Chapter 3.

• *Be sure you need a health care provider.* Could your problem be solved by lifestyle changes?

• *Know the limits of your insurance coverage.* Some insurance plans cover only certain kinds of treatment or the services of certain doctors. If you're interested in alternative care, find out under what terms it is covered, if at all. If you do not have any insurance coverage, look into low-cost clinics or hospitals. (See "Community Health Care" on page 572 and "Hospital Care" on page 583, both in the Resource Directory.)

• *Start by collecting names.* Most people choose their health care providers by word of mouth and convenience. When you ask friends, family, current health care providers, or phone-referral services for recommendations, ask why they are suggesting that person. The reason may or may not be an important one for you. Talk to the nurses in the relevant department of your local hospital, if you can, or call an organization concerned with the condition for which you want care. (See the Resource Directory starting on page 541 for organizations, which are listed by topics, that give referrals. They can usually give you names not only of traditional doctors, but of alternative practitioners as well.)

• *Find someone who fits your preferences.* If gender, race, and sexual preference matter to you, that narrows your possibilities. You may prefer a woman health care provider, especially if you perceive your ailment as embarrassing. There are more women doctors now than ever — by the early 1990s, one in five practicing obstetrician/gynecologists, for example, was a woman. But women physicians are not always easy to find. Furthermore, the fact that a health care provider is a woman does not guarantee that she will listen more, or be more caring, or be less likely to perform operations that are often optional, such as hysterectomies and cesareans — but some research does suggest just that.

Both African-American women and lesbians sometimes meet prejudice from health care providers because neither group is considered part of mainstream America. If you're African-American and want an African-American physician, you will need to search, as African-American physicians comprise only three percent of the total number of doctors in the United States. (See "African-American Women's Health" on page 610 in Recommended Reading and also on page 552 in the Resource Directory for leads to physician referrals. If you prefer a lesbian physician, contact the "Lesbian Health" organizations on page 585 in the Resource Directory. See also "Lesbian Health" on page 610 in Recommended Reading.)

• *Don't overlook women-run clinics.* Nearly all women-run and Planned Parenthood clinics dispense birth-control information and devices and provide other services, including pelvic exams, Pap smears, and tests for sexually transmitted diseases. Some provide abortions as well.

These clinics are staffed by nurses, nurse practitioners, occasionally nurse-midwives, and physicians. Some women report that staffers are usually conscientious and tend to give more information to patients than a typical doctor might. Women-run clinics often offer nutritional counseling and help with emotional health, too, and sometimes practice both traditional and alternative treatments. (See "Women's Health Centers" on page 598 in the Resource Directory.)

• *Look for a person with "heart."* Your process of healing can be enhanced or inhibited by your health care provider. Does she act like she thinks you can get better? Does she make you feel good about yourself, or is she arrogant? Does she know your name, appear to be familiar with your history, and seem prepared for your visit? Is she empathetic — can she put herself in your shoes? Does she listen to you and treat what you say as important? Is your health care provider irritated when you don't agree with a suggestion? If so, research shows that she may become less vigilant about your treatment.

You decide if your relationship with this person is positive or negative, realizing that a positive experience leads toward healing, and a trusting relationship means mutual cooperation. If your current health care provider leaves you often in tears with comments that are "for your own good," know that you are free to go elsewhere.

• *Respect your vulnerabilities.* If you don't have a high tolerance for pain, find a doctor who will prescribe painkillers if you need them. If you're embarrassed about your weight, find a health care provider who isn't judgmental about this issue. If you feel awkward talking to a doctor while you're sitting half-naked in an examining room, find a doctor who will talk to you in her office after you're dressed.

• *Choose a health care provider who will tell you as much as you want to know.* Whether you get the amount of information that you want determines your satisfaction with your physician more than most other issues. Often women and their doctors have different perceptions, with physicians believing women are getting more information than the women themselves believe they are getting.

It's up to you to know when you've received enough information about your condition, a drug, or a procedure that your health care provider will perform. Surveys have shown that most people want more details, not fewer, though some doctors want to shield women from negative information for fear that it will make the patients feel worse, not better. You decide how much you want to know.

• *Try to find someone who isn't always in a hurry.* What is the scheduled length of appointments? How many patients are booked for each hour? The closer appointments are (15 minutes or less, for example), the more likely it is that you'll wait and/or be rushed out. Even worse, overbooking can cause errors in medical judgment.

• *Decide whether a group practice is okay with you* (if you have a choice). Group practices can offer many conveniences, but you won't always get to see your favorite doctor. How do you like the other people in the group? If you don't like one of them, can you see someone else instead?

Before you decide on a health care provider, schedule an interview, not an exam — especially if this will be a long-term arrangement, for example, for pregnancy or chronic illness. It's important to interview health care providers in advance of a physical exam because you may not like this person and may not want to pursue the relationship. Also, you'll feel more objective if you haven't experienced the vulnerability of a physical exam. Take someone with you, either your partner or a friend. The other person can hear things you missed and keep notes on the items you overlooked.

At this initial appointment, clarify right away how you want to be addressed and how the doctor prefers to be addressed. This is especially important if you're going to see this person more than one time. It affects both how we feel about ourselves and the other person. If you are offended by how you are addressed, speak up; if still not satisfied, find another health care provider.

Whether you see this person once or many times, these suggestions may help you make the most of your partnership:

• *Keep as well informed as you can.* Ideally you'll be up to date on your particular health care issue (if you know what the symptoms mean) before you walk into that office.

• *Describe your symptoms in specific detail.* "My head hurts right here and has for 14 hours" is more helpful than "I've had a headache forever." You may want to keep a record or journal of your symptoms.

• *Write down your pertinent medical history in advance.* Make a list of your allergies, previous operations, and any medications you're taking and give that to the health care provider. (You'll save time and money with this step, since most office visits are billed by the amount of time spent with you.) Be knowledgeable about your family history, too.

• *Organize your thoughts before you go.* Write down your questions for office visits. Having a list helps both you and the professional cover *your* important points.

• *Ask what her policy is about phone calls.* Under ordinary circumstances, how soon could you expect a call back? Is there a fee for phone conversations? If you don't think of a question until later, or if health issues come up between appointments, you need to know this person's telephone rules.

• *Ask for self-help suggestions if your health care provider doesn't automatically offer them.*

• *Don't say you will do things you know you won't do.* Say what you will do, then work from there.

• *Don't agree to procedures, tests, or medications you don't think you need.* That's especially true if your physician performs the tests or dispenses the prescription drugs right there in the office. On average, the work of independent labs is more reliable than the tests (blood, urine, and so on) performed in the typical doctor's office.

• *Be aware that physicians order more tests if they have the test equipment in their office, or if they have a financial interest in a medical lab to which they refer you.* Studies in the early 1990s showed that doctors who have their own office x-ray and ultrasound machines use them more often and charge more for those tests than radiologists do. Similarly, when patients are referred to outside labs that are owned by the prescribing doctor, more tests and procedures of all kinds are recommended. In 1992, it became illegal for physicians to refer to their own medical labs, but only when caring for Medicare or Medicaid patients. (Several states have followed up with similar laws that extend to *all* patients.) Ideally, your health care provider will tell you if she has a financial interest in the suggested lab and will also advise you of other available labs. If you're not automatically given this information, however, ask for it.

After your physician's explanations, if you have any lingering doubts about the need for a test, consider getting a second opinion (see Second Surgical Opinion Program on page 596 in the Resource Directory).

I f you are given several options to consider or if you disagree with your health care provider, here are some comments you might make:

"This is an important decision for me. I need to think about it and discuss it with my partner (daughter, mother)."
"Let's review all the options, including wait and see."
"I want to read a full description of this procedure or test (or the patient insert, if it's a drug) first."

Your health care provider will cast an educated eye on your problem, perhaps make a diagnosis, and is likely to recommend treatment options. But the gospel of good medical care regularly changes, and good physicians give conflicting advice. So you may as well decide for yourself what the best treatment plan is for you.

Choosing the Places

Hospitals are not equal in price, safety, or "heart," so it makes sense to shop around — although most women do not. The majority go to a hospital within one mile of their doctor's office, often on their doctor's advice. (A few doctors take advantage of this and get a fee from the hospital for each patient brought in.) Some women find it's easier to let the physician choose, especially after seeing hospital ads, which many people find confusing, "mushy," or useless.

Before deciding on a hospital:

• *Compare hospitals for price.* For-profit hospitals (often owned by hospital chains) generally charge about 15 to 20 percent more, including higher prices for drugs, coronary care, and the use of the newborn nursery. It's suspected that more unnecessary medical testing is performed at for-profit hospitals, although teaching hospitals are usually the first to switch to new, more expensive technology. On the other hand, teaching hospitals can also be the places where new medical guidelines are first put into practice. The rate of cesareans (which cost more than vaginal births), for example, is now usually lower at teaching hospitals than at other hospitals, as a direct result of a national effort to reduce the number of these operations.

• *Compare hospitals for safety.* Many studies show that hospitals do not necessarily police themselves well, and death rates, especially for exotic operations, vary enormously from hospital to hospital. In general, death rates are lowest in large hospitals in big cities. Choose a hospital that specializes in your particular condition or often performs the procedure you need.

• *Compare hospitals for "heart."* Religious-affiliated hospitals have a reputation for lots of heart and less hardware. Teaching hospitals usually offer resident experts and the latest in high-tech medical procedures. That's important if you have a rare disease or need an unusual operation. It may not be important if your reason for hospitalization is more ordinary. Teaching hospitals also have a reputation for impersonal care, though individual hospitals vary. They have student nurses, interns, and residents, many of whom will want to learn on you by giving you yet one more exam or one more needle prick, whether you need it or not. You can refuse, of course, though many women don't, either because it seems to be too much trouble to say no or because they are unaware that they can.

Because we're influenced enormously by our environment when we're sick or vulnerable, look for a hospital that has a caring staff where you are assigned to one nurse, rather than to a team of nurses or doctors.

• *Compare hospitals for their nurse-to-patient ratio.* Unless you have hired a private duty nurse for your care, you will share a nurse each shift with at least four (and sometimes eight or more) other hospital patients. Your hour-by-hour comfort is not her job, although you may be fooled into thinking that it is because your stay probably costs more than $1,000 a day. Nurses are not there to make sure you're comfortable. A nurse's job is to perform certain procedures with each person under her care. These include dispensing medication, monitoring a variety of tests, and record-keeping—all of which are affected by how many patients she has that day and how many emergencies arise.

Nurses often wish they could do more, but they don't have time. Nursing shortages nationwide into the 1990s have left a majority of hospitals short-staffed. It's in your best interests to choose a hospital with the lowest nurse-to-patient ratio because most of the time the hospital staff members you'll see are nurses, not doctors. To find out, call hospitals, request the floor on which you would be staying, and ask what their ratio generally is. The nurses on duty will have some idea.

THE HOSPITAL STAY

You can make your hospital stay safer and briefer with these steps:

• *Arrange for a room with a view.* Some facilities have a window in all patient rooms. It has been documented that people who have a window view of trees, for instance, recover with fewer complaints and take fewer pain relievers.

• *Bring along things from home that make you feel good.* Favorite books (especially joke books), new nightgowns, things that smell good (such as scented soap), and special photographs can reduce your anxiety.

• *Contact the hospital's patient representative or health advocate if you have any questions.* Her number is usually on the pamphlet given to you when you enter the hospital. (About half of U.S. hospitals have these representatives.)

• *Pay attention to whether hospital workers wash their hands in your room before they attend to you.* Outrageous suggestion, right? Why do you need to notice this? Because many of the iatrogenic (doctor- or hospital-caused) infections that patients contract are from illnesses passed around on the unwashed hands of the staff. Amazingly, 1992 research in intensive care units confirms that this is still a problem. So, if someone doesn't wash her hands in your room, it might be wise to say in a matter-of-fact tone of voice that you'd feel better (and would be glad to wait) if she did.

Bring a Friend

Nearly all of us become helpless when we walk through hospital doors for treatment, even if for only one day. Some hospitals invite patients to bring someone to help, but not all U.S. hospitals are enthusiastic, although it's common in some cultures for whole families to come and stay with the sick person. With today's intense competition among hospitals for patients, you're likely to find a cooperative facility. If you can't find a hospital that readily accepts your helper, or if your insurance plan binds you to a hospital that won't accommodate your friend because of those ubiquitous hospital regulations, you can make an appointment with the hospital administrator and plead your case for an exception to the rule. (If that person is reluctant, then make an appointment with the head of the hospital board.)

If you have to suddenly go to a hospital in an emergency and it's not possible to arrange in advance to have a friend with you, have a staff member call a friend for you when you get there. If you're going to be in the hospital for a few days, arrange for several people to take turns to be with you, and have a cot in your room for your helper. Your helper can calm you when you're upset or confused. She can help common sense to prevail and can serve as a buffer with the staff, making sure you're getting your questions answered. Your friend or relative can ask questions for you in a persistent way that may be beyond your capabilities if you're sick or medicated.

Your helper can make sure the test or drug you're getting is the one prescribed by your physician. (Studies show that hospital staff members often change orders on tests, and recording errors sometimes occur with prescriptions.) If you're in a teaching hospital, your helper can check with you before any staff members perform extra exams. Or in the days after surgery, when the nurse comes in and says it's time for your pain pill or shots, you can decide for yourself if you want that or not, because it's a lot easier to speak up when there's a friend there with you.

The hospital nurse assigned to you will likely appreciate your helper, too. On your arrival in your hospital room, ask which nurse is in charge of your care. Ask her what you can expect from her during your hospital stay. Introduce her to your helper and explain that your friend will be staying with you. Review with the nurse any allergies you have or medication you're taking. (See "The Hospital Stay" on page 610 in Recommended Reading.)

YOUR LEGAL RIGHTS

When you enter a hospital as a patient, generally speaking, you give up privacy (nurses are likely to go in and out of your room while you're clad in a backless gown) in exchange for your care. You also give up a certain amount of self-determination (what time procedures or tests are performed or when you eat) and are controlled instead by hospital schedules. Ideally, your desires and hospital actions will not be in conflict. However, that's not always the case, so it's wise to know what your hospital rights are by law. All of the following rights are, of course, easier to enforce if you always have a helper with you.

You have the right at all times to refuse treatment or exams by your physician or any other hospital staff member (remember those exams by student nurses in teaching hospitals mentioned earlier?). You have the right at all times to refuse any medication, any medical test, any procedure, any surgery, or hook-up to any machine. (See "Court-ordered Cesareans" on page 272 for an exception to this rule.) However, sometimes you will have to give up something yourself for this right. For instance, laboring women in most hospitals will not get epidural anesthesia unless they're willing to be attached to the electronic fetal monitor for the duration of their labor.

You are entitled to *informed consent*. This means that your doctor must tell you everything about a medical procedure or drug before you accept it. With this right, it's important to know that you, not doctors, decide if you've been told everything you need to know. You decide how much detail you want, and then ask for it if the explanation you get is incomplete. (See "Do Your Homework About Prescription Drugs" on page 74 and "Don't Be Seduced by Medical Technology" on page 71 for sample questions.) If you're in great pain, in labor, or in the hospital because of a serious accident, it may be impossible to truly receive informed consent because you are unable to comprehend what you're being told. Avoid this dilemma by having your helper ask questions, take notes, and discuss options in a reasonable way.

You also have the right to leave the hospital any time you want. (Once again see "Court-ordered Cesareans" for the exception.) If you decide to leave against your physician's orders, and if it's a concern to you, you may want to check with your insurance company before you leave to make sure they will still pay your bill. You also have the right to contact your lawyer or your local Bar Association if you believe your rights have been violated. (See "Your Legal Rights" on page 610 in Recommended Reading.)

And, finally, you have the right to inspect and copy your doctor's office or hospital medical records in some states but not others, though many hospitals and doctors are cooperative regardless. (See Isaacs on page 610 in Recommended Reading for a state-by-state list.)

SURGERY

Millions of women have surgery every year, and for many it's one of the most stressful events they experience. Most of these procedures are elective, that is, your life is not threatened if you don't undergo the surgery. Women are more likely than men to be hospitalized inappropriately and have unnecessary surgery. Three of the most commonly performed unnecessary surgeries, according to many researchers, are the cesarean, dilation and curettage (D & C), and hysterectomy. (See "Cesarean Birth," on page 267, "Dilation and Curettage" on page 313, and "Hysterectomy and Oophorectomy" on page 354.)

Some experts believe the United States has twice as many surgeons as it needs at a time when new drugs and procedures have replaced many traditional surgeries. Physician surpluses lead to extra procedures, especially the elective kind, and higher costs.

Being prepared for surgery on all levels, mentally, emotionally, and physically, increases your sense of control, and that reduces your risk for side effects (including excessive bleeding) and can hasten your healing. If surgery is in your future, here's what you can do to make sure it's both necessary and as safe as possible:

• *Check out the alternatives.* When your physician suggests that you have surgery, you can ask what other choices you have. Look up your condition in the alphabetical section of this book. You can also check the Resource Directory for self-help organizations that may provide information on alternatives or referrals to physicians who treat an ailment like yours non-surgically or in a simpler procedure.

• *Get a second opinion.* Your insurance company may require this anyway. A second opinion is especially important if the physician who recommended surgery to you is also the surgeon who would perform it. You may find you don't need the operation after all, or that the procedure doesn't require a hospital stay and can be handled on an outpatient basis. You may even find a doctor who charges less.

Another reason to get a second opinion is that treatment options are changing so rapidly that it's difficult for any one physician to keep up with all of them, especially when the diagnosis, for example, is cancer. Doctor No. 1 might tell you that there is no treatment for you, and Doctor Nos.

2 or 3 may tell you of a treatment that may save your life.

Avoid going to a colleague of your doctor for your second opinion. Peer pressure may force the second doctor to agree with the first, especially if both doctors are on the same hospital staff. Good resources in your town for finding a second-opinion referral can be pathologists (they examine tissue removed during surgeries and biopsies), surgical nurses, anesthesiologists, and recovery-area nurses, because they work with all the surgeons. (Call the hospital and ask for these people. Hospital staff members are generally proud of their facility and are often cooperative with questions like this.) If possible, go out of your geographic area for a second opinion, as physician opinions may vary on surgery depending on what part of the country you live in. (For more information, see Second Surgical Opinion Program on page 596 in the Resource Directory.)

• *Discuss all the options with all the doctors you consult.* Each one will probably contribute a new piece of information. When you get several opinions and they're all different, one may appeal to you more than the others. Go with that one. But if it's not clear what you should do, consider going back and asking each physician what each thinks of the other opinions.

• *Choose an experienced surgeon*, one who is board certified in the field that specializes in your problem. (See the discussion of the National Practitioner Data Bank on page 305 if you want to find out about your prospective surgeon's history of malpractice suits.)

• *Choose an anesthesiologist who is board certified, too*, and who regularly performs regional anesthesia. This is an option for scheduled surgery only, but even with that most women don't know to ask, or don't realize it's important. (Women who have emergency surgeries ordinarily get whoever is on call.) Ask your surgeon or hospital staff nurses for an anesthesiologist referral, or call the offices of the anesthesiologists who work at your hospital. Regional anesthesia—as opposed to general anesthesia, which puts a person in a drug-induced coma—is preferable for many women, though it is not appropriate for all procedures.

• *Ask friends who've had the operation what you can expect.* If you know someone who has already had the operation you'll be having, ask her the same questions you asked the doctor and anesthesiologist. Some of her answers are likely to be different than theirs, especially regarding the experience of pain and the length of time for recovery, because she's had the personal experience and they probably have not.

• *Ask to room with someone who has had surgery and is recovering smoothly.* Her success may rub off on you. If you are having a scheduled operation, mention your preference to the head nurse or whoever makes the room assignments when you check in (or call before you arrive). If your surgery is an emergency, have your helper ask for you when you are in the recovery area and haven't yet been moved to a room.

• *Prepare physically for surgery.* Quit smoking, or at least cut down to increase your body's oxygen. Avoid other recreational drugs, including alcohol. (Most surgeons recommend that you quit taking the Pill four to 12 weeks in advance of surgery.) Increase your intake of all vitamins, especially vitamins C, A, zinc, and B, in the weeks before and after surgery to help your body cope with the stress of both the procedure and all the drugs that will be used, as well as to help the body's recovery afterwards.

• *Plan your meals.* If hospital food won't meet your nutritional needs, plan to have someone bring you the appropriate food. (If you drink caffeinated beverages daily, be aware that you might get caffeine-withdrawal headaches and fatigue if you avoid these drinks entirely during your hospital stay.)

• *Plan for the aftermath of surgery.* If you're having outpatient surgery, have someone drive you home, and have someone stay with you for at least a day. Find out in advance what physical therapy exercises and/or relaxation techniques will ease your recovery and help you to manage the pain. (See techniques for relieving stress beginning on page 54.) Emotional let-down, anger, and unwelcome dependence are common after surgery. Plan in advance to get help from your supporters after you get home.

Before the procedure, resolve your doubts about surgery. Women who are thoroughly informed about the benefits, risks, and alternatives have realistic expectations and experience less anxiety and more satisfaction. Arrange a preoperation briefing with your surgeon and ask:

• *How long will this operation last?*
• *What exactly is involved?* What will be repaired or cut or removed?
• *What kind of improvement can I expect?* What percent of women improve after this particular surgery? Be specific about what you want to see improved. Otherwise, your surgeon's opinion about what is successful may be different from yours.
• *How much pain can I expect immediately after the operation and days or weeks later?* What kind of pain medication does your surgeon recommend? Do you know of any nondrug techniques that will help lessen the pain?
• *What are my chances of survival without the operation?* What would happen if I didn't have it? If you know surgery is necessary, it's easier to tolerate.
• *What will happen if I don't have or postpone the surgery?*
• *What are my chances of survival with the operation?*
• *What are the possible complications?* Expect a positive outcome, but don't

close your mind to the procedure's inherent risks. This only makes them harder to accept if they do occur.

• *What are the chances of failure of this operation?*

• *How will the surgery affect my life-style?* The procedure could make life easier or harder—or both.

Another issue to resolve ahead of time is the matter of blood transfusions. Research shows that if, when, and how much of a blood transfusion you might get varies among doctors and hospitals for the same procedure with people in the same condition. Ask prospective surgeons how they make their decision. Donate blood for yourself in advance if there's a good chance that you will need a transfusion. The safest blood to use for a transfusion is your own, not only to avoid blood-borne diseases, but to avoid weakening your immune system.

Although blood banks now test more successfully for viruses like HIV (AIDS) and hepatitis, no blood supply is 100 percent safe. (One expert estimate is that HIV testing fails to detect the virus in one in every 61,000 units of blood; another expert estimate is failure occurs in one in 10,000 units of blood.) If you decide to donate your blood, your physician will give you a prescription to take to a blood bank, usually for several pints of blood. Your physician will give you guidelines on how you can plan ahead so that you have enough time to gather a sufficient amount in the time you have between the gathering of the blood and your operation. (See "Anemia" on page 158 for suggestions on how to avoid becoming iron-deficient after donating blood.)

Ask the surgeon how long your hospital stay will be. Ask about recuperating in a surgical recovery center outside the hospital. If your surgeon recommends this, ask how your care will be managed there and how it differs from the hospital's routine. (Be sure to find out if your insurance company will pay for this out-of-hospital center.)

Talk to your anesthesiologist as well. Ask her what kind of anesthesia you will have and what its effects will be.

Tell both your anesthesiologist and your surgeon if you are taking any medications, smoke or drink alcohol, use recreational drugs, or are allergic to any drugs or substances. Be sure they're aware of any lab tests you had in the previous year to avoid unnecessary duplication. Ask them both what suggestions they have for you to prepare yourself better for surgery. Think twice about hiring a surgeon or anesthesiologist who won't take the time to meet with you.

Ask your surgeon and anesthesiologist to please keep their remarks positive during your procedure. (1992 research shows that surgical patients recovered quicker and left the hospital sooner if they were played tapes with positive therapeutic suggestions while they were under anesthesia.) Many people who've had surgery remember the conversations of the operating room staff during the procedure, or on some level they remember the positive or negative tone of what is said, regardless of how deep their state of anesthesia was.

Sometimes these remarks are not pretty. ("Look at those terrible stretch marks" or "This is the worst cancer I've ever seen.") The operating room staff means no harm by these comments, and probably think patients can't hear them. However, these remarks may provoke anxiety or induce nightmares in you later, and that ultimately affects your speed in healing. An alternative to a positive-suggestion tape is to wear headphones tuned to soothing music during the operation. Check with your surgeon and hospital personnel before you enter the hospital about using headphones or any other special arrangement.

I f you attend to all these issues before surgery, you'll be in much better shape afterwards. Most of us don't have surgery that often, so we aren't aware that there is a right way to go about it until we've done it the wrong way.

COMMON MEDICAL TESTS

Most U.S. women have had at least one of the following tests or exams as a form of preventive medicine. Having them will not guarantee an illness-free life, and those women who don't have them won't necessarily get sick. None of the tests is performed or interpreted accurately all the time. It's not always clear which women would benefit from these tests at what age, and some medical experts suspect that financial reward sometimes has more to do with test recommendations in certain age groups than women's needs. There are, however, individual women who have benefited from all of these tests.

DO-IT-YOURSELF BREAST EXAM

If you want to avoid lung cancer, you don't smoke or spend a lot of time with people who do. But how to avoid breast cancer isn't as clear, so there are several tests and exams that are recommended for early breast cancer detection. The first is the self-exam.

About 80 percent of breast cancers are discovered by women themselves when they notice that there's something obviously and persistently different about one of their breasts. It would seem logical then that monthly breast self-examination, following specific instructions, would lead to earlier detection and a higher cure rate. But research doesn't seem to show that.

Although the American Cancer Society continues to urge all women to perform breast self-exams monthly, most women don't. And most of those who do apparently don't do it according to directions — in particular if those directions came from written material (which is why I haven't included an illustration or instructions for this exam). A common error is not examining the underarms, one of the most common sites of breast cancer. Nor is there just one recommended "right" way to perform a manual breast exam.

If you want to examine your breasts regularly in a systematic way, learn to do it with confidence. Find a health care provider who will not only teach you how to do it correctly, but will also give you several follow-up sessions for review.

You might reduce any cancerphobia (see "Cancerphobia" on page 242) you have by remembering that at current rates nearly 90 percent of all women will *not* have breast cancer. Also, if you're acquainted with your breasts at all, you're likely to notice any major changes. (See "Breast Health" on page 611 in Recommended Reading.)

MAMMOGRAM

This is an x-ray picture of the breasts used to search for early signs of breast cancer that show up as shadows on the x-ray. The enthusiasm for mammograms is due to the potential for physicians to detect cancer too tiny to feel in a manual exam at an early stage when it's believed to be least likely to spread. (Breast cancer is the most commonly diagnosed cancer among U.S. women and is the second leading cause of death from cancer.)

The American Cancer Society recommends a mammogram every one to two years for women in their 40s, and a mammogram each year after age 50. Reflecting the wide disagreement about the appropriate age for screening, the U.S. Preventive Services Task Force, the Canadian Cancer Society, the United Kingdom's Breast Screening Program, and now the U.S. National Cancer Institute only recommend an annual mammogram for women over 50 because research shows this reduces the risk of dying of breast cancer by 20 to 30 percent. However, no routine mammograms for women under 50 are recommended by these groups because worldwide research does not show any value for this age group.

The women who appear to benefit the most from mammograms are those who have already been treated for breast cancer and those who have symptoms of breast disease. These include a lump, nipple discharge, new retraction of the nipple, dimpling of the skin on one area of the breast, or persistent breast pain. The other category of women thought to especially benefit from mammograms are those who have a family history (meaning two or more first-degree relatives, that is, mother, sister, daughter) of early (before age 40) breast cancer. This group, however, only accounts for five percent of all diagnosed breast cancer. In fact, it's difficult to say who should have a mammogram and who shouldn't. Despite the medical community's frequent listing of breast cancer risk factors, *three out of four women with diagnosed breast cancer have no known risk factors.* That not only shows how much we don't know about breast cancer, some would say it's a good

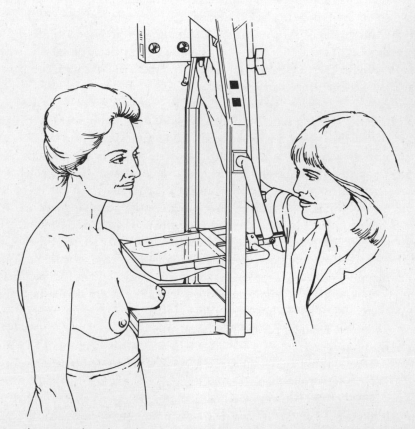

Your breast is placed on the machine and gently compressed, though it may be painful, between the x-ray plate below and a plastic cover above.

MAMMOGRAM MACHINE

argument for getting routine mammograms, regardless of personal history.

As with any procedure, decide for yourself if and when a mammogram is appropriate for you. When you've decided, here are suggestions on obtaining mammograms:

• *Call the National Cancer Institute (NCI) hot line or your local American Cancer Society office to find a facility accredited by the American College of Radiology (ACR).* (See "Mammography" on page 587 in the Resource Directory for the NCI toll-free number.) Mammograms are performed in hospitals, doctors' offices, outpatient clinics, and traveling vans. They are not all equal in quality or safety. (See "Tests That Involve Radiation" on page 111 for questions to ask.) The same mammogram may not be interpreted the same way by several radiologists, in part because of training, skill, and experience, but also because there is a lack of standardization, which affects the quality of the interpretation you're given. Mammograms are one of the most difficult x-rays to read. Once you've found a good place, it might be wise to always have future mammograms there, so that they will have comparable quality. Read on for another option if that's not possible.

• *Always ask for your mammogram x-ray for your own records — for two good reasons.* One, it makes sense to have a copy of each mammogram so that your current physician can evaluate any changes in your breast tissue. A mammogram left in a doctor's office is of no value in determining the ongoing health of your breasts if you change doctors. Many of you will have mammograms over several decades, and at least some of you will move to other states during those years or have other reasons for changing doctors.

After you have obtained the phone numbers of approved centers, call and ask each one about keeping your mammogram. At some centers you can pick up the mammogram after the radiologist has read it by signing out your mammogram on their medical records sheet. Other facilities may prefer to send your mammogram on to your next physician. If that's convenient, fine. If it's not, see "Your Legal Rights" on page 610 in Recommended Reading for the next step.

The other reason to get a copy is safety. If you have copies of all your mammograms, you'll avoid unnecessary retakes. There is no safe level of radiation exposure, although researchers agree your risk for damage from radiation reduces as you get older, particularly past age 55. Best estimates are that there's a 1-in-25,000 risk that a mammogram performed correctly on ideal equipment will cause breast cancer. However, not all women get mammograms performed on ideal equipment, and some women have previous radiation exposure that should be taken into consideration. (See "X-Rays" on page 608 of Recommended Reading for information about radiation's cumulative effect.)

• *Ask the technician to explain each step of the procedure to reduce your anxiety and increase your comfort.*

• *Plan on getting your test a few days after your period when your breasts are least likely to be tender,* since it's important that the breast be compressed tightly for a few seconds. Mammograms are difficult to perform because positioning has to be exact.

• *Avoid any products (such as bath powder or deodorant) or jewelry (such as a necklace) on the day of the test that might show up and cause possible distractions on the film.*

• *Return to your physician if you receive an "all's well" report from a mammogram but find a breast lump afterwards.* There's a chance you may have cancer. If you are told to wait and see because the recent mammogram did not indicate any suspicious lumps, one option is to say that you don't want to wait, another is to discuss the matter with a different physician. The reliability of mammograms has improved over the years, but no one claims they are 100 percent accurate. Of all women with diagnosed breast cancer who got mammograms, about 20 percent went undetected. This is known as a false-negative — it suggests the absence of cancer when in fact a cancer is present. This error occurs more often with very dense breast tissue, which is more common in younger women.

• *If you have breast implants, find a facility and a technician experienced with taking mammograms of breasts like yours and who can make a custom adjustment of the equipment for you.* Usually, three or more x-rays of the breast (instead of the usual two) are appropriate, because it is more difficult to view a breast that has an implant and perhaps scar tissue, too. Be sure to remind the technician every time you have a mammogram that you have breast implants to avoid the risk of implant rupture. (See "Breast Implants" on page 302.)

• *If you are using estrogen replacement therapy (ERT), tell the mammography technician.* The breasts of one-fourth of women who use ERT have increased density that can be difficult to interpret.

• *Consider what the next step is if you are told that you have a suspicious mammogram.* After an initial screening mammogram indicates a suspicious lump, ordinarily a set of diagnostic mammograms (which show more detail) follows. If that set is unclear or suspicious, then there are at least two more options. A biopsy, the usual next choice, is the removal of tissue that is examined under a microscope. Tissue can be removed with a surgical knife or aspirated with a needle.

If you have a biopsy, ask how long the procedure takes, how reliable is it, will you be awake, what side effects might there be including a scar, and how soon will you get test results. Biopsies carry risks for scarring, infection, allergic reactions, and anesthesia complications, along with often intense anxiety caused by the fear of cancer.

A newer alternative to the biopsy is magnetic resonance imaging (MRI), a diagnostic technique that does not use x-rays or other radiation. It can provide a more accurate and detailed picture of the breast. MRI is unlikely to take the place of all mammograms because it ordinarily costs eight to ten times more than a screening mammogram.

If you have cancer, you'll need to decide what to do next. (See "Treatment Options" on page 236.)

It's also possible to go through a number of diagnostic tests and discover that you don't have cancer. It's important to know that many women who have false-positive or suspicious results leading to biopsies end up with lingering, nagging fears that they *almost* had cancer when, in fact, what happened was a misinterpretation. They didn't *almost* have anything.

• *Don't rely on a mammogram to prevent breast cancer, because, of course, it can't.* It is an early-detection screening exam. To increase your odds that breast cancer won't happen to you (or to avoid a recurrence if you already have had breast cancer), adopt an anticancer life-style. (See "The Anti–Breast Cancer, Healthy Heart Diet" on page 28, "Preventive Measures You Can Take" on page 235, and "Mammogram" on page 611 of Recommended Reading.)

PELVIC EXAM

The intent of the routine pelvic exam is to check the health of your reproductive system, and the exam often starts with questions. You'll be asked about your menstrual and pregnancy history, the date of your last Pap smear, whether you've had vaginal infections or surgery of any kind, and a few questions about your family's disease history. Then, while you're on your back with your feet in stirrups at the end of the examining table, your external labia, your vagina, and your cervix (the mouth of the womb) will be examined.

The Pap smear — a test to detect abnormal changes in the cells of the cervix, named after the physician who devised it, Dr. Papanicolaou — is taken at the time your cervix is examined. The last step in the process is when your health care provider places two gloved fingers into the vagina while pressing the other hand on your lower abdomen to check for enlargements or abnormalities in the pelvic organs. Then she will place one finger in the vagina and another finger in the rectum, with the other hand again on the lower abdomen, to check the shape and contour of organs.

The women who benefit the most from having a pelvic exam are those who are uncomfortable or in pain in their pelvic area, those who think they may be pregnant, those who take the Pill or are on estrogen replacement therapy, those who use the cervical cap, and those who have specific reasons to have annual Pap smears, such as a family history of cervical cancer. (See "The Pill" on page 181, "Estrogen Replacement Therapy" on page 337, "Cervical Cap" on page 205, and see "Pap Smear" below).

Before your exam, tell your health care provider that you'd like to save any discussion for after the exam when you've had a chance to put your clothes back on. (Come prepared with your written list of questions.) You'll hear more of the examiner's comments and you'll feel more comfortable asking questions when you're upright and clothed. If your health care provider is unwilling to do this, reevaluate whether this is the right person for you.

You can make a pelvic exam more comfortable if you find a health care provider with whom you feel comfortable. Request that each step of the procedure be explained and that the speculum, the instrument that is inserted into your vagina, be warmed before it's put into your body. Consider asking for a mirror so that you can see your vaginal walls and cervix yourself; this could be the start of your learning how to do your own vaginal exam. (See "Do-It-Yourself Vaginal Exam" on page 107.)

PAP SMEAR

In this procedure, a sample of cells is taken from the cervix and used to identify early precancerous cells of cervical cancer, and perhaps endometrial cancer (see "Cancer" on page 231) or genital warts (see "Sexually Transmitted Diseases" on page 493). The cells are placed on a slide and sent to a lab where they are examined. It's not a perfect test, but it's the best available for its purpose, and its use has saved the lives of many women by the diagnosis of cervical cancer in its early, treatable stages.

Some physicians recommend that all women have an annual Pap smear. Newer recommendations, however, suggest that, after three negative tests, once every three years is just as effective. Pap smears are especially valuable for DES-daughters (women whose mothers took diethylstilbestrol, or DES, during their pregnancy — see "Diethylstilbestrol" on page 309), women who have genital warts, women with a past history of cervical cancer, and women who have multiple sex partners or who have a partner who has multiple sex partners.

Women who have had hysterectomies in which the cervix has been removed, which is the case most of the time in the United States since the 1960s, ordinarily do not need Pap smears.

Estimates of Pap smear inaccuracy range from 20 to 40 percent. These inaccuracies include both false-negatives (missing cancer when it's present),

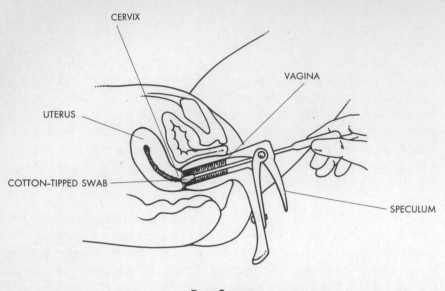

CERVIX

VAGINA

UTERUS

COTTON-TIPPED SWAB

SPECULUM

PAP SMEAR

and false-positives (believing cancer is there when it's not). The person who takes the smear may do it incorrectly, or the lab technician who evaluates it may be undertrained or overworked. A Pap smear sample is not easy to take well, and the most accurate health care providers are both very careful and very experienced. Some of the best and worst Pap smear samples come from physicians. (It's not just labs that complain about the skill of physicians in taking Pap smears. The American College of Obstetricians and Gynecologists does too.) In addition, even when the Pap smear is accurate, there may be some confusion about whether you have a problem and how to treat it.

You can improve the accuracy of your Pap smear by doing the following:

• *Get the test when you're not menstruating.*

• *Empty your bladder before the exam for both your personal comfort and an easier view of the cervix.*

• *Avoid a vaginal douche, vaginal lubricant, tampons, or vaginal contraceptive for at least 48 hours before the test.* (A Pap smear collects cells from the cervix that these products might remove.) Some also recommend that you avoid intercourse for 48 hours prior to a pelvic exam or Pap test. (See "Douching" on page 222 for a discussion of problems associated with this practice.)

• *Reschedule your test if you've had a yeast infection within the past month* (see "Yeast Infections" on page 533), as that may alter the Pap results.

If you're told that your Pap smear results are positive, which suggests you may have cancer, you have several options. One is to have repeat Pap smears, but these could be misleading because of the high false-negative rate of this test. The most reliable option is a *cone biopsy* (a surgical technique in which a section of the cervix is removed for examination). A colposcopically guided Pap smear, in which the cervix is visually examined using magnifying lenses, may be useful as well. (See "How to Improve the Accuracy and Safety of Your Tests" on page 110.)

DO-IT-YOURSELF VAGINAL EXAM

This is an at-home exam in which you can view your genitals and cervix (the neck of the womb). This exam acquaints you with your body and alerts you to vaginal symptoms. It helps you learn what's normal for you, and shows you what your body looks like inside. It's not a substitute, however, for pelvic exams performed by health care professionals, nor are all women interested in learning how to do this self-exam.

Ideally, have a health care professional show you how to do a self-exam, while explaining to you what are normal vaginal and cervical conditions and what are not. Or — if you positively can't find a health care professional to help you — choose a woman who is experienced with this procedure and with whom you feel comfortable.

You'll need a plastic speculum, which can be bought at many Planned Parenthood clinics and doctors' offices, pharmacies and hospital supply stores; a hand mirror, preferably one that can stand alone; a flashlight; and perhaps lubricating jelly (such as K-Y, but not Vaseline or cold cream) to make insertion of the speculum easier. After you've gathered your supplies, here's how to do it:

• *Find a private place.*
• *Feel unhurried.*
• *Get into a reclining position* on a firm surface (on a firm bed, on a rug on the floor) with your back against something firm (a chair, the arm of a couch).
• *Dab a little lubricating jelly on the tips of both blades of the speculum* before inserting it.

The woman most likely to be interested in this self-exam is comfortable touching her body and is probably curious about the signs of ovulation, or

Position

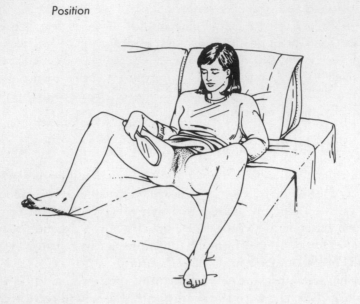

The tools

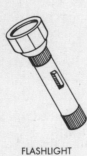

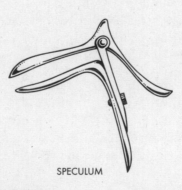

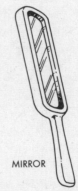

FLASHLIGHT   SPECULUM   MIRROR

Do-It-Yourself Vaginal Exam

any unusual vaginal symptoms she may have. Women who have chronic vaginal infections can benefit by learning what to look for as an early warning for possible flare-ups. (If you discover any bumps, sores, or blisters, contact your health care provider.)

CHOLESTEROL TEST

Most experts say your cholesterol should be checked only if there are sound clinical indications, such as women who already have had a heart attack or heart disease, or those who know they have a high level of cholesterol (probably in the 240 range). If you are getting your cholesterol checked, here are suggestions to provide the most accuracy:

- *Fast for at least 12 hours before the test* to get the most accurate reading.
- *Have your high-density lipoprotein (HDL) cholesterol checked also, and have a triglyceride (a blood fat) measurement, too.* (It's a better indicator of heart disease for women past age 50 than is cholesterol.)
- *Get cholesterol measurements taken several times and then average the results* (particularly if the results of the first test are troublesome). Many doctors do this automatically because an individual's cholesterol level is not stable and may vary by as much as 10 to 20 percent. There's also a high error rate with these tests that can be due to the person performing the test, the handling of the sample, or the calibration of the equipment used. In addition, certain conditions affect your cholesterol measurement. Pregnancy, for one, will often double your cholesterol levels.
- *Have your test made at a large lab,* not at your M.D.'s office, for the most accurate results. Beware readings given to you at shopping center health fairs or grocery store promotions.
- *Do not let the person who draws your blood "milk" your finger (which is not going to happen at a reputable lab),* as that can dilute the sample and lead to a false low measurement.

BONE MEASUREMENT TEST

The densitometer works by passing a beam of radiation through bone to measure bone fracture risk. Some machines are sensitive enough to detect a 1 to 8 percent loss of bone (1 to 1½ percent of bone loss per year is typical in women after menopause), whereas x-rays require at least a 30 to 40 percent loss before osteoporosis is detected.

There are two kinds of densitometer. The *single beam densitometer* measures bone at the wrist and may be the one most used, although some believe it is the least effective in measuring your risk for osteoporosis, the bone-thinning disease (see "Osteoporosis" on page 431). The *dual beam densitometer*, or dual-photon absorptiometer, measures bone at the spine and hips. This procedure costs more and takes longer.

Other means, less common, used to measure bone loss are quantitative computed tomography (QCT) and bone biopsies. QCT, a fancy version of computerized axial tomography (CAT) scanning, is technically difficult, gives a much higher radiation dose than the densitometer, is more expensive, and is not readily available. Bone biopsies are usually reserved for distinguishing between osteoporosis and osteomalacia (abnormal bone mineralization, usually associated with poor metabolism of vitamin D, or vitamin D deficiency).

The newest measurement tool to evaluate bone density is *dual-energy x-ray absorptiometry (DEXA)*. It is perhaps more accurate, more precise, and safer (less radiation) than the single- and dual-beam densitometers and QCT.

If you want a bone scan, find a facility that provides them, preferably DEXA scans, with experienced technicians. (Perhaps you'll only need one scan for an accurate measurement at menopause to predict future fracture risk.) Otherwise, if you have a single- or dual-beam densitometer reading, just one scan won't tell you all that you need to know. The scan numbers only have value in comparison to each other. Even if over time your densitometer readings indicate lowered bone density, this still doesn't mean you'll get bone fractures.

The best use of any bone measurement equipment is for women who want to make up their minds about the use of estrogen replacement therapy. Several densitometer scans over a period of years will help them do that (or perhaps just one DEXA scan at menopause). However, you don't need a bone scan to know that you should exercise regularly and eat a calcium-rich diet to prevent osteoporosis.

HOW TO IMPROVE THE ACCURACY AND SAFETY OF YOUR TESTS

We think of tests as being objective measurements of evidence, but in fact tests are subject to many variables and have a wide range of accuracy. Here are some guidelines to help ensure you get the most accurate test results you can.

Tests That Involve Radiation

When you're having a mammogram or bone scan, find three people with experience and training: the physician who prescribes the test, the technician who performs it, and the radiologist who interprets it. Their experience will reduce your chances of having unnecessary radiation exposure, an inaccurate machine, and/or a misread diagnosis.

To get as little radiation as possible, ask the technician how many rads (the units by which absorbed radiation is measured) you are getting when you're using the mammogram machine or the densitometer. Machines vary enormously and emit a range from 0.1 rad with newer mammogram machines to 20 rads with older machines or those that are not calibrated well.

Specific questions for mammograms are:

- *Is your equipment used for mammograms only?*
- *Does your facility perform at least 10 mammograms per week?* (Any less than this is believed to indicate too little experience on the part of the technician.)
- *Is the machine calibrated annually?*
- *Was the machine inspected in the last year and did it receive state approval?*
- *Are you voluntarily accredited by the American College of Radiology?* In 1992, only 31 percent of mammogram facilities met the quality standards set by the American College of Radiology.
- *Are your medical technicians certified, and do they have specific training in mammography?* These technicians, due to their extensive training and experience, are ordinarily more accurate in administering these tests than any other specialists, including physicians.

Lab Tests

If you're having a test that will be evaluated at a lab, ask your health care provider what lab is used, and why it's used. The lab where your test is sent may be understaffed, and as labs are rarely checked for quality, there is no uniform accountability. If your test is for a Pap smear or a cholesterol screening, call the lab and ask if they are voluntarily accredited by the College of American Pathologists or licensed by your state. If the lab is licensed by the state, you can call your state health department and get further information.

One fourth of all tests are performed in physician offices, and they are on average the most inaccurate lab tests of all. However, that may change as the U.S. government plans for the first time ever to implement regulations for reviewing physician-office testing equipment.

HOME TESTING KITS

Home testing kits can increase your self-reliance, save you money, and result in earlier detection of some health problems, especially if you're reluctant to visit your health care provider unless you positively know you have a problem. You can get blood pressure monitors, urine test strips for diabetes and urinary tract infections, and even an instrument with which to examine your child's ears. You can buy do-it-yourself vaginal speculums, ovulation detection kits, and pregnancy tests, perhaps the most popular of all home kits. (See "Making the Diagnosis" on page 447.) A self-administered Pap test may be available in the future, too.

Home health care is not new, but the tools available to us are. Parents, especially mothers, have always provided the bulk of health care for the family through temperature-taking, hand-holding, and common sense. Now we have access to diagnostic tools as well. If you use these kits, follow directions precisely, although they may seem tedious. No test, whether performed at home or in a doctor's lab, is 100 percent accurate, but following directions to the letter is your best insurance. Read the package insert, and pay attention to expiration dates and ideal storage temperatures, too. Call the 800 number with the kit if you have any questions, and keep accurate records.

Find a health care provider who will advise you about home kits and work with you when you obtain test results at home. For example, if you have chronic bladder infections, after you recognize the early symptoms, your first tool for diagnosis can be the home test. Then you can discuss the results with your health care provider.

At-home kits are not the last word in accuracy, diagnosis, and treatment, just as one lab test or one physician's opinion is not always enough. Be aware that these tests can produce false-negatives or false-positives just as more sophisticated tests can.

After using a home test kit, decide what your options are. Most home kits are used for early detection of something that will need a health care provider's attention or to evaluate a chronic condition. If the test is something you do frequently, like the urine test for urinary tract infections or a blood-pressure reading for hypertension, you are probably in regular contact with your health care provider. If you're using a test to evaluate a new development, you may want to use your home test, look at the results, gather your questions, and go see your health care provider. (See "Home Testing Kits" on page 611 in Recommended Reading.)

CHAPTER 5

WOMEN IN SPECIAL CIRCUMSTANCES

Mainstream health care is designed for white, middle-class, middle-aged-or-younger, able-bodied, well-insured women who have traditional ailments and diseases, especially those that can be evaluated with state-of-the-art tests. That makes all other women unusual, uncommon, and sometimes uncared for in the U.S. medical system.

WOMEN WHO ARE POOR

Although many health differences show up when women's racial groups are compared, nearly all of those differences between minority and nonminority women are a result of economic factors, and this is true from birth through old age. Higher rates of infant death, AIDS, sexually transmitted diseases, heart disease, some forms of cancer, even a threefold higher rate of dying in a hospital, for instance, are associated with poor minority women, whether they are African-American, Latina, or Native American — and the rates are higher for poor white women as well.

Poor and/or single women and their children, as well as rural Americans, usually have the least access to the health care system. This is partly because they, particularly Latinas, are the least likely to have health insurance. Nearly one third of the estimated 35 million people in the United States without health insurance are under age 30, and the least insured of any age group are women over age 45.

When uninsured women do get medical attention, they usually wait the longest in emergency rooms, their conditions are often in more advanced stages, which makes recovery more difficult, and they are the most likely to suffer a medical injury due to substandard care. In addition, they also may face racial or class prejudice, especially if they do not speak English as a first language. If you are uninsured, have a low income, and need medical care, see "Community Health Care" on page 572 and "Hospital Care" on page 583, both in the Resource Directory. If you are a single mother, see "Single Mothers" on page 595 in the Resource Directory.

There are other groups of women who may or may not be poor and who belong to all races who have special needs. They are women who are caregivers or disabled or who have a "social" condition, such as being abused.

WOMEN WHO ARE CAREGIVERS

Most caregivers for a disabled spouse, parent, infant, or friend are women. Typically, women spend at least 18 years helping elderly parents, and that number of years will increase as more people live longer. These women care for the young and the old, the mentally ill and retarded, and the physically handicapped. Caregivers often pay not only financially, but with their health and careers as well.

If you're a caregiver, don't forget to take care of yourself. Caregivers who are calm and rested handle difficult situations better than those who are upset and fatigued, and those who get a break from their responsibilities are far less likely to get sick themselves. In addition, the morale of the sick improves enormously when the caregiver is optimistic. With that in mind:

• *Take time off from caregiving.* Arrange "sitting" times, whether for babies or the elderly, with other relatives or family friends. (Mothers of twins, triplets, or children close in age especially need to plan for help.) Others may be reluctant to offer because they don't know what you want, but if you ask them and are specific (I need your help next week for two hours), they may be glad to assist.

• *Find out what resources your community or your employer offers*, including home health care workers and adult daycare. Your company may offer benefits, including counseling, resource directories of housing and daycare options, and help with funds for the care of elderly parents. Call the senior center or the health department in your town to find out about the variety of federal and private programs for disabled people and those past age 65, including subsidized housing and transportation, as well as hot-meal programs. Also, investigate insurance policies for long-term care.

• *Join a support group of other caregivers.* This is essential for morale and is also an excellent source of information.

• *Maintain your own health.* Be sure to eat well and to exercise. (See "How to Stay Healthy" on page 25.)

• *Inform yourself about the disease or condition of the person for whom you are caring.* That will help protect you both from mistakes made through ignorance. Explain to your family, including children and friends, what the disease or condition is so that their comments and efforts can be helpful rather than a source of further frustration. Don't assume that everyone knows.

• *Plan ahead.* Although it's easy to get caught up with the everyday-is-a-crisis care, it's important to think ahead and to make arrangements for next month or next year. If you're caring for an elderly parent and know that it's possible that you will place her or him in a nursing home in a few years, or if you have a severely retarded child who will need at least daycare in a few years, investigate now, or ask a friend or family member to do it for you. Waiting lists are long, and arrangements vary enormously.

• *Consider hiring a private care manager.* This person will do many of the things that you or others might do if you had the time — arrange for home health care, find a nursing home, help with governmental assistance applications, and so forth. Fees are high, so shop carefully. Local welfare or health agencies, as well as the social work staff of your local hospitals, may recommend individuals or tell you what to look for in a private care manager. Many of the qualified people have training as geriatric social workers or nurses. Ask private care managers whether they have experience with a situation like yours and how much time your particular case would take.

Remember that you don't have to be a saint. It's normal to feel a wide range of emotions — embarrassment, frustration, self-pity, sadness, and satisfaction, among others — when you are a caregiver. To let off steam, talk to a friend, meditate, or go see a counselor. (See "Caregivers" on page 557 in the Resource Directory and also on page 611 in Recommended Reading.)

WOMEN WHO ARE DISABLED

Disability may range from difficulty in walking several city blocks or lifting objects to paralysis, which requires the help of other people on a regular basis. In the United States one in six people has such a functional limitation. How much your health care is affected depends on the nature and severity of your disability.

Some steps you may be able to take to cope better are:

• *Become the expert on your condition.* That's true for most women about most ailments in general, but particularly for you. No one else will know more about your history of symptoms, medications and treatments, though it may be difficult to keep track of all this. It may be helpful to have one primary physician who coordinates with all the specialists, if, like most disabled people, you have several health care providers.

• *Choose health care providers who have experience with people with your disability.* Reflecting society at large, many doctors and nurses are biased against, as well as ignorant about, the disabled, and this prejudice may lead to poor care, inadequate diagnoses, and your feeling insulted.

• *Choose health care products that are compatible with your life-style.* Birth control, for instance, to be effective must be a method you can physically manage, because that's your best guarantee that you'll use it. If you're limited in movement, you may find some methods like the diaphragm and the cervical cap difficult to use. Or the heavier periods that you may have with the IUD may be more than you can cope with. Many disabled women find the Pill the easiest to use; however, if your disability keeps you immobile, that may put you at a higher risk for side effects from the Pill. (See "Birth Control" on page 162 for more information.)

• *Find a support group for yourself*, whether family and friends or a mutual self-help group. These groups provide information and friendship, as well as social gatherings, including opportunities for dating.

• *Keep physically fit* to reduce stress, tension, and depression. Ask a physical therapist to show you appropriate exercises. (See "Disabled Women" on page 574 in the Resource Directory and also on page 611 in Recommended Reading.)

WOMEN WHO ARE ABUSED

Abuse can be physical, mental, or emotional; it ranges from outright violence to verbal put-downs, humiliation, and subtle domination. No one knows how many women are abused, but it's estimated that battering is the single major cause of injuries to women, and that women are twice as likely to be harmed if they are pregnant. Emphasis is often put on physical abuse because of the evidence of visible scars, but many women are subjected to mental and emotional belittling that is just as devastating. Abused women are married and single, college and high-school students, heterosexual and lesbian, young and elderly, rich and poor, members of all racial groups, and may or may not have come from an abusive background.

An abused woman has survival skills, strength, and persistence that are shown in her ability to live through the experience. She also has a jealous, angry, or badgering partner who repeatedly makes derogatory comments about women, who was likely abused or witnessed abuse as a child, and who is often a regular drinker. He is the dominant of the two, and the one who manages the money. She believes that he is omnipotent, and she fears him. In addition, she feels isolated, she has given up her independence, and she feels frightened for her own or her children's safety, and she feels sad most of the time. Many times she rehearses what she will say to her partner.

The abused woman feels chronic anxiety, shame, guilt, vulnerability, and depression and has low self-esteem that sinks even further with the gradual wearing down of her defenses. She may prefer a quarrelsome relationship and may not like calm men, whom she may consider boring. Because she was drawn to her partner's macho, fighting, kiss-and-make-up style (whether physical, mental, or emotional) from the beginning, she may equate with love the adrenaline-driven excitement and release of anxiety that she and the abuser create together. An abused woman is 15 times more likely to be an alcoholic, nine times more likely to abuse drugs, and also at a greater risk of suicide.

The woman most likely to stay in an abusive relationship believes she has nowhere else to go. She believes this relationship is forever, or she thinks she can't afford to leave. She may have friends and perhaps family who are also abused. Battered women fear being on their own, unable to take care of the children. They may believe that the known (abuse relationship) is better than the unknown. They don't want to go public and expose family problems or face the humiliation of being accused of being a masochist, a lover of pain and domination. Abused women are often accused of masochism, but that's not why women stay in abusive relationships. They stay because they're exhausted and emotionally and physically hurt. Abused women don't seek out pain, but they learn to endure it.

An abused woman may want to protect and "rescue" her abuser from his dark and cold side and may feel a "traumatic bonding" with his warmer side. She believes, like many terrorist hostages, that she deserves the abuse and that it is her fault resulting in an overwhelming passivity, all of which may be intensified if she was abused as a child. She believes that the abuser will hound her and her children if she leaves, and because of that, she finds it easier to stay.

If you decide to stay with an abusive partner, recognize your reasons and take steps to alleviate the situation. For instance, although 40 percent of physically abused women don't call the police, you will reduce by one third your chances of being abused again in the next six months if you have the batterer arrested. Rarely does any form of abuse, whether physical, mental, or emotional, totally stop. If staying is better than leaving, you must seek support for yourself. Find ways to rebuild your self-esteem. Call your local health department social services section, and ask if they provide low-cost or free counseling.

The woman most likely to leave permanently an abusive relationship (women on the average leave and come back seven times before they leave for good) has deep faith in the idea of a better life, knows her life is as important as her abuser's, overcomes her self-hate, and believes she has a right to be treated with respect. She knows she has alternatives and makes plans she can accomplish, including one to keep the abuser from finding and maiming her (though in fact wife killers are a very small percentage of all wife abusers).

She wants to protect her children, although this is also a reason some women give for staying with an abusive partner. She experienced frequent, severe beatings, instead of infrequent beatings or mental or emotional abuse. She makes new friends who think battering is *not* okay, and she understands that many women are in her situation and that she's not alone or odd. She knows she's not responsible for her mate's behavior or for helping him to learn how to be nonviolent.

When you decide to leave your abusive relationship, here are steps that have worked for other women:

• *Don't wait for a professional to make the diagnosis that you've been abused.* In spite of the growing awareness of domestic violence, physicians and other health care workers correctly diagnose it less than 5 percent of the time (although efforts are now being made to correct this). More often than not, when examined in emergency rooms, abused women are blamed for their problems, perhaps even being labeled hysterics or neurotics. Women who suffer from emotional and mental abuse fare no better. Most medical schools do not teach any courses on physical, emotional, sexual, spousal, or elder abuse, nor do most of these schools have any instruction about battered women or dating violence.

• *Be your own expert.* If you think you've been abused, you have. Now decide what you are going to do next. Get support for your new way of thinking. Avoid friends and family who reinforce the old abusive life-style. Begin to plan your exit by becoming informed. Hide some money, and keep in one place important documents, such as birth certificates for you and your children, your bank account book, and social security cards. Find out your rights. One source may be your local health department. Call and ask for the department that answers questions about domestic violence.

• *Discover what resources you have in your community.* Many communities have "safe houses" where abused women can find friendship and safety, as well as a temporary home for themselves and their children. (See organizations listed under "Abuse" on page 546 for a local referral, or call your company psychologist — if your company has a domestic violence program — for information.)

Making a phone call to any of these resources, especially a women's support group, doesn't mean that you have decided to leave your situation now or ever, but the trained counselors, many of whom are former abused women, will describe for you some of your options in a noncritical way.

Women who turn to the clergy and medical professionals for counseling seldom report receiving as much help as they do when they turn to women's groups. (See "Abused Women" on page 611 in Recommended Reading.)

If you're a friend of a battered woman, give her the phone number of your local safe house. Don't abandon her. Remind her of her talents and skills. (See Statman on page 611 in Recommended Reading for a book you can give to her.) If you witness a battering, experts suggest that you not intervene, because you don't want to be the second victim. But it's good to announce that you are going to call the police and then do it.

A NOTE TO MOTHERS OF TEENS

We don't want to be abused, nor do we want our daughters abused, yet millions of women are abused every year. Many battered women have said that they wish they could have recognized the signs of violence early on in the relationship before both the involvement and the abuse escalated. Now you can give your daughters (and your sons) the information you perhaps did not get. Since abusive relationships start as young as junior-high age, you can teach your daughter now about how she can avoid selecting an abusive boyfriend, a lesson in preventive health more valuable than many others.

Tell your daughter about the warning signs that indicate a potentially abusive relationship. She should avoid boyfriends who push beyond playfulness, pinch, or hurt, or generally bully others (whether with physical force or words); sooner or later he'll do the same to her. Also worrisome are boyfriends who are possessive and jealous, who want to make all the decisions, and who believe that they have a right to own and control her. Explain that this kind of boy does not have her best interests at heart even though he claims he does.

Remind your daughter that nothing ever happens just once. Tell her that although she may believe he was mean only once, or insulted her profoundly only once, or hit her only once, or forced her to do something sexual only once, it's never true. Given time, it will happen again. If your daughter likes a boy, but she's not sure if he's playful or if he's mean, ask her how his behavior makes her feel. Does it make her feel enhanced or diminished? Did this boy witness abuse as a child or was he abused himself? Research indicates that many men who become abusive partners have a personal history of abuse or witnessed abuse as children (although most abused children do not grow up to be abusers themselves).

If your daughter is especially kindhearted and has a lot of "rescue" energy (that tendency to want to help injured or helpless creatures or "fix" needy boyfriends), she should use it in moderation and not waste it on a boy she hopes will learn to behave better, if only she has enough patience and kindness. Her efforts, no matter how well intentioned, will not solve his problem.

You can speak with your son, too, about his attitudes toward women. Help him be clear about the meaning of the word *rape* and understand that sexually pressuring a date is always unacceptable, that women never owe men sex, and that no woman wants to be raped, just as your son doesn't want to be raped or assaulted.

RAPE, INCEST, AND SEXUAL HARASSMENT

Women react to assaults differently than men do, and it doesn't matter what kind of assault it is. A man might lash out, and because of his physical strength, believe that he will overcome his attacker. Women, on the other hand, typically are more passive, trusting, and helpless and blame themselves more readily (just as most of the rest of the culture blames them, too).

Society doesn't like victims, whether they are the homeless, damaged wartime veterans, or abused women, and mainstream medicine doesn't offer much support to women who've been raped or who are victims of incest, although both are noticed more by the medical profession than they once were. Even employers are now beginning to be held accountable for sexual harassment on the job.

RAPE

No one knows for sure how many women have been raped, and statistics may vary depending on where you live. But one study in an urban area showed that one fourth of all women had their first sexual intercourse as a result of rape, and it's estimated that perhaps as many as one woman in four will either have a rape attempt made on her or be raped in her lifetime.

Date rape, or acquaintance rape, is forced sex with someone you know. It's estimated that 90 percent of these rapes are not reported. (Fewer than one in four women who were raped were raped by strangers, according to the 1992 U.S. National Women's Study.) Date rape can happen at any age, but it's believed that it occurs most often to women ages 15 to 24. (See "Date Rape" on page 611 in Recommended Reading.)

If you've been raped, call the rape crisis center in your town. (You'll find the number in the phone book, or call the police and get it.) Ask them to have someone meet you at the hospital emergency room immediately, so that you can be examined—don't shower or bathe before the exam—and any evidence can be saved. Talk with the rape crisis counselor about birth control, if you weren't using any, and ask her about the pros and cons of using "morning-after" contraception (see "Morning-After Birth Control" on page 218) and the spermicide, Nonoxynol-9, to prevent possible transmission of the AIDS virus (HIV). Since an unknown number of women contract a sexually transmitted disease (STD) through rape, and since many STDs don't have obvious symptoms, it is wise to have tests immediately. If left untreated, STDs may damage your pelvic organs and other parts of your body. (See "Sexually Transmitted Diseases" on page 493.)

Take pride in yourself for surviving, and get support from loving persons in your life. One woman called her family after she was raped, and seven of them came and stayed in her home for two days, surrounding her with positive attention. Women who have been sexually assaulted may need at least six months to recover and often have nightmares, anxiety, and sleeplessness. If that happens to you, consider professional counseling. Sometimes the issue of betrayal can interfere more with recovery than the assault itself. Donate some of your time to work at rape crisis centers. Research has shown that you may recover sooner from possible long-term emotional effects if you talk about this and help others who have the same problem.

If you're considering filing charges for rape, plan for success. Go to the emergency room immediately to obtain evidence and a written medical record. Get counseling from the rape crisis center people, as well as from lawyers who are experienced and successful in rape cases.

INCEST

Incest is sexual experiences with relatives, and it occurs most frequently between brothers and sisters, then fathers and daughters. But it can also involve sex with other family members. Like rape, incest has nothing to do with love, rather it has to do with power and lack of respect. It's estimated that one third of women were sexually abused as children, although most of these incidents are not reported. It's also common for children to tell others that they've been abused but not to be believed.

If you were a victim of incest, you may experience depression, anxiety, a sense of isolation, low self-esteem, and anger. In addition, symptoms such as substance abuse, fear of intimate relationships, chronic pelvic pain, and frequent illnesses may appear. Many victims of incest believe that the crucial aspect of abuse is not what occurred, which was often many years ago, but how what occurred still affects their lives today. They suggest that you seek support groups and/or find the right therapist for you. (See "Abuse" on page 546 in the Resource Directory for helpful organizations, "Finding a Therapist" on page 607 in Recommended Reading, and "Incest" on page 612 in Recommended Reading.)

SEXUAL HARASSMENT

Sexual harassment, an unwelcome sexual advance, can be verbal, nonverbal, or physical. It can be a pat on the rear, a lewd comment about a part of your body, an unwanted visual undressing. What most women call harassment, many men call flattery. Sexual harassment has caused many women to feel like second-class citizens, resulting in low self-esteem.

Although society at large is more aware of sexual harassment today than it was years ago and women employees have been successful in lawsuits filed for it, it still occurs all the time. The National Organization for Women estimates that half of all working women experience some form of sexual harassment, and the Pentagon reports that the same is true for two out of three women in the military.

If you are being sexually harassed, don't wait for someone else to solve the problem for you. You are the best person to handle it. Here are some suggestions:

- *Avoid known harassers.* Don't work for them, don't take classes from them, and don't try to be "friends" with them.
- *Keep written records of incidents of harassment.* You can use these to support your formal complaint or lawsuit.
- *Don't keep this to yourself.* Tell your friends and family. If it happens on the job, tell the harasser you are going to tell others, including the boss. And then do it. If the boss is the harasser, tell his boss. Use established complaint procedures at your school or place of business. Report the harassment to your state's Civil Rights Commission and get information as well about the laws in your state. Consider legal action if all else fails. (See "Nine-to-Five Hotline" on page 546 in the Resource Directory for their hot line number.)
- *Confront the harasser if you believe it will give you more control.* Responding to comments from a construction crew is not going to help much, since they don't think their comments are effective unless you respond. That means that making comments back to them is reinforcing their behavior. However, if your harasser is someone you work with, confronting him is likely to have better results, if only because U.S. companies are held responsible for harassment. Be specific when you confront a harassing colleague. Tell him what he did wrong, how you felt, and what you want him to do. You could say, "I don't like it when you tell me that my suit shows off my nice rear. It makes me feel cheap. Stop doing it." That's more concrete than telling him he says rude things. (See "Sexual Harassment" on page 612 in Recommended Reading.)

BLAMING THE VICTIM

If you've been a victim, whether of incest, rape, date rape, or sexual harassment, don't let someone else decide whether you were raped, had an incestuous relationship, or were harassed. Most men deny date rape, especially if you have been dating for a while, if you let him fondle you, if you weren't a virgin, or if you "led him on."

In any rape, many others will accuse you of doing something wrong — whether wearing the wrong clothes, being in the wrong place, or walking outside at the wrong time. Young girls have even been accused of "asking for it" from adult relatives. That's called *blaming the victim*, and it's a time-honored way for abusive men to avoid taking responsibility for their behavior. If you're not sure about that, ask yourself if men who are raped or sexually harassed or who were part of an incestuous relationship in child-hood are blamed for the assault.

Remember that you are *not* to blame, and you're not alone. If you decide to have therapy, find a therapist who has experience being helpful to other abused women.

PART II

THE ALPHABETICAL GUIDE

ABORTION

WHAT IT IS

Abortion is the removal of the embryo or fetus from the uterus. It is the most commonly performed surgical procedure in the United States.

TYPES AVAILABLE

Legal abortion is performed by:

• *Vacuum aspiration*, also known as suction dilation and curettage (suction D & C) or vacuum curettage, is used for 99 percent of U.S. abortions. This procedure was introduced in the United States in 1967 and is the simplest. It takes 10 to 15 minutes and is used after seven weeks and up to 16 weeks after a woman's last menstrual period (LMP). LMP is used to determine the length of a pregnancy, when in fact, fertilization doesn't occur until two weeks after LMP. That is, a ten-week abortion occurs when the fetus is eight weeks old.

First the uterus is examined, then a speculum (a tonglike instrument) is inserted to hold the vagina open, and then the cervix is cleansed. After a local anesthetic is injected, the opening of the cervix is enlarged with a dilator (narrow tube), and the tube of the aspirator, a machine that has a vacuum-producing motor, is inserted into the cervix, and the contents of the uterus are removed. Then the lining of the uterus is scraped with a curette to make sure all the placental tissue is out.

• *Intrauterine instillation*, sometimes called a saline abortion, accounts for about 1 percent of U.S. abortions. Performed with a local anesthetic, this procedure can be used up through 20 weeks or more after a woman's LMP. An ultrasound scan is also often used with second trimester abortions to make sure of the gestational age of the fetus. During intrauterine instillation, a small amount of solution that stimulates contractions is placed within the uterus. Laminaria are small, narrow sticks usually made of seaweed that are inserted into the cervix in advance. As the laminaria swell, the cervix is gradually opened so the contents of the uterus can later be expelled. Instead of the 10 to 15 minutes for vacuum aspiration, this procedure can take many hours.

Other procedures that can terminate early pregnancy include menstrual extraction, a simple vacuum-suction technique (see "Menstrual Extraction" on page 219); "morning-after" birth control (see "Morning-After Birth Control" on page 218); and the abortion drug RU486 (see "RU486" on page 219), which is not yet available in the United States.

POSSIBLE COMPLICATIONS

Complications occur in less than 1 percent of all legal abortions, according to U.S. government research. Among possible complications is infection. About half of all providers of abortion in the United States give women antibiotics after an abortion to prevent infection.

Other possible complications are: the presence of blood clots in the uterus, which are treated with a followup D & C procedure (see "Dilation and Curettage" on page 313); continuing pregnancy, which occurs in less than 1 percent of abortions and is more likely to occur with an abortion performed earlier than six weeks from LMP or performed by someone with little experience; cervical or uterine trauma; and excessive bleeding.

Maternal death occurs in less than 1 percent of legal abortions, a rate that continues to drop. The maternal death rate is related to the abortion procedure that is used and how far pregnancy has advanced; it is even lower for abortions that are performed in the first 12 weeks of pregnancy.

Women who have a legal, infection-free abortion by vacuum aspiration

are *not* prone later to miscarriages, infertility, ectopic pregnancies, premature births, or low-birth-weight babies. But what about those women who
have more than one abortion? According to 1992 research, there is no
increased risk for at least one of those problems — a subsequent low-birth-
weight baby — after a second abortion by vacuum aspiration, and very little
risk after a third or fourth. The risk for other problems after two or more
vacuum aspiration abortions is unknown due to lack of research.

Those who have had a second-trimester abortion, however, by uterine
instillation may have (research is neither adequate nor definite) an increased
risk for premature or low-birth-weight babies. As with all surgical procedures, however, outcome is due in part to the skill of the physician performing this kind of abortion. Because of the lack of comprehensive research,
no one knows what the consequences are, if any, of instillation procedures
on future reproduction.

HOW TO DECIDE

You have your own beliefs about abortion. Everyone does. You may
believe it's murder. You may believe it's last-resort birth control. You may
believe it's okay sometimes, but not others; or it may be another woman's
preference, but not yours. Two thirds of women consistently report in U.S.
research that abortion, with some exceptions, should be decided by the
woman. Whatever our beliefs, abortion makes most of us feel uneasy and
ambivalent.

Of women choosing abortions, 12 percent fear the fetus was harmed
by medications or other conditions, while 1 percent were told that the fetus
had a birth defect. Most women who have abortions, however, experienced
an unplanned pregnancy.

What you do about an unplanned pregnancy may change from time to
time in your life. You can be sure at any time that you have lots of company:
55 percent of all U.S. pregnancies are unplanned, and the percentage soars
to 82 among unmarried teens. (In fact, it's estimated that 45 percent of all
U.S. women will have an abortion in their reproductive lifetime.) Many
women become supporters of abortion after they are faced with an unwanted pregnancy, or someone near and dear to them is. On the other
hand, many women who thought they supported abortion became opposed
to it after having children of their own.

Many opponents of abortion believe that at least some women have
abortions nonchalantly. No doubt some do, but there's no research that
confirms this and it certainly isn't what women say who have had abortions.
More than a few opponents of abortion also believe that most women who

have abortions have three or four. And some do. Although there's under-reporting of the total number, surveys show that a majority of all U.S. abortions are first abortions. Of the remaining number, most are reportedly second-time abortions.

---

*M*y husband, who was very upset, and my 15-year-old daughter both encouraged me to get an abortion, but I just couldn't. Because of my age (40), I got an amniocentesis. I definitely didn't want to raise a defective child. Motherhood was exhausting enough for me without adding that. I believe women have the right to an abortion and I would go with my daughter if she ever needed an abortion, but it's not for me.

*W*e love kids. We've raised seven of our own and put up with all the inconveniences and ups and downs. I still feel like I'd do anything for my kids. I have to tell you, then, how surprised I was when my unmarried 19-year-old daughter told me she was pregnant. My surprise was in my reaction. I didn't welcome that baby. It was an intruder. My husband felt the same way. Nature intervened two weeks later and my daughter had a miscarriage. Had that not happened, we would have supported her through an abortion. Which for me is an amazing thought, since I had all those kids and always considered abortion the wrong thing to do.

*I*n my 20s I had friends who had abortions, and though I never would have had one myself, I believed they had a right to that choice. Now that I have kids of my own, I strongly believe abortion is always wrong.

A lot of people think an abortion is something a woman does casually, like changing the color of her hair. But I defy anybody to tell me that she has had a casual abortion. There is nothing casual about it. It's a horrific decision to make.

If you're trying to make up your mind about whether or not to have an abortion, don't let any individual or any group pressure you one way or the other. Find a doctor or a clinic that supports your views. An American College of Obstetricians and Gynecologists' poll indicated 84 percent of these doctors support a woman's right to abortion, but most refuse to perform abortions in late pregnancy, many refuse to perform them at all, and now fewer physicians are trained in medical residency programs to perform these procedures.

Similarly, the abortion opinion of political parties and organized religions is mixed, with separate groups in each that are for and against. In national polls, most people of all religions support a woman's right to an abortion. That finding is reflected in who gets an abortion, too. Women of all religious persuasions, including those who usually consider themselves antiabortion, have abortions. Catholics, for instance, who represent about one fourth of the U.S. population have one third of the abortions.

If you are pregnant and considering an abortion, listen to yourself before you listen to anyone else about what you should do.

EMOTIONAL PROS AND CONS OF ABORTION

There's much concern that women who choose an abortion often regret the decision later. Is that true? Sometimes. Some women regret having an abortion, just as some other women regret having the baby. Feelings are typically mixed. That's normal. Pregnancy is frequently full of emotion and ambivalence, and so is abortion.

I had the abortion, and if I had it to do over again, I would have done the same thing. Yet I'm left with nagging feelings about my future. Will I ever have a baby or was this my only chance?

I am a single, well-educated, middle-income white woman who had an abortion last month. I am a woman who told a friend (not so long ago) that "I could never choose abortion." I am a woman who respected another's right to choose abortion, but I ached to know how lightly the choice was made by some. I am a Christian woman who loves and delights in God and life and freedom. In fact, I am a Protestant clergywoman. I am neither irresponsible nor promiscuous. In fact I taught birth control in a women's clinic after college. I know how to use my diaphragm. It failed. It's as simple as that.

Many who are opposed to abortion believe that women are severely traumatized by the experience. It is common for most women to feel anxious and depressed before an abortion procedure — but not afterwards when they generally feel relief. Among those who choose abortion, studies do not indicate widespread, long-term emotional problems, and for adolescents, abortion seems to be more maturing than harmful. In 1989,

C. Everett Koop, then U.S. Surgeon General, who personally is opposed to abortion, published a report after a review of more than 250 studies that found no conclusive evidence one way or the other that abortions are psychologically harmful to women.

If you are scared to have an abortion because of the emotional consequences, you also need to consider the long-term emotional effects of bearing a child from an unplanned pregnancy. Either way you won't avoid emotion.

Therapists who report long-term emotional problems after abortion may be reporting the problems of a select population: women who come to see them. They cannot know about all the women who don't go to therapists. Most women when asked their opinion after an abortion, report mild feelings of guilt, regret, or remorse (which are not psychological disorders), which diminish rapidly and are replaced with relief, satisfaction, and happiness.

The further along in a pregnancy an abortion is performed, however, the more "body" grief there may be. (See "Pregnancy Loss and Body Grief" on page 490.) Body grief may be part of the reason why some women, particularly those who have had more than one abortion, feel compelled to give birth with all future pregnancies.

I had an abortion at 12 weeks and was surprised at the milk my body produced. I knew I was finished with the pregnancy, but my body wasn't yet.

Your reaction to an unplanned pregnancy is very individual, and you're entitled to that. If you can't decide what to do, seek counseling. If you need more counseling after you've made up your mind, by all means get it. Be aware of the profile below of the woman who is most likely to have serious emotional trouble with an abortion. If you see yourself in the description, seek support so that whatever you decide, you have access to people who are sympathetic, which will help you accept full responsibility for your decision. (See Gardener and Townsend in "Abortion" on page 612 in Recommended Reading for more information about abortion and emotion. If abortion is not for you, see "Abortion Alternatives" on page 545, as well as "Adoption" on page 550 and "Single Mothers" on page 595, all in the Resource Directory.)

Here is the profile of the woman most likely to have emotional trouble after abortion: She is young, unmarried, and in her first pregnancy. (As the young and unmarried group represents three fourths of all women who get abortions and studies do not indicate that most of that group has emotional problems later, bear in mind that the more a woman resembles this *entire* profile, the more likely she is to have emotional problems later.)

She's somewhat passive, alone, with no social network, and from a religious background strongly opposed to abortion. She may prefer to have the baby and feels pressured by family or boyfriend to have an abortion. She feels bad, inferior, undeserving of consideration, and may have a history of emotional difficulties. She believes she felt fetal movements (which usually occur at 18 to 20 weeks) although she probably had her abortion by 12 weeks, and experiences more physical pain than is expected. She is ill prepared, ill informed, and anxious.

I was being a good little girl [eldest of 8 children whose parents were active in the antiabortion movement]. I was going through with the abortion to solve everybody else's problems.

If I knew what I know now, I never would have had my abortion. I was 18 years old, married, and I already had two children. My husband was unemployed . . . and we were on welfare. I talked with my husband and he said, "Choose. It's either me or the baby."

On the other hand, the woman who has a positive emotional outcome after an abortion receives counseling prior to the abortion, which allows her to express her feelings and perhaps her ambivalence; she is cared for by considerate personnel who believe she has a right to her choice, she feels support from an important person or people in her life, and she either is naturally good at coping with difficult decisions or got sufficient help so that she felt good about her decision.

How to Get the Safest Abortion

• *Don't even consider an illegal abortion.* They are not safe. In fact, illegal abortion accounts for about half of maternal deaths worldwide.

• *Do not do anything to yourself to try to induce abortion.*

• *Take all the time you need with a counselor to consider the pros and cons of an abortion for you.* It's common to have at least one hour of counseling in advance of an abortion, so that you can discuss your decision and readiness to abort, in addition to having the procedure explained.

• *Choose your abortion provider and/or facility carefully.* Two thirds of U.S. abortions — many of which are covered by insurance — are performed in abortion clinics, while the rest occur in general clinics, hospitals, and doctors' offices. To get started, see "Abortion" on page 544 of the Resource Directory and call the 800 hot line number listed there to find a reputable abortion provider near you. You can also look up "Abortion" or "Reproductive Services" in the Yellow Pages of the phone book, but be aware that some antiabortion groups list themselves under these headings as well. (In the future, these nonmedical abortion-alternative groups will likely be listed under "Abortion Alternatives" in the Yellow Pages.) If you are willing to share your situation with your doctor or friends, ask them for information.

If you go to an abortion clinic staffed primarily by women who have strong empathy for your situation, you are likely to be handled with consideration and respect. Occasionally women obtain abortions from doctors who are not comfortable doing abortions, or are not comfortable with the women having them. Avoid negative, judgmental, nonsupportive people, because their attitude will probably affect how you feel.

• *Have someone with you during the preliminary counseling and the abortion procedure.* This is someone who is there just for you — a friend, family member, or your partner. You will feel more secure, and any discomfort you will experience will be lessened by her or his presence, and any negative feedback from others will be minimized. Shop around for a clinic that welcomes or allows you to bring a friend who will be with you. Some clinics will encourage you to bring someone with you. If there's no one you want to bring, find a clinic that will provide someone just for you. Many abortion clinics do not allow men in the room where the abortion is performed, but surveys show that most of the men involved wanted to be there.

• *If you think you might have been exposed to any sexually transmitted diseases (STD), discuss tests for STDS with your abortion provider before you have the abortion.* If you test positive and are treated before the procedure — not after — it will reduce your risk for infection later.

• *Get a RhoGam injection after the abortion and before you leave the clinic if your blood is Rh-negative.* Rh refers to a blood protein that is present in the blood of most people. It's possible that if an Rh-negative mother gives birth in a subsequent pregnancy to an Rh-positive baby, then that newborn could be born with severe anemia requiring blood transfusions. RhoGam prevents the pregnant woman's body from manufacturing the troublesome antibodies that cause this problem.

• *Go to an emergency room or see your physician immediately if wheezing results from antibiotics, especially along with hives.* Together these are symptoms of anaphylactic shock, a rare, life-threatening allergic reaction.

• *Contact your physician or clinic if you develop any of the following after your abortion:* soreness and/or cramps, heavy bleeding (some bleeding will occur for several days), fever, nausea or vomiting, foul-smelling vaginal discharge, rash, hives, or asthma (possible reaction to antibiotics).

• *Go to your follow-up appointment.* You'll be scheduled to return in a week or so for a checkup. This may be an easy appointment to pass up because you probably will feel good, but it's important to get your uterus checked at this time. Ordinarily, sexual intercourse can be resumed after two or three weeks, so this is a good time to discuss that. (Depending on the circumstances, some women swear off sex — at least for the immediate future — while others do not.)

• *Expect your menstrual period within six weeks or so.* If it doesn't arrive, contact your health care provider.

I was 18 years old and it is a pain I will never forget. I didn't tell my mother about it, because I did not want to hurt her. I went through my abortion alone, no parents, no boyfriend.

My grandmother had an abortion when they were illegal, but I never thought it would happen to me. After my third child was born, my husband had a vasectomy and five months later I had an abortion. It was bad enough when my husband's operation failed, but the worst part was the phone calls from my husband's doctor, telling me the operation couldn't have failed, therefore, I was a whore. Years later my unmarried daughter told me she was unexpectedly pregnant and would I please come and be with her for an abortion. I said, "Of course." I didn't want her experience to be like mine. It wasn't easy for me to be there, but I wanted to help her. That was more important than any memories it would dredge up for me. Since my daughter's abortion, she and I are closer. She said it meant a lot to her that I was there. We're closer, better friends, more genuinely loving and caring.

ABORTION AND THE LAW

Abortion has existed at least since recorded time, and it was legal in the United States until the 1860s. Statistics show that in the 1930s, the illegal abortion rate was the same as the legal abortion rate today, about one quarter of all pregnancies. Abortion became legal again in 1973 with the U.S. Supreme Court ruling on *Roe v. Wade,* one of the most liberal abortion judgments in the world, allowing women to have abortions for any reason up to the seventh month of pregnancy. Although more than 50 other countries have legal abortion, most have restrictions limiting abortions to the first trimester, except for unusual circumstances.

Several U.S. Supreme Court rulings since 1989 have allowed states to regulate abortion procedures with specific restrictions. These rulings did not make abortion illegal, nor did they create a law for the whole country. In certain states, these restrictions include: requirement for minors to get parental or court approval, 24-hour waiting period, obligatory explanation by doctor of abortion's risks and benefits, and prohibition of public employees from performing abortions or prohibitions on abortions at public hospitals (i.e., those that receive federal funds).

Also, states may mandate medical tests at physician discretion to determine the possibility of fetal survival for any fetus thought to be at least 20 weeks old — about 1 percent of U.S. abortions take place at 20 or more weeks. (Testing for fetal viability — such as the maturity of the lung — is of questionable value, since babies under 26 weeks seldom survive outside the womb. Moreover, there are no 100 percent reliable tests to determine fetal age. Ultrasound determines gestational age with an error rate of two weeks and the use of amniocentesis for fetal viability is not effective until at least 28 weeks.)

It is yet to be determined how much more each state can further regulate abortions, including the scope of the rights of fathers. If your state limits abortions, or if you live in an area where abortions are not available, remember to check the "Abortion" listings mentioned earlier for referrals.

Regardless of the evolution of its legal status, abortion will remain a volatile, emotional issue in the foreseeable future. Because of that, some women who have had abortions suggest that you be very cautious about telling your abortion history to those who keep written records of your medical background. (Sometimes people other than your physician or clinic have access to your medical records through national computer networks.) Similarly, there are women who have given up their infants for adoption who have also learned through experience to be cautious about passing along that information to avoid unsolicited value judgments.

ABORTION AND TEENS

More pregnant U.S. teens give birth than have abortions, and in the states where teens are required to get parental approval for an abortion, the teen abortion rates have dropped. The higher up the educational scale the pregnant teenager's family is — regardless of religious affiliation — or the more accessible abortion facilities are to her, the more likely it is that she will have an abortion.

International research shows that the United States has the highest teen pregnancy rate among 37 industrialized countries, although the rate of sexual activity among teens in those countries with the exception of Japan, which has a lower rate, is reportedly the same. Countries with low teen-pregnancy rates generally have liberal attitudes toward sex, easy access to low-cost birth control without parental approval, and comprehensive sex education. (See "A Note to Mothers of Teens" on page 169.)

Similarly, abortion rates around the world are linked to the availability of contraceptives. In Latin America where abortion is illegal and birth control is not readily available in most countries, 20 to 25 percent of all pregnancies are illegally aborted.

ACQUIRED IMMUNE DEFICIENCY SYNDROME (AIDS)

WHAT IT IS

AIDS is an illness in which the AIDS virus (called the human immunodeficiency virus, or HIV) destroys the body's immune system and allows otherwise controllable infections to invade and overcome the body and cause additional diseases.

SIGNS AND SYMPTOMS

Women's early signs of AIDS are usually different from men's. Gynecologic symptoms, like cervical cancer, yeast infections, and other vaginal infections, sexually transmitted diseases (such as genital warts, herpes, chancroid and gonorrhea), and pelvic inflammatory disease may be the first sign of AIDS in some women. (See "Vaginal Infections" on page 532, "Sexually Transmitted Diseases" on page 493, "Cervical Cancer" on page 234, and "Pelvic Inflammatory Disease" on page 441.) Most women who have these symptoms do not, however, have AIDS.

The disease begins, probably in the organs of the immune system, long before any symptoms are apparent. The first step is contracting the HIV virus through the blood of another person or through seminal fluid, which carries sperm. Once the the HIV virus is in your bloodstream, your body then produces antibodies to fight it. It is these antibodies that can be detected in blood tests. In newer, experimental tests, pieces of the actual HIV virus are visible sooner than are the antibodies.

Sometimes years can pass between the time of infection and the appearance of symptoms. (Seven years is the average time for HIV infection from transfusions to show up, for example.) You will ultimately develop AIDS, although some research suggests that a tiny fraction of people infected with HIV (less than 1 percent) may successfully defeat the virus. The interval between infection and signs of the disease sometimes shortens if a pregnancy intervenes, though not always.

The traditional forerunners of AIDS are blood abnormalities and AIDS-related complex symptoms, such as weight loss, night sweats, fever, fatigue, diarrhea, pneumonia, and persistently swollen lymph nodes. All of these individually can be symptoms of other diseases, and at least two of them — fatigue and weight loss — can also be symptoms of pregnancy in some women.

Symptoms of full-blown AIDS include pneumonia and a dozen other infections, cancer, and dementia. People with AIDS are also especially susceptible to tuberculosis, a contagious, chronic wasting disease. By the time people have well-developed AIDS, they are often hospitalized frequently. Many survive several months with AIDS and a few live a decade. Both women and men who are treated aggressively, however, tend to live longer than these estimates. In fact, some people have lived for 14 years or more after an HIV diagnosis. (See "Treatment Options" on page 142.)

White males, rather than men of other races or women, are more likely to be long-term survivors of AIDS, if they are not IV-drug users. That may be due to genetic factors and their socioeconomic advantages, including better health to start with and more options for treatment, such as a choice of hospitals and access to a wider variety of AIDS-delaying drugs.

PREVENTIVE MEASURES YOU CAN TAKE

HIV is transmitted best through blood and is ordinarily not an easy virus to "catch." It is not transmitted through saliva during passionate kissing or by shaking hands or from the bites of insects. Nor will you get it from a toilet seat or from casual contact with an infected person at your school or workplace.

Once the HIV virus is in your bloodstream, you become a carrier and can pass the virus on to others, either through blood (sharing intravenous-drug needles or receiving blood transfusions), sex (vaginal or especially anal intercourse), or pregnancy. Between 1980 and 1989, 79 (less than 1 percent of all U.S. women with AIDS) lesbians were diagnosed with AIDS, and nearly all of these women were IV-drug users.

More than one half of U.S. women who contract AIDS do so through heterosexual sex, and this fraction increases each year. (Worldwide, AIDS is transmitted heterosexually 75 percent of the time.) Perhaps because there is more virus in semen than in cervical fluid and semen remains in the vagina for days giving the HIV virus time to work, U.S. women are 10 times more likely to contract AIDS from men through sex than the other way around. It's believed that men may contract the HIV virus through sexual contact with vaginal secretions or menstrual blood.

Some people still think of AIDS as a gay men's disease. Although the highest proportion of U.S. men with AIDS are homosexual, AIDS is an equal-opportunity illness. It's a very real health threat for women, even though the number of U.S. women with AIDS is still considered small (nearly 25,000 in 1992). To minimize your risk of getting AIDS:

• *Don't use illegal IV drugs.* Until 1992, the most common way U.S. women contracted the virus was through sharing contaminated needles.

• *Don't have sex with a partner who is an IV-drug user,* since IV-drug users are at high risk for AIDS. Of the women who contracted AIDS heterosexually, about 60 percent had partners who were IV-drug users.

• *Don't have sex with a male partner who is bisexual,* since his contact with gay men puts him at high risk for AIDS.

• *Don't have sex with a hemophiliac.* Hemophiliacs, who are always male, have an inherited condition that causes them to bleed excessively, which requires frequent blood transfusions. Almost every U.S. male with this disease born before 1985 has been infected by contaminated blood with HIV.

• *Don't have sex with a male partner who "sleeps around."* He could contract AIDS and give it to you.

• *Be celibate or be monogamous with a monogamous partner who does not have the HIV virus.* If neither you nor your partner is at high risk, your chance of contracting AIDS each time you have intercourse is one in five million. If you use a condom, your chances diminish to one in 50 million. Monogamy seems to be the rule now for many adult U.S. women and men, if studies on sexual behavior can be believed. A government study found that most adult Americans had only one sex partner, or none, in 1988. People who've been tested for HIV, whether or not they test positive, are more likely to practice safer sex. However, many teens, including college students who are theoretically well informed about AIDS and its transmission, have multiple partners and don't use condoms. The number of teens with AIDS is still small, but that number grew 40 percent between 1987 and 1989.

• *Build up your immune system.* (See "How to Stay Healthy" on page 25.) Some experts estimate that of 100 to 300 people who have the HIV antibody in their bloodstream, only one has symptomatic AIDS. It's believed that one of the reasons most of these people have not gotten sick yet is their still healthy immune systems.

• *Use your own donated blood if you plan to have elective surgery.* Although the risk of contracting AIDS via a blood transfusion may be extremely low now because of new testing procedures, no one claims all U.S. blood is 100 percent safe. (See "Surgery" on page 95 for more information about using your own blood for elective surgery.)

• *If you are planning to use artificial insemination, have it performed with frozen sperm that has been tested several times,* preferably over a period of several years, for the HIV virus. (See "Artificial Insemination" on page 371.) A small percent of women have contracted the HIV virus via blood transfusions or artificial insemination.

Some researchers think uncircumcised males are at higher risk for AIDS, because it's believed they are more likely to contract a sexually transmitted disease, but this conclusion is controversial. Whether or not your partner is uncircumcised, you'll want to practice safer sex.

---

*H*ow could I have known [that he was bisexual]? He didn't tell a soul, not even his family. I didn't find out until several years after we split up. His doctor called to tell me he had died of AIDS. So I ran down and took an antibody test. And there it was: I was HIV-positive.

I am a 36-year-old happily married, white female, who has never had syphilis, gonorrhea, or chlamydia, has never used crack, never been an intravenous-drug user, never had a blood transfusion. I test positive for the human immunodeficiency virus. Clearly, I contracted the virus through heterosexual contact.

HOW TO HAVE "SAFER" SEX

Since it's not likely that men are going to tell you if they are bisexual, IV-drug users, or have multiple sex partners, you need to protect yourself. In fact, it's probable that the only person who will tell you he's been tested for HIV is someone who has tested negative. (HIV-infected women don't necessarily tell their male partners either.)

If you have unprotected sex (no condom) with a man who has the AIDS virus, it's estimated that your chance of contracting the virus yourself is one in 500 each time. But that's just a statistical average. A few women, particularly — but not always — those who already have a sexually transmitted disease (STD), have reported contracting the virus in this situation after just one sexual encounter. Investigators have discovered that some strains of the virus are more infectious than others.

Safer sex means using either latex male condoms (*not* lambskin) that include spermicide (Nonoxynol-9), or the Reality female condom. Other barrier contraceptives (such as the diaphragm or cervical cap) may be effective in preventing other sexually transmitted diseases, but not HIV. (See "Birth Control" starting on page 162 for more information about all of these contraceptives.)

Safer sex means no anal sex because there is more likelihood of bleeding, resulting in a twofold increased risk for transmission of the HIV virus, or any sexual practice (such as having sex during menstruation) that results in the mixture of your blood with the blood or semen of your partner. The use of condoms will enormously reduce your risk for STDs, too, which are a precursor for AIDS in women. (See "How to Use a Male Condom with Pleasure" on page 194 and "Acquired Immune Deficiency Syndrome" in Recommended Reading on page 612 for more information about safer sex.)

If you are already HIV-positive, safer sex will help protect your partner. However, neither of you needs an AIDS diagnosis for you both to practice safer sex.

TREATMENT OPTIONS

There is no effective AIDS vaccine, and an all-purpose AIDS vaccine is unlikely because the HIV virus quickly mutates, creating new viral strains. Nevertheless, by the early 1990s about 30 vaccines were being tested. While new AIDS drugs continue to be developed, by 1992 the FDA-approved AIDS drugs in the United States were zidovudine (AZT), dideoxyinosine (DDI), and zalcitabine or DDC, which is used in combination with AZT.

Other drugs include alpha-interferon, fluconazole, and aerosolized pentamidine. (See "The AIDS Clinical Trials Information Service" on page 547 in the Resource Directory for more information about AIDS drugs.)

Until large research trials were performed in the 1990s, it was thought that AZT delayed the progression from HIV to full blown AIDS in symptomless people. The same has been thought of DDI as well, although it's not clear that DDI can delay the progression either, because of insufficient research. AZT is toxic for many people who use it, it may lose its effectiveness over time, it helps some and not others, and currently costs thousands of dollars per year. Sometimes, as with DDI and DDC, it is covered by insurance. In 1989 the U.S. government began to pay for AZT for some low-income people. (See "The AIDS Drug Assistance Program" on page 547 in the Resource Directory.)

Today nontraditional treatments are used by growing numbers of people. Some use experimental drugs and treatments available in other countries. Other options are: acupuncture (especially for pain relief), acupressure, massage, herbal therapies, meditation, visual imagery, megavitamin therapy, and a macrobiotic diet. (See "Acupuncture" on page 82, "Acupressure" on page 56, "Meditation" on page 59, and "Alternative Medicine" on page 82.)

AIDS TESTING

Now that early drug treatment may postpone the development of AIDS symptoms for many months, sometimes years, there are benefits to finding out sooner, rather than later, that you are HIV-positive. Some experts would encourage women, especially those who are at risk for AIDS, to be tested because of these options. (Don't wait for your physician to suggest testing, however, because many don't—especially if you're white and middle-class. If you know you're at risk for AIDS, it's up to you to get the test.)

Others suggest testing only if it would make a difference in your behavior. For instance, if you are pregnant, test positive, and subsequently have an abortion, then the test altered your behavior. In the same circumstances, if you decide to keep the baby and take AZT to reduce symptoms, then the test has altered your behavior.

To get the most reliable AIDS test results:

• *Know that one test is not necessarily enough.* Testing negative for AIDS once isn't a 100 percent guarantee that you are HIV-free. Since the HIV antibodies can lie dormant on account of a six-month "window" of time (rarely, a "silent" HIV infection will last even longer) between the moment of contamination and the time when the HIV virus is apparent through testing, you could get a false-negative result. If you test negative yet you have good reason to believe you might have been exposed to the HIV virus during the previous six months, get another test for your piece of mind.

• *If you test positive, immediately repeat the test at least once.* Errors in processing at labs and misinterpretations by staff are not uncommon, especially if the experimental five-minute AIDS test is used in an emergency room. Although some errors are falsely negative, the most common error is the false-positive result (you're told that you have the virus, but you really don't have it), particularly if you are a low-risk woman. People with liver disease, such as hepatitis, and women who have had several pregnancies are more likely to get a false-positive result. It's important to know this in advance, because we all tend to believe that *our* test results are correct, even though we know no test is error-free each time.

If you want to avoid any possible discrimination, keep your test confidential by obtaining it through a clinic where a number is your only identification. However, this may be difficult in an increasing number of states that no longer provide anonymous testing. Many states, however, may have one clinic for anonymous testing. Call your local or state health department for this information.

Speak with an AIDS counselor if your test has been confirmed positive through several samplings. Discuss the effect this will have on your life, your body, and — if you're pregnant — your baby. Talk with a counselor at length about this, because feeling alone with the news may make you feel worse than you already do knowing that you have the virus. Ask the counselor how you can obtain AIDS-delaying drugs, such as AZT, and how those with whom you have had sexual contact can be notified.

When pregnant women have AIDS, the women who keep the pregnancy do so often because of their desire for a child, religious beliefs, and/or family pressure. If you're pregnant and choose to keep the baby, talk with an AIDS counselor about that and find a doctor who has experience working with pregnant women who have AIDS. If you can't find someone with that experience, find someone who is willing to learn about it. (See "Acquired Immune Deficiency Syndrome" on page 547 of the Resource Directory for organizations to help you both find support for yourself, as well as perhaps referrals to knowledgeable doctors. See also "A Note About AIDS Babies" on page 500.)

A few of my very sexually active friends decided not to have the AIDS test. They were practicing safe sex all the time now and couldn't see what difference it would make. But I have kids, and I needed to know for their future.

A friend was plunged into depression when her first test result came back positive and she didn't dare believe the second test result, which was negative. She has taken the test a third and fourth time (with both results negative) yet has become convinced that she still may be infected with the virus.

AIDS OVERVIEW

AIDS in the United States occurs more frequently in men, although women are the fastest growing infected group. By 1991 AIDS was one of the five leading causes of death among women aged 15 to 44. Of the more than 315,000 people who were diagnosed with AIDS by 1993, almost 12 percent were women. No one knows how many women have AIDS or the HIV virus that causes it, because so few of the U.S. population have been tested for it. Most experts believe that many existing AIDS cases are unreported.

Future estimates of the number of people who will develop AIDS vary, but some experts believe that more than one million people in the United States are already infected with the HIV virus. The highest known AIDS rate in the world is in the New York City – northern New Jersey area with one in four men aged 25 to 44 having the HIV virus. In the United States, the majority of men with AIDS are white, while half of the known AIDS-infected women are African-American or Latina and live in New York, Miami, or Newark.

AIDS is a global disease, and known cases are found in increasing numbers wherever people live. The spread of AIDS has not been stopped in any community or country. In 1990 it was estimated that three million women and five million men had the HIV virus. The World Health Organization in 1991 said there may be as many as 30 to 40 million by the year 2000, and most of the AIDS-infected worldwide will be women.

In Western countries, women contract AIDS the same way they do in the United States. But in Africa in particular, where AIDS is more widespread, women are far more likely to contract the virus heterosexually. That's due to several factors, one of which is that women are more likely to have sexually transmitted diseases. Also, blood transfusions, which are more common in parts of Africa than elsewhere, are sometimes performed with unsterile equipment. A third reason for the high AIDS rate in Africa is the traditional custom among an estimated 80 million African women of infibulation (stitching up of the vulva) and the removal of the clitoris. These practices of genital mutilation not only may cause infection and severe blood loss at the time they are performed, but also can cause bleeding during sexual intercourse later, which increases the potential to be exposed to the virus.

Alzheimer's Disease

What It Is

Alzheimer's is a progressive disorder that destroys the brains cells used for memory and reasoning, causing mental deterioration, personality changes, and eventually death.

Signs and Symptoms

Alzheimer's disease follows a course that can be roughly divided into four phases. People with Alzheimer's in:

Phase 1:
• Have less energy and enthusiasm, the beginnings of memory failure, depression, and mood swings
• Are slow to react and learn new things, but are easily angered
• Prefer the familiar in their lives, while relatives aren't positive that there's something wrong with them

• Cannot on occasion remember common nouns, such as "book" or "bird";

Phase 2:
• Have a lessened sense of smell
• Speak more slowly and misunderstand easily
• Seem to have forgotten how to calculate numbers
• Misplace objects and accuse others of stealing them
• Have more and more difficulty making decisions
• May be awake and restless at night and will sleep during the day
• Are insensitive to others — a once cheerful, caring person may become sullen and grouchy
• Often repeat words and stories, including frequent rambling, and actions — such as putting on a hat and going to the front door dozens of times a day;

Phase 3:
• Don't recognize family members
• Can't remember recent events, but may be able to recall things from childhood
• Have trouble with once-easy daily tasks, such as dressing, bathing, or eating
• Are given to bizarre or coarse behavior;

Phase 4:
• Will likely be placed in a nursing home — if at all possible
• Recognize no one, not even themselves in a mirror
• Are uninterested in their surroundings
• Are totally helpless and feeble
• Wander if given the opportunity
• Are both bowel- and bladder-incontinent
• Can't walk well
• Unable to speak
• Develop body emaciation, urinary tract infections, and a tendency toward pneumonia.

Someone who has Alzheimer's may survive 20 years. Women live longer with the disease than men, but this may be because women are more likely to live to be very old. Usually the length of time from onset of the disease to death is from five to eight years, especially with genetically linked Alzheimer's.

MAKING THE DIAGNOSIS

Diagnosis is only certain with an autopsy that reveals the telltale tangled nerve endings in the brain. However, a variety of tests can be used to rule out Alzheimer's in the living. Disoriented or forgetful behavior in the aged can have many other causes, some of which can be successfully treated (see "Other Causes of Senility" on page 156).

Alzheimer's was named for a German neurologist, Alois Alzheimer, who in 1907 described the symptoms in a 51-year-old woman. It seems to be a twentieth-century phenomenon, possibly because fewer people before the twentieth century lived into their 70s and 80s. This disease affects about 10 percent of the U.S. population past the age of 65. The actual incidence of Alzheimer's in older people depends on the age group. Between 65 and 74, the rate is 3 percent in some research, however, the rate is up to 20 percent for those past 85. As our population ages, the number of affected people will grow. In spite of that, at current levels nearly 90 percent of the population will *not* develop Alzheimer's.

Many Americans say they fear getting Alzheimer's. They wonder if every memory lapse and lost thread in a conversation is an early sign of the disease. No, they are not. We all experience those distractions from time to time, but the symptoms of Alzheimer's do not include these occasional lapses. The disease follows a specific, steady path and sooner, rather than later, the symptoms become profound.

Typical medical tests and procedures performed to determine the cause of senility are a detailed medical history; a complete physical; a neurological exam; a mental-status examination (series of questions); several blood tests; thyroid test; a spinal tap or lumbar puncture to check for infections of the nervous system; a biopsy of nasal nerve cells; an electroencephalogram (EEG), a test that records electrical activity in the brain; and a computerized axial tomography (CAT) scan, a kind of x-ray of the brain.

Other tests are a positron-emission transaxial tomography (PET) scan or single-photon-emission computed tomography (SPECT), which are newer versions of a CAT scan; psychiatric evaluation; occupational therapy evaluation; and neuropsychological testing (evaluation of memory, reasoning, coordination, writing and more).

Although a simple blood test for a protein found in people with Alzheimer's may be available in the future, currently, a diagnosis in the living can be made only by ruling out other conditions and undergoing a battery of tests. These cost anywhere between several hundred dollars and several thousand, depending on which tests are used and where they are performed.

CAUSES

No one knows for sure what causes Alzheimer's, but some researchers believe it is a group of related disorders that have different causes.

Genetically linked Alzheimer's is estimated to trigger 10 to 15 percent of all cases. Your risk for the disease is about 20 percent if you have a sibling or parent who develops Alzheimer's before age 65. Your risk doubles to about 40 percent if you have both a sibling and parent with the disease. Heredity is apparently not a factor, however, when Alzheimer's first shows up past 65 — it's this late-onset Alzheimer's that effects an estimated four million people in the United States.

Alzheimer's also occurs frequently in people over 50 who have Down syndrome, the most common cause of mental retardation (see Down syndrome on page 454). In addition, although the connection is not clear, some research suggests that elderly women who have had heart attacks are more likely to develop Alzheimer's.

Another suspected cause is the ingestion of aluminum. Researchers seem to agree that aluminum in the body is not good for anyone, but while there is a lot of evidence to support the connection between aluminum and Alzheimer's, experts are not in agreement that avoiding the ingestion of aluminum prevents the disease. Everyone is exposed to aluminum in the environment, but nearly 90 percent will not develop Alzheimer's.

Aluminum is a metal found naturally in soil and water. (It was first processed in 1888, making it a twentieth-century metal.) It is sometimes added to drinking water (many municipalities add aluminum to the water supply for purification), and it is in hundreds of everyday products, such as antacids, beer and soft drink cans, and nondairy creamers.

Autopsies performed on Alzheimer's victims show a two-times higher-than-normal concentration of aluminum in four areas of the brain. Some researchers say a healthy brain will not absorb aluminum no matter how much of the metal is ingested. Others say that the presence of aluminum in our daily lives makes it easier for harmful substances to enter the brain. Aluminum has been shown to sometimes trigger hyperactivity and learning disorders in children, and in the 1960s, many people using kidney dialysis machines showed symptoms of Alzheimer's that were ultimately traced to the aluminum used in both the equipment and the treatment water. "Dialysis dementia" disappeared when the water and method of treatment were changed.

TREATMENT OPTIONS

There's no cure, and no treatment that alters the outcome. The drug tacrine (THA), which was approved for use in the United States in 1993, increases the levels of acetylcholine, a chemical that carries messages among nerve cells in the brain. The manufacturers of THA claim it may reverse memory loss due to Alzheimer's in some patients, and some caregivers of Alzheimer's patients who have used the drug agree. THA also has a variety of side effects, including liver damage, and remains controversial. Along with THA, there are other experimental drugs to slow Alzheimer's mental degeneration which are also being tested.

PREVENTIVE MEASURES YOU CAN TAKE

• *Avoid ingesting aluminum.* If ingested aluminum proves to be one of the culprits for some of the people who have Alzheimer's, staying away from aluminum may help save your brain from destruction, especially if you have a family history of the disease. It also may contribute to your general health regardless.

• *Avoid over-the-counter health care products that contain the word aluminum* in any combination of words in the list of ingredients. Examples of these products are antacids, analgesics (buffered aspirin), and antiperspirants, antidiarrheal products, and douches. Examples of ingredient combinations are aluminum hydroxide, bismuth aluminate or dihydroxyaluminum, among others.

• *Don't use aluminum foil to save food when the foil comes into direct contact with the food,* especially with high-acid foods like tomatoes. Use glass or plastic containers or other kinds of wrapping material.

• *Likewise, avoid commercial food products covered by aluminum foil,* including many frozen dinners and dairy products, such as some brands of yogurt, cream cheese, and ricotta cheese, as well as some dried fruit, cereals, and candy packages.

• *Don't buy beverages in aluminum cans,* such as those used for beer or carbonated beverages (especially those stored for a while), and avoid aluminum-coated waxed containers of fruit juices. Choose glass or plastic containers instead.

• *Look out for sodium aluminum phosphate,* an additive used in products such as baking soda, baking powder, self-rising flours, most pancake batters, frozen doughs, many cake mixes, pickles, maraschino cherries, nondairy creamer, and processed cheese (especially the individually wrapped kind).

• *Don't use aluminum cookware*, because it leaches aluminum into your food, increasing the amount of aluminum you take in each day by an estimated 9 to 17 percent. Use stainless steel, glass, iron, well-glazed pottery, tin-lined copper, or nonstick pans (but only those that still have their surface intact, as many are made of aluminum underneath the coating). If you eat out often, be aware that aluminum is the cookware of choice in most restaurants, although some chefs use stainless steel for some sauces to avoid the metallic taste or gray color caused by aluminum residue.

• *Maintain a healthy immune system* (see "How to Stay Healthy" on page 25).

• *Exercise regularly.* When you work out, lactic acid is formed in your muscles, which helps remove toxic metals from your body.

• *Eat foods that help remove metals from your body.* Foods that are rich in the amino acids cysteine and methionine "grab" toxic metals in your body and remove them. Some of these foods are onions, garlic, chives, red peppers, beans (limas, pintos, kidneys, soybeans), seeds (sesame, pumpkin, sunflower), English walnuts, and asparagus. Foods rich in calcium and magnesium may be helpful as well.

• *Add foods rich in choline, an amino acid associated with memory retention.* The richest sources are: brains, liver, yeast, wheat germ, kidneys, egg yolks, and granular lecithin. Choline and lecithin, which are available in tablets, may relieve depression, and lecithin may also dissolve excess cholesterol in the body. As we age, the body's ability to absorb and use vitamins and minerals usually decreases so that malnutrition, an overall factor in Alzheimer's, becomes more common. Some nursing home operators routinely give choline to their elderly residents.

WHAT TO DO AND HOW TO COPE IF YOU'RE THE CAREGIVER

Since women continue to be the primary caregivers in families, it is likely that if Alzheimer's strikes your family, you will be at least one of the caregivers, if not the primary one. In this case, you need to know how to cope with and plan for a situation that may last for a number of years. Following are some important guidelines:

• *Make sure of the diagnosis.* Not all senility is caused by Alzheimer's and many other forms are treatable if the cause is diagnosed (see "Other Causes of Senility" on page 156).

• *Ask the physician what tests will be given and how much each will cost.* If the person with the possible Alzheimer's has insurance, don't assume that it will pay for these tests. However, if the person is at least 65, or disabled at any age, she or he is eligible for Medicare. This government-funded insurance program pays 80 percent of the medical fees for Alzheimer's testing. Other insurance programs may pay for expenses incurred in a hospital, but not necessarily those in a doctor's office or clinic.

• *Consider going to a doctor who has special interest and extensive experience in dealing with senility.* In one study, two thirds of the cases were misdiagnosed two or more times. Your relative's family doctor may or may not be the right person to make the diagnosis, because the causes of senility are varied and a diagnosis for Alzheimer's is arrived at only by eliminating all other possible causes.

• *Find out if local medical schools have special units for evaluating and treating senility, or consult an Alzheimer's organization for suggestions of who to contact in your area.* (See "Alzheimer's Disease" on page 612 in Recommended Reading and on page 554 in the Resource Directory.)

• *Learn to cope day to day.* Treat the person with dignity and respect, for their sake and yours. Focus on what they can do, not on what they can't do. Don't argue. Agree and distract. The feelings, not the facts, are what matter.

• *Understand that this person will never again be the woman or man you remember.*

• *Be as calm as you can in your dealings with this person.* Know that the undesirable behavior of someone with Alzheimer's, just like the crying of an infant, is not an attempt to "get even" with you.

• *Realize that this person may be as frightened of what's happening as you are upset in watching it happen.* Avoid bringing up issues from the past, which of course require memory, and talk instead about pleasant events in the present.

• *Keep life simple for the person with Alzheimer's as much as possible.* Travel and visitors can confuse and irritate her or him.

• *Find help for yourself so that you don't feel isolated and powerless.* This support will perhaps allow you to find meaning and value in taking care of this person and transform a potentially devastating experience to one of personal growth.

• *Contact an Alzheimer's support group.* They'll have day-to-day coping suggestions for you. (See also "Caregivers" on page 611 in Recommended Reading, and on page 557 in the Resource Directory.)

• *Understand this person's financial situation.* Talk with members of an Alzheimer's support group, perhaps other members of the family, or an attorney about obtaining a power of attorney, which is a written statement legally authorizing you to act for another person. Make financial arrangements now, if possible, that will not leave you penniless later because of the cost of institutionalized care.

I try to be positive and extend them [people with Alzheimer's] dignity, even though they may not be able to do very simple things and even have to be shown how to sit down. I find that if I am polite and understanding and respectful because of what they were as human beings before the disease came to them, that they're still capable of responding.

When I last saw my Grandpa, he was 82 and I was 13. He was coloring in a coloring book and pleased that he was staying in the lines. Once I realized that in his head he was only a child like some of the kids I babysat, it was easy to sit and color with him. He said he liked me, but I knew he didn't know I was his granddaughter.

She [Aunt Jenny] was like a mother to me, and there was no way I could live with putting her in a home. Her forgetfulness wasn't really a problem, but when she started staying up all night, yelling at the kids for no reason, and refusing to bathe, I knew we were in for trouble. Children are trying enough, but eventually they learn how to take care of themselves. But here was Aunt Jenny, a woman I'd always looked up to, coming apart piece by piece right before my eyes. It was very wrenching for me, and painful and confusing for everyone else in my family.

For two or three years Mary had known that her memory was slipping. First she had trouble remembering the names of her friends' children . . . She would find herself groping for a word she had always known, and she worried that she was getting senile . . . The bathroom was not where it was yesterday. Her hands forgot how to button buttons. . . . Mary was glad when her family came to visit. . . . She was glad when they didn't try to remind her of what she had just said or that they had come last week, or ask her if she remembered this person or that one.

It was during this trip that both the doctor and I realized that Phil was changing. He would ask our friends where I was, and then tell them he wasn't going to leave the room until he found me. But I was in the same room and not out of his sight at the time!

I became profoundly depressed when I had to quit my job and stay home to take care of my mother-in-law who had Alzheimer's. The fact that I never liked her didn't help much. I rallied and got help after I spoke with an Alzheimer's support group.

CAREGIVING OPTIONS FOR PEOPLE WITH ALZHEIMER'S

About half of the elderly in nursing homes have Alzheimer's, but two thirds of people with this disease are cared for at home by family members. This probably happens because either the Alzheimer's is in the early, more manageable stages, or because the family can't afford to pay for a nursing home. Current options specifically for people with Alzheimer's are:

• *Nursing homes.* Ask your friends or members of an Alzheimer's support group who have had experience with nursing homes for suggestions on what to look for and what to avoid in a facility. There are now some nursing homes just for people with Alzheimer's. Nursing homes often cost at least $25,000 a year, although those patients who qualify for Medicaid do not have to pay anything. Medicaid is a state-administered program for people with low incomes, and it pays for some expenses not covered by the federally administered Medicare program. If you are interested in this option, contact the health department in your county to reach the Medicaid office. Ask them well in advance, years if possible, how your family member could qualify for Medicaid and receive free nursing home care. (See "Nursing Homes" on page 613 of Recommended Reading.)

• *Adult daycare centers.* These may be a good option for people in the early stages of Alzheimer's, but they may not be for those who refuse to leave home, who are confused by new places and strangers, or who have become entirely unpredictable. Costs at these centers vary enormously from no charge or a few dollars (which is rare) to $125 per day.

• *Home health care.* Health care workers, who are usually women, provide care for the person in the home. Their fees vary, depending on the needs of this person, the health care worker's training, which varies a great deal, and where you live.

My wife got sick just about the same time I retired. All I was doing was taking care of her. I thought I should get some exercise, so I joined a senior citizens' exercise group. I take my wife to a daycare center the day I go to that group.

Other Causes of Senility

Senility or dementia (Latin for "out of one's mind") can be caused by any of 60 disorders, but Alzheimer's accounts for 60 to 80 percent of all senility in people past 65. The second major cause of senility in the United States is a series of small strokes. Unlike Alzheimer's, these can be revealed by a neurologic exam or other tests. Also, the senility caused by Alzheimer's is constant, whereas the senility caused by strokes is sporadic.

Other causes of senility are serious brain injuries (those suffered by boxers, for example) that required physician evaluation, a so-called slow virus, infections, or the aging process itself. Overmedication, which is likely on the increase due to greater prescription drug use by the elderly, is another cause of senility. Older people's bodies have more difficulty tolerating the toxicity of drugs, and older people may take more combinations of drugs than people at any other age. Some people's senility goes away when drugs are removed or are correctly balanced. (See "Prescription and Over-the-Counter Drugs" on page 609 of Recommended Reading for books (particularly Wolff's) that describe the potential problems of specific drug combinations.)

My father who was in his early 80s was irrational and given to bizarre behavior. We took him to a doctor who diagnosed Alzheimer's disease. We were devastated! My mother was distraught, and my husband and I worried about our responsibilities. I spoke with a friend shortly after who had had the same thing happen in her family. She suggested that we take my father to the university hospital nearby, and it's the best thing we could have done. A doctor there took a full history and evaluated all the medication my father took, including pills for his heart. This doctor told us that my father did not have Alzheimer's. That, in fact, he was reacting to the combined medications he was taking. It seemed too good to be true, but he turned out to be right. We are all relieved and thrilled now to have my "real" father back with us.

Another cause of senility is depression. This can come at any age from sitting around doing nothing, thinking nothing, and eating very little—

which is not an uncommon description of a day in the life of many older people. Depression is more common in the elderly, and its effects may give the impression of senility.

Neurologic ailments, including Huntington's disease and Parkinson's disease, can cause senility. These diseases often cause tremors or involuntary shaking of the head or limbs, among other symptoms.

Vitamin deficiencies and/or malnutrition may cause senility, too. Older people, especially those who live alone, often eat poorly, and their bodies don't absorb nutrients as well as they did when they were younger.

A thyroid problem may cause mental confusion. This, too, can be tested for and corrected.

Chronic infections, like pneumonia, are especially devastating to older people and may produce inattentiveness and mental confusion. Treating infections successfully can restore mental capacity.

ANEMIA

WHAT IT IS

Anemia is a shortage of oxygen-carrying red cells (hemoglobin) in the blood. Anemia is not a disease itself, but rather a condition that has a variety of causes. Average hemoglobin levels range from 12 to 14.2 g/100 ml, although what's normal varies from person to person. Blood tests can reveal anemia when hemoglobin registers below the level of 12.

SIGNS AND SYMPTOMS

Women who are mildly anemic feel tired, with perhaps a few of the following symptoms. Those with a more pronounced deficiency may have a greater number of illnesses in general and have more of the following symptoms:

- Bone-weary fatigue with any exertion.
- Depression, headaches, heartburn, and irritability.

• They may experience fainting spells; hair loss, especially in young women; coldness or tingling in hands or feet; sensation of rapid or fluttering heartbeat; and itching.

• Often they have pale lips and complexion; poor appetite; poor memory and decreased attention span (even mild anemia can handicap work or school performance); sore, shiny tongue, with perhaps sores in the corner of the mouth; sore gums; brittle nails; a craving for ice or other non foods, such as dirt or clay; and little interest in sex.

CAUSES

The most common cause of anemia in women is a diet that is deficient in iron, and/or the B vitamins folic acid and B_{12}. The body needs iron to make hemoglobin. When iron intake is inadequate, iron-deficient anemia is the result. Similarly, a deficient supply of certain vitamins will lead to the production of red blood cells that carry less oxygen.

Excessive bleeding—from menstruation, especially heavy flows or occasionally uterine fibroids (see "Uterine Fibroids" on page 522); or from taking large amounts of aspirin, ibuprofen, or other nonsteroidal anti-inflammatory drugs; or gastrointestinal bleeding from malignant polyps or bleeding ulcers—can also cause anemia. Chronic diseases like rheumatoid arthritis, hepatitis, and tuberculosis are associated with anemia, as are certain inherited conditions such as sickle cell anemia and thalassemia.

Anemia is more common among women than men and is most likely to show up in those who are black, poor, young or old, those who are pregnant or nursing, and women who have heavy menstrual bleeding. (Women typically lose about two pints of blood every year from menstruation.) Women who use an IUD for birth control (see "Intrauterine Device" on page 208) are also more likely to be anemic, because this device causes heavier menstrual flows.

Pregnant women are usually warned about anemia (particularly the kind caused by a folic acid deficiency), but often they are the only ones. Mild anemia is typically ignored by other women, especially young women. They think the symptoms are merely the signs of a busy life, and not related often to a diet rich in fast food and poor in foods that build health.

Other women who are at risk for anemia are those who drink a lot of alcohol, which interferes with vitamin absorption; women who follow low-calorie diets, which do not supply the daily requirement of iron, folic acid, or B_{12}; and vegetarians who don't get their daily requirement of B_{12} (which is most commonly found in meat).

TREATMENT OPTIONS

Treatment for anemia depends on the type involved. When anemia is caused by a disease, it's important to have a medical evaluation. When anemia is caused by an improper diet, treatment may consist of either dietary changes (see below) or dietary changes plus iron supplements, such as ferrous sulfate or ferrous gluconate.

The possible side effects of (and perhaps indication of too much) iron supplements may be constipation, diarrhea, indigestion, cramps and/or nausea, and a black-colored stool. These side effects are often eliminated with dose adjustment.

The iron from these preparations, like the iron from iron-enriched cereals, is not absorbed as well as it is from foods that contain it naturally. But absorption from supplements is improved when it's taken with liver and vitamin C in the same preparation (or with citrus juice). That's why some women take a good multivitamin pill instead.

---

*M*y hair was falling out, my nails were breaking, and I needed more makeup to cover my paleness. I thought that was the price I had to pay to work two jobs and go to school part-time. A friend set me straight though by explaining it probably had a lot to do with what I wasn't eating. She was right. I made a few changes, and it didn't take long for my body to respond. But I found it was easy to fall into my old fast-food habits when I didn't pay attention.

HOME REMEDIES YOU CAN TRY

• *Eat foods that are rich in iron and the B vitamins daily or at least twice a week.* The lists that follow are from Jean Carper's *Total Nutrition Guide;* each is organized with the richest source first, down to the poorest. You'll note that liver shows up on all three lists. (See "Anemia" on page 613 in Recommended Reading for Carper's and other books.)

1. *Foods high in iron:* Liver — all types ("organic" is best — see discussion of "organic" food on page 27); brewer's yeast; beef steak; pumpkin, sunflower and squash seeds; beef kidneys; sorghum molasses; fish roe (caviar); oysters; soybeans; liver sausage; wheat germ; pine nuts; dried lima beans; clams; potatoes with skin; cashew nuts; sardines;

dried apricots; peaches; raisins; prunes; dried kidney beans; cod; turkey; and chicken.

2. *Foods high in folacin (folic acid):* sunflower seeds; soybeans; spinach; turnip greens; liver; asparagus; brussels sprouts; whole-grain cereals; hazel nuts; collards; cashews; parsnips; avocados; almonds; dried beans; corn; beets; wheat germ.

3. *Foods high in Vitamin B$_{12}$:* organ meats, especially kidneys and liver of all types; liverwurst; liver pate; milk, especially nonfat dry milk; seafood, especially shellfish; meat; and most cheeses.

• *Avoid caffeinated tea, in particular, and coffee at meal time*, since they interfere with iron absorption from food. Wait an hour or two after meals to drink them. Some recommend herbal teas as a substitute, but it's not known whether or not they interfere with iron absorption.

• *Avoid antacids, phosphates* in ice cream, candy bars, baked goods, beer and soft drinks, *and the additive EDTA*, which is found on the ingredient lists of many canned and processed foods, because they block iron intake.

ANOREXIA: *see* Eating Disorders

Birth Control

What It Is

Birth control is the prevention of pregnancy.

The process of conception begins with ovulation, a process that occurs every month and that lasts up to 48 hours. During that time a woman's body releases an egg (ovum) from one of her two ovaries. In the hours after

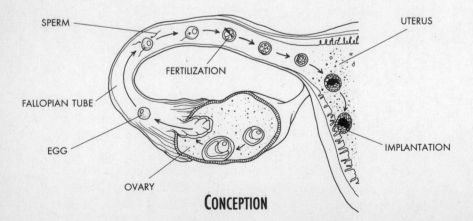

CONCEPTION

its release, this egg is held in one of her two fallopian tubes. If unprotected intercourse occurs, the sperm travel upward through the vagina, the cervix, and the uterus and into the fallopian tubes. It is there that the sperm may fertilize the egg. If the egg and sperm do not meet at this time, the egg disintegrates and the woman's body sloughs off the now unnecessary uterine lining about two weeks later.

TYPES AVAILABLE

The methods of birth control available in the United States today are:

- Sterilization for both women and men
- The Pill
- Barrier contraceptives (condom — male and female, diaphragm, Today sponge, cervical cap, spermicides)
- IUDs
- Natural family planning (also called periodic abstinence, fertility awareness, or rhythm)
- Implants (Norplant)
- Depo-Provera

Other birth control options that are less common (and in some cases less reliable) include:

- Morning-after contraceptives
- Withdrawal
- Douching
- Breastfeeding

(See "Abortion" on page 127 for another option.)

U.S. BIRTH CONTROL HISTORY

Birth control's widespread acceptance, nearly universal availability, and range of choices have only been available in the United States since the 1960s. Before that, with the exception of the practice of withdrawal, contraceptives were only for a privileged few.

Earlier in this century, birth-control advocates were sentenced to jail terms for violation of obscenity laws. In the 1920s, Margaret Sanger had to smuggle diaphragms into this country from Germany via Canada, because birth-control devices were illegal here. Prior to the late 1950s, reflecting the culture at large, it was a rare doctor who recommended birth control to women.

Today, birth control is considered respectable and sensible and is used by married and unmarried alike. (In most of the world, however, a wife still needs her husband's approval to obtain contraceptives, and usually single women have no access at all.) U.S. women are having sex earlier and marrying later, making birth control a vital issue for a large part of the population. Average first-time brides are 24 years old (the oldest age this century), and at least three out of four had sex as teenagers.

Nearly all forms of birth control have their roots in the past. Although rare, women's sterilizations were reported in ancient Greek times as were plant-based oral contraceptives, and vasectomies were performed in the 1890s. IUDs, barriers, and abortions date back thousands of years. Today's versions are easier, safer, and more reliable, though now as in the past, no form of birth control is 100 percent effective, trouble-free, and safe, except for total abstinence.

Women's attitudes about contraception are based on feelings about sex and the body, physical health, age, plans for future pregnancies, life-style, income, education, career, race, and location. Among women answering government surveys, all of these considerations are more influential today than are religious beliefs. Despite their church's official opposition to any birth control other than natural family planning, for instance, only 3 percent of church-going Catholics use that method. (There are some patterns that emerge along religious lines, however. Protestants are more likely to choose sterilization, Catholics select the Pill, and Jews prefer the diaphragm.)

Young, single women and women who live in the South prefer the Pill. Married and formerly married women and those in their 30s most often opt for sterilization. Women who have gone to college and women who live in the Northeast are more likely to use barrier methods. Today, most women change their birth-control methods several times over the course of their 35 or so reproductive years, perhaps using the Pill in their 20s and moving to barrier methods or sterilization later on. If a 20-year-old woman married and remained so for 25 years, her uncontrolled fertility would result in about 12 children, or 10 more than most women say they want.

Most people feel strongly about sex whether they consider intercourse sacred or casual. Similarly, most women have strong feelings about birth-control methods. Some oppose those that invade the body (IUD or surgery) and prefer those that don't (barriers). Others embrace the "chemical" (the Pill) and avoid the "natural" (periodic abstinence). Which method is best for you is entirely up to you.

Along with increased use of birth control, sexual abstinence has come back in vogue for some. AIDS has made that difference for millions of women, while a change in life-style has for others.

When things go wrong (there's a contraceptive failure or side effects, or both), we take the consequences all by ourselves. We can file suit against the manufacturer of an IUD, for instance, as 300,000 women did, but that doesn't repair the damage to our bodies. We can use barrier contraceptives because they don't have long-term side effects, but thereby run a greater risk for an unplanned pregnancy and its consequences. Or if we use no birth control, with the exception of the 8 percent of U.S. women who are infertile, we can count on nine out of 10 of us getting pregnant.

It may be easy to feel impatient with our imperfect system of birth control, but birth control has always been imperfect. As with all health issues, we need to take responsibility for what we are doing, or not doing. Ready or not, we are in charge of our own sex lives and birth-control choices.

In the 1920s I went to New York from the Midwest to visit my sister. She took me to a clinic where I got my diaphragm — surely one of the happiest moments in my life. I was tired of being pregnant and didn't care what people thought. Of course, I never told anyone except my husband. People gossiped plenty where I lived and they didn't need any more fuel for the flames.

When I first had sex, I didn't use birth control because "Nice girls shouldn't have to." To do so would be to face that I was going against strong parental directions. Once I faced my initial guilt over having sex, I felt a strong responsibility to myself not to have an unplanned pregnancy. Since I conquered my guilt I have never had sex without birth control.

My mom never used birth control. She had 10 kids and several miscarriages. She spent her whole life until her late 60s taking care of people. First it was the kids, then it was her parents, and finally my dad. After I married, she kept asking me when I was going to have kids. I told her that I was on the Pill and if I ever had kids, it wasn't going to be for a long time because I was building my career. She was upset with me.

Most of my friends don't take men to bed the way they used to. We're all afraid of diseases — chlamydia, herpes, but mostly AIDS. I don't want any part of that. Celibacy is just fine for me now.

*A*t age 20, I gave up my virginity. At 22, I took it back. My purpose was not so much to give up sex as it was to regain my sense of self, which had been bent out of shape by the contradictory pressures I felt.

HOW TO DECIDE

Have you ever had an unexpected pregnancy? If so, you have lots of company. More than half of U.S. pregnancies each year are unplanned. (Over a reproductive lifetime, about two thirds of us will have an unintended pregnancy.) And, no, it can't all be blamed on carelessness or that alleged hidden desire to be pregnant. Contraceptives sometimes fail regardless of how faithfully and carefully they are used. Contraception is not perfect, and manufacturers of birth-control products do not claim otherwise. For some conscientious users, contraceptive failure happens only once. Some "superfertile" women become pregnant several times even while using the most effective forms of birth control.

Ignorance is a factor in contraceptive failure particularly in carrying out details of some contraceptive methods — inserting a diaphragm correctly each time, checking the string on an IUD, or taking birth-control pills each day at about the same time. Some women don't use birth control because they believe it's their "safe" time, that approximately 14-day period between ovulation and menstruation.

Akin to "swept away" with love or lust is the expression "It won't happen to me." Yes, you *can* conceive that one time you didn't use a contraceptive. Teens do 15 to 20 percent of the time. And then there's the everyday risk-taking among people of all ages. If you don't think you'll get pregnant, you're more likely to take a pregnancy risk. You'll take a chance "this time." And when that works, you're led to believe it will work other times, too. But don't count on it.

To avoid an unplanned pregnancy, choose a contraceptive that works for you. First, you have to like it. It's better to periodically change birth-control methods than to let dissatisfaction lead to total nonuse.

Be aware that contraceptive needs vary in your life, not only based on your current level of fertility, but also on your circumstances and personal preferences. If red-hot passion, which can and does come at any age, overwhelms any possibility of a time-out for barrier contraceptives like condoms and foam, don't pretend to rely on them. Know yourself, and plan in advance to use something else. Stop using a method that doesn't work for you anymore, especially if you know you used it correctly.

Know that motivation matters. Women who are postponing pregnancy are more likely to have an unplanned pregnancy than those who are not having any more children period. Don't wait until you're in Cupid's clutches to decide which group you're in.

If you're told that you have a condition that keeps you from conceiving, and therefore do not need to bother with birth control, you may want to get a second opinion.

---

*M*y husband was sure I had been careless about using my contraceptive when I got pregnant. But I know I used it correctly each time. Sometimes things just don't work. I must admit before this happened to me I thought women who "accidentally" got pregnant were just careless and didn't want to admit it.

I had my first son because my diaphragm was clear across the room in a drawer and I knew it was my safe time.

I went out with a man last night. Like a dummy, I went totally unprepared for sex. I wanted to take my diaphragm, but I was afraid that he might think I sleep around. I couldn't tell him to use a rubber, it sounded like I'm a little too hip about sex.

*I*t was time for a change, but not chance. When I find myself wanting to be a little careless, I know it's time to change contraceptives. I learned that about myself in my 20s.

I used a diaphragm for 15 years with two husbands and never got pregnant. Then I married husband No. 3 and conceived using my diaphragm. My doctor told me that it would never happen again. That wasn't true—I was pregnant 18 months later.

*W*hen I got pregnant, I was furious. I went to my doctor and said, "I thought you told me I couldn't get pregnant because my uterus is tipped." He claimed that he said it would be difficult for me to get pregnant. Either I need to listen better, or he needs to talk more clearly. Meanwhile, I'm pregnant and 44 years old.

The chart below will give you an overview of the most popular birth control methods used in the United States today and their failure rates, followed by a brief summary of the eight leading birth control methods worldwide.

U.S. CONTRACEPTIVE METHODS

Methods	(Percent)	Failure Rates with Average Use	(Percent)
1. Sterilization	39.2	1. Norplant	0.05
Women's	27.5	2. Sterilization	0.7
Men's	11.7	Men's	0.2
2. Pill	30.7	Women's	0.5
3. Condom (male)	14.6	3. Depo-Provera	0.4
4. Diaphragm	5.7	4. IUD	4.0
5. Natural family		5. Pill	6.0
planning	2.3	6. Condom (male)	16.0
6. Withdrawal	2.2	7. Diaphragm	18.0
7. IUD	2.0	8. Cervical Cap	18.0
8. Spermicides	1.8	9. Natural family planning	19.0
9. Sponge	1.1	10. Withdrawal	24.0
10. Other methods	0.4	11. Sponge	24.0
		12. Spermicides	30.0
		13. No method (chance/fate)	85.0

These charts are based on 1992 information from The Alan Guttmacher Institute. The newer contraceptives — cervical cap, Norplant, and Depo-Provera — are not included in the list on the left, because the percentage of U.S. use for these methods is not yet available. The female condom is so new, it doesn't appear on either list.

BIRTH CONTROL IN OTHER COUNTRIES

To see how the United States compares to the rest of the world, here are the eight top contraceptive methods in other countries. Worldwide, the most popular method is sterilization, as it is here. The IUD is No. 2 (China alone claims 45 million users), followed closely by the Pill as No. 3. Abortion, recently the most common form of birth control worldwide, is now No. 4. Condoms are No. 5. The Japanese use them the most, surpassing any other method in that country. (The Pill and the IUD are not available in Japan.) Withdrawal is No. 6 and vaginal contraceptives (such as spermicides, diaphragms, cervical caps, and sponges) are No. 7. Rhythm or natural family planning, method No. 8, is used exclusively by 3 percent of the world's population.

A NOTE TO MOTHERS OF TEENS

Most parents like to believe that their daughters and sons will wait until they are on their own, far from home, responsible for their actions, and so on, before they become sexually active. In today's real world, over half of teens have had sex before leaving high school. To further complicate matters, half of unmarried sons and daughters live at home until age 24 if they're not living in a college dormitory. (In 1992, on average, women college students had more than five sexual partners and male students had eleven sexual partners before they finished an undergraduate degree.)

At least one third of all teens did not use birth control the first time they had sex. The good news is that this statistic is a substantial improvement over the recent past. One million U.S. teenage girls, or 10 percent, get pregnant every year, and this is the highest teen pregnancy rate in the industrialized world. (In 1990, after an 18-year decline, there was a sharp increase in U.S. teen births.) Sex and teens are not necessarily a bad mix, but they are a volatile and unpredictable combination. When abstinence is not the rule, then perhaps birth control ought to be.

What is your part in all this? You and your children's father have several options about what role you will take in your children's sex life. No matter what your position is — for or against teen sex — your children will benefit from your spoken concern about their well-being. Much to the amazement of many parents, teens care intensely about their parents' opinions, even though they may not always agree with them. Studies show that parents are still the best teachers of values.

When surveyed, teens say they wish they could talk to their parents about sex, although that seldom happens. Surveys show that only one third of U.S. teenagers had actually discussed birth control with their parents. Sex Ed 101 doesn't happen much at home. Most of a teen's information, a mixture of fact and fiction, comes from friends. Examples: You can't get pregnant if you do it standing up, or nobody gets pregnant the first time. (Actually 20 percent of teens conceive the first month and some of them the first time. In fact, teen fertility is so powerful 11 percent of Pill-using teens conceive — a rate nearly twice that of adult women who use the Pill.) And demonstrating the need for more AIDS education, some students believe the Pill protects them from this disease, and they can tell if people have AIDS just by looking at them.

If the average age for first intercourse is 17, do you want your children to learn about sex and contraception only from other 17-year-olds? And though there's some research that suggests *comprehensive* sex education classes reduce teen pregnancy and delay sexual activity, those classes are not available to at least three fourths of teens. Many teens are dumbfounded when an unexpected pregnancy happens to them. Many parents are equally dumbfounded to discover that their teens are sexually active or a daughter or son's girlfriend is pregnant.

If you're like most other women, when you were a teenager, your mom didn't discuss sex and birth-control options with you. Unless, of course, you're going to count the times she said, "Don't!" when the subject came up. Perhaps when you were that age, there were not nearly as many kids having sex as there are today. Your teen sexual experiences and opportunities were most likely quite different from those of your sons and daughters. Keep in mind, too, that today the risk of AIDS and other sexually transmitted diseases means teens need more factual information than ever.

What is the No. 1 reason teens give for having sex? Raging hormones, right? Wrong. Only 4 percent gave pleasure as the reason in one large survey, and only 10 percent said they were in love. Peer pressure (everyone else is doing it) and curiosity were the main reasons. Choosing to be sexually active is no small step in a person's life, no matter what the age or reasons. Next to your kids themselves, who could care more than you, the parent?

One of your options as a parent is to say nothing to your children about sex, and hope for the best. But the younger they are, the more dangerous that is. Younger teens not only conceive easier, they often don't know they're pregnant for months because their world is not on that page of life.

You might think that because they regularly attend church or synagogue your children will be opposed to premarital sex. A 1989 Christian Broadcasting Network survey of church-attending college students, however, showed that 70 percent did not believe sex before marriage was wrong.

As a parent, you have three choices. You could play the odds and do nothing. If three fourths of teens are having sex, that means one fourth is not. Maybe yours is one of the one fourth; therefore, your daughter or your son's girlfriend is not going to get pregnant (or your children are not going to contract a sexually transmitted disease). But know that the odds are weighted against you.

A second option is to discuss your concerns about your child's sex life with someone else: your mate, your friends, or your minister, priest, or rabbi. But that alone is not going to solve the problem, because your kids can't read your mind any better than you can read theirs.

Then there's the third choice. Talk with your teens. That means, if you're doing it effectively, you're listening a lot. And your conversations about life and love, sex and birth control, maybe even dope and booze, aren't all going to happen in two or three let's-go-out-for-a-hamburger sessions.

Of course, your kids may not agree with you or follow your wishes. Or maybe you're a single mom who dates and you're not sure what you should be doing sexually, much less what your kids ought to be doing. But studies repeatedly show your teens are looking to you for guidance, no matter how aloof they may seem at the time. This is true regardless of how many doubts you may have about their honesty on the subject of sex and personal experience.

If you don't want your daughters or sons to be sexually active while still teenagers or still in high school or still living at home, speak with them. Even if it's okay with you that your teens are sexually active while still living with you at home, there's still plenty to talk about, including birth control. If you haven't offered an opinion, they may believe you don't have one. You may not feel comfortable initiating these conversations, but this may get easier with practice.

You don't have to be an expert on all of this. Who is? You probably don't have all the answers in your own life, much less all the answers for your children. But having all the answers is not the point. The real value of these conversations is that your teens have someone to talk with who has more facts and more experience and who also cares deeply.

In one large survey, college students gave lots of wrong answers to questions about their bodies, fertility, birth control, and sexually transmitted diseases. Who else is going to tell them if you don't? Giving them a book to read, or saying, "Let me know if you have any questions about things" is not going to be as helpful as you hope it might be.

They may not know, for instance, that celibacy is a valid, acceptable option, especially in these days of sexually transmitted diseases and AIDS. They may not know the right words, like "If you loved me, you'd wait," to help them avoid sex. (A 1992 study showed that "resistance" skills for young men was the most effective deterrent to too-early, risky sex.) If all your children's friends can't wait to get rid of their virginity, don't expect your kids to get peer pressure at school promoting sexual abstinence. You may want to talk with them about choosing contraceptives and sexual partners, about what their options are if they get pregnant, and about how not to be taken advantage of — a conversation for both sons and daughters.

All of us have found our way through the world of love and sexuality, making decisions along the way, and your children will, too. The kids are all right, but these days they need all the help they can get. And who better than you, Mom?

We talk a lot about sex and birth control. It's very spontaneous, sometimes prompted by TV or the newspaper. I'm assuming both children [ages 18 and 22] are virgins, of course.

I used to think that my teenagers would figure out sex by themselves, like I did. But now that they have friends with chlamydia and gonorrhea and know about others who are getting tested for AIDS, we talk about sex.

I don't care how many teenage girls get pregnant, I'm not going to talk to my daughters and sons about sex. If their mother does, fine. But not me. Of course, I hope that our family doesn't have unexpected pregnancies and VD. Frankly, I don't think my kids would run that risk. I didn't when I was their age. Oh sure, sure, you're getting ready to tell me that times have changed. Well, I'm saying I haven't.

It [sex] is such an uncomfortable subject that the conversation lingers with them [my parents] a long time, so they think they talk about it more than they really do.

When I was growing up, the topic of sex was "hush-hush." It was never talked about in my family. I regret that it was not. I think I would be a different human being today if we could have talked about it. I didn't know as a child that sex was for making babies; I learned from my peers that it was something dirty to do.

When I was 17 my boyfriend talked me into going all the way. I knew from what my mom said that I better get some birth control. So I did. And I got pregnant right away even though I used my diaphragm. At school they told us to use birth control, but they never told us that it doesn't work sometimes. I think they should emphasize that more at the clinics, too. I had an abortion several months later.

My sex manual was The National Geographic. I knew a lot about anatomy as displayed in New Guinea, but closer to home I was on shaky ground.

One of my daughter's eighth-grade classmates got a vibrator for Christmas and told all the girls about it. These girls are only 13!

*M*y 16-year-old son barely talks to me. Most of his communication these days sounds like grunts, not words. And the Surgeon General thinks I should sit down and have an enlightening conversation with my son about condoms and AIDS. I think I'll send my son to Washington.

*O*ne girl told me that when her mom has a date Friday night and he's in the kitchen eating breakfast Saturday morning, how can she preach about premarital sex?

*T*alking to my 17-year-old daughter about sex was the worst conversation I've ever had. She didn't help me a bit and acted like she was bored to tears. When I told her what I thought she should do and not do, she asked me, "Are you done yet, Mom?"

I am a 17-year-old virgin by choice. . . . I was very lucky because my parents talked to me about sex very openly. Sex education and birth-control information do not encourage promiscuity. At least with the facts you know what you're getting into.

STERILIZATION

WOMEN'S STERILIZATION (TUBAL LIGATION)

What It Is

Sterilization is an operation in which the fallopian tubes are cut, tied, or burned, preventing eggs from entering the uterus.

Effectiveness

Tubal ligation is 99.5 percent effective. Surgeons claim that the less than 1 percent of operations that are failures are usually due to surgical error, pregnancy prior to surgery, or regrowth of the fallopian tubes.

Types Available

In U.S. women, sterilization is performed almost entirely by one of the following two methods:

• *Laparoscopy*, the most popular sterilization method, is performed through an incision in the abdomen. A laparoscope is a thin, lighted instrument that brings the fallopian tubes into view through a small incision just below your navel. A needle will be inserted under your belly button to fill the abdomen with gas to allow the organs to move slightly for better viewing. The surgeon then inserts a small instrument either through the original incision or through a second tiny opening. Fallopian tubes are then either banded, cauterized or clipped. The gas in the abdomen is then released and the incisions are sewn shut. (Small bits of tissue can also be collected for a biopsy for other reasons when this procedure is performed.)

Laparoscopy may be performed in an operating room or as outpatient surgery, often with only local anesthesia. It is the procedure of choice when you have not given birth for at least two months, and your internal organs

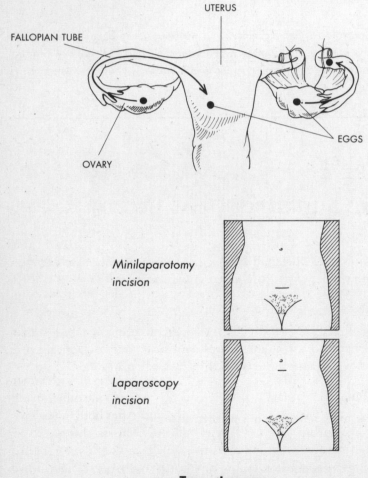

TUBAL LIGATION

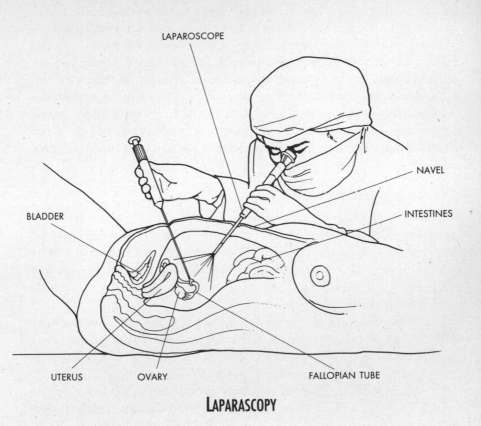

LAPAROSCOPE

NAVEL

INTESTINES

BLADDER

UTERUS   OVARY   FALLOPIAN TUBE

LAPARASCOPY

are back to their prepregnancy size and location. When local anesthesia is used, your operation time is shorter, recovery is quicker, you'll feel less abdominal pain later, and — most likely — it will cost less than the alternative.

• *Minilaparotomy* is performed by making a two-inch incision in the abdomen, moving each tube gently to the incision, reaching in with either a hook or a finger, lifting out a loop of tube (first one, then the other), tying each tube, and removing a segment out of each tube. After both tubes have been "tied," the incision is closed with stitches. This is the preferred method for postpartum sterilization, that is, within days or the first month after giving birth, because the uterus and fallopian tubes are high in the pelvic cavity.

Until the late 1960s, tubal ligation required a large abdominal incision and a long hospital stay and recovery. Prior to this time, a woman couldn't be sterilized unless two other doctors, in addition to her own, gave their approval. And that's not all. In many states, a husband's permission was required, too, and if the woman was under 25, she needed to have had five babies already. If she was older, then fewer babies were necessary. For many years a hysterectomy for "female troubles" was a way around sterilization rules, but today's surgical procedures are far safer than a hysterectomy, which costs four or five times more and has a complication and death rate at least 10 times greater. (See "Hysterectomy and Oophorectomy" on page 354.)

How to Decide

Women of all ages are sterilized, including single women in their 20s. However, the woman most likely to use sterilization is married and past age 30, has three or more children, and perhaps has had a cesarean birth. (Convenience is surely a factor here: a woman having a cesarean, and almost 25 percent of U.S. birthing women do, already has an abdominal incision and is anesthetized.)

Sterilization is not recommended for women who have had extensive internal scarring from previous abdominal operations. Tubal ligation can be performed on those who are obese (generally 20 to 30 percent more than desired weight), but it is technically more difficult.

Advantages to sterilization are that it's permanent, it's extremely effective, it requires a one-time-only expense, it's immediately effective (unlike a vasectomy — see page 179), and it gives freedom from having to do anything about birth control again, which is probably why some women report they have better sex afterwards.

Disadvantages of sterilization are the abdominal pain for a few days, along with dizziness, nausea, bloating, and fatigue, although in a few days, you'll likely be back to your normal routine. Ectopic (tubal) pregnancy is a rare complication as are infections, damage to bowels, perforation of the uterus, or excessive bleeding. (See "Ectopic Pregnancy" on page 488.) Death and serious complications occur even more rarely, but when they do, anesthesia is the leading cause.

It is unknown how often the controversial "post-tubal-ligation syndrome," which includes pelvic pain, spotting, and cramps, occurs, though some research shows it may take up to five years for menstrual symptoms to occur. However, as many as half of women report changes in their menstrual cycle, including an increase in bleeding, irregular cycles, and cramps. Part of the explanation for immediate menstrual changes may be that many women had used the Pill previously, which usually reduces menstrual symptoms, so that reports of increased bleeding and pain may be due to going off the Pill.

Some women who became sterilized in their 20s have hysterectomies later and those women who've been sterilized with cautery techniques (burning the tubes closed, instead of tying them off) have higher hysterectomy rates as well. (Cautery sterilization can interfere with the blood supply to the ovaries, which may affect their function. Hormonal output could decrease, causing irregular ovulation. The end result might be an abnormal pattern of uterine bleeding that can lead to a hysterectomy.)

Endometriosis (an often painful condition in which tissue normally found in the uterus is found in other nearby parts of the body, causing irregular and painful menstruation or pain during sex) occasionally occurs following tubal ligations. However, sterilization most often occurs in the age group of women who are most likely to be diagnosed with endometriosis, so this factor may not be a cause. (See "Endometriosis" on page 329.)

Another disadvantage of tubal ligation is that unlike barrier methods, it offers no protection against sexually transmitted diseases.

Sterilization Reversal

About 10 percent of U.S. women report regret after sterilization, but the woman most likely to do so was in her early 20s at the time of the operation or now has a new partner, or perhaps she lost a child or was sterilized after a cesarean or an abortion. About half of these women seek surgical reversals. The best candidates for a reversal are healthy women in their 20s or 30s who ovulate regularly and who have a fertile partner.

To reverse sterilization, a major operation that takes one to four hours is required in which the remaining parts of the fallopian tubes are sewn together after all damaged parts have been removed. Sometimes diagnostic laparoscopy is used first to evaluate how much of the tube is left.

Reversal success (pregnancy resulting in live birth) depends mostly on the sterilization technique used, rather than how long it's been since the procedure was performed. The most successful reversals are performed by very experienced surgeons and have followed sterilization procedures where only short lengths of the fallopian tubes were destroyed (pregnancy is far less likely when the joined tube is less than four centimeters long) and were closed with clips or rings. For instance, reversals of laparoscopic sterilization using clips in some studies shows an 84 percent pregnancy rate. Reversals of sterilization procedures that destroy more of the tubes or that burn the tubes are far less successful and can be as little as 30 percent successful.

The most serious complication is an increased risk of ectopic pregnancy (2 to 5 percent) within a year or more after the reversal surgery. This is apparently due to the two ends of the joined fallopian tube not being the same size.

Y*ou have everything figured out in your 20s . . . you never, ever figure you'll be divorced. In your 30s you find out how your circumstances in life can change. Looking back, which is always easier in these cases, I wouldn't make such a permanent decision.*

How to Prepare

If you currently take the Pill, it's suggested that you quit at least one month before this surgery, or any surgery, and use another form of birth control. Women who have the surgery by doctors who perform less than 100 sterilization operations annually have a higher complication rate. If you definitely don't want to be unconscious due to general anesthesia, search to find one of the many surgeons who has experience with using local anesthesia on an outpatient basis for this operation. (See "The Hospital Stay" on page 92 and "Surgery" on page 95 for more information about both preparation for surgery and recovery.)

MEN'S STERILIZATION (VASECTOMY)

What It Is

A vasectomy is the surgical cutting and tying off of a small portion of the vas deferens, the two tubes that transport sperm into the penis, leaving a man sterile. A newer method, called the no-scalpel vasectomy, uses a puncture tool instead of a surgical cut.

It's performed by injecting a local anesthetic into the skin of the scrotum so that a small cut can be made in order to reach the vas deferens. When the physician, usually a urologist, reaches the tube, she cuts it and ties the ends. Then she repeats the same procedure on the vas deferens on the other side of the scrotum. A man's body still produces sperm, but after this operation, sperm is no longer ejaculated. Instead, it is absorbed into his body. A man will still have orgasms and ejaculate, however. Sperm accounts for only 1 to 3 percent of semen.

The most common complications of vasectomy—and they appear only less than 2 percent of the time—are swelling, pain, and skin discoloration. The no-scalpel method has even fewer incidences of complications. After a vasectomy, it's important to rest for several hours and strenuous exercise should be avoided for a day or two.

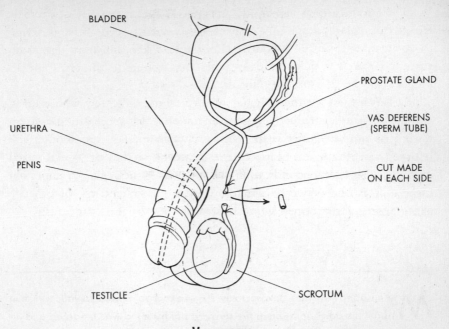

VASECTOMY

Effectiveness

Male sterilization is 99.8 percent effective, using either the traditional surgical procedure or the no-scalpel method. However, it does not provide immediate sterilization. Sperm usually remain through 20 ejaculations. It's also possible for the vas deferens to reconnect, or a man may have a third or fourth vas deferens. That's why monthly semen checks are important until the sperm count is zero at least twice. Most physicians and clinics recommend that men bring in semen samples at three and four months. It's rare for sperm to survive longer than three months, but occasionally sperm has survived five months. To be safe, other birth-control methods should be used for at least five months to avoid pregnancy.

How to Decide

Although vasectomies are cheaper, easier, and safer than women's sterilization, twice as many U.S. women are sterilized as are men, and nearly all are in white men. In general, men who know what to expect, who talk with other men who've had vasectomies, and who get their questions answered in advance of the operation experience no trauma from having a vasectomy. Approximately one in five U.S. men past the age of 35 has had a vasectomy.

The advantages of vasectomy are that it is permanent, it's extremely effective, it requires a one-time-only expense, it gives freedom from having to do anything about birth control after the first 20 ejaculations, leaves no scar, and there's a quick recovery after the 20-minute surgery (only 10 minutes for the nonsurgical puncture).

Disadvantages are the difficulty of reversal for those few who want it, and the rare surgical failure when the operation is not successful. Based on a study of monkeys a few years ago, there was some concern about a link between vasectomy and heart disease. However, studies of vasectomized men since then show no indication of such a link. A newer as yet unproven association is one between vasectomy and a subsequent risk of prostate cancer, particularly in men who had vasectomies 20 years previously.

---

*M*y husband just had a vasectomy six weeks ago. I tried to talk with him about his decision to have the surgery, but his mind was made up and he wouldn't consider my feelings about it. I felt that at 25 it was too soon to choose a permanent method of birth control. Even though I don't want any more children at this point, I realize I may change my mind in five or 10 years. . . . I believe the decision in a matter like this should be made between both partners, not just by one.

*O*nce my husband understood that his sex life wouldn't change for the worse — only for the better — because I wouldn't be afraid of getting pregnant anymore, he decided to get a vasectomy five years ago. He's had no complaints, and neither have I.

Sterilization Reversal

Reversals of men's sterilization are generally more successful than the reversals of women's sterilization when measured in pregnancies. Under the best of circumstances, men's reversals have a 50 percent success rate. However, the outcome depends on many factors.

Among them are how long it's been since the vasectomy was performed (the longer it's been, the more unlikely a reversal will be successful) and the type of procedure used (as with women's sterilization operations, some are more difficult to reverse). In addition, some men develop anti-sperm antibodies that attack sperm, thus making it difficult to impregnate even though the reversal operation itself is a success.

The reversal operation costs many thousands of dollars and most insurance plans will not cover the expense. With men's reversals, it's normally many months, sometimes years, before the sperm count is adequate to create a pregnancy. Like women, men who want to reverse sterilization were probably in their 20s when they had the vasectomy and have since changed partners.

Since it was 10 years since my vasectomy, the specialist warned me that a reversal might not be successful. Even if it was, it could take years. I wanted to try anyhow. About a year later Tina got pregnant, and my third son was born nine months later.

THE PILL

WHAT IT IS

The Pill is a drug made from synthetic hormones that prevents pregnancy by suppressing ovulation and inhibiting implantation of a fertilized egg.

The Pill mimics pregnancy, which is why some side effects it causes sound a lot like symptoms of pregnancy, including weight gain, breast tenderness, fatigue, and nausea. The estrogen in the Pill inhibits ovulation by stopping the development of the egg in the ovary and also prevents implantation of the fertilized egg (if one gets by). Progestin or progestogen are common names for the synthetic version of progesterone. The progestin in the Pill creates a thick cervical mucus, which prevents the sperm from reaching the egg, and also inhibits implantation.

EFFECTIVENESS

The Pill is 94 percent effective (although it's only 89 percent effective for teens). Some medications and conditions can contribute to Pill failure (see failure rates of contraceptives in chart on page 168).

TYPES AVAILABLE

All Pills are based on a 28-day cycle. Pills come in forms that can be taken one per day for each of those 28 days, or one per day for three weeks and no pills for one week, or one per day for 28 days, in three different colors for different hormone levels during the month.

When the Pill was first released in 1960, there were only a handful of brands and limited combinations of hormones. Today's Pills contain one fourth to one twenty-fifth of the original amount of progestin and one fifth to one half of the original amount of estrogen. They are packaged in more than 50 brands and combinations of shape, size, color, and number of Pills per pack.

HOW TO DECIDE

Certain women are at risk for complications associated with using the Pill. If you are trying to decide whether the Pill is right for you, first read the following section on "Who Shouldn't Take the Pill." If after reading this material you're still in the running, review the next section on "Advantages and Disadvantages" before making up your mind.

WHO SHOULDN'T TAKE THE PILL

Women who should not take the Pill are those with any of the following conditions: pregnancy; clots in veins; smoking, especially age 35 or older; history of stroke or heart disease; and history of lupus, since the Pill can trigger flare-ups (see "Lupus" on page 391). Other women who shouldn't take the Pill are those with liver disease of any kind, including hepatitis and jaundice, or those with a history of breast cancer or cancers of the reproductive organs. Although some breastfeeding women use the Pill, it is not recommended. Pill hormones get to the baby via mother's milk, and can cause a folic acid (one of the B vitamins) deficiency in both mother and infant. More importantly, these hormones reduce the amount of B_6 in the milk. The Pill also reduces the amount of milk nursing mothers produce, which may be the reason that nursing mothers on the Pill breast-feed for fewer months. (See "Breastfeeding As Contraceptive" on page 223.)

Certain other women should use the Pill with extreme caution and perhaps as a last resort only. They should also find a physician or clinic who will follow them closely. They are women with the following conditions: severe headaches, especially migraine (see "Migraine Headache" on page

419); high blood pressure; diabetes or strong family history of it; family history of death of parent or sibling due to stroke or heart attack about or before age 50; and chlamydia, a sexually transmitted disease that can cause infertility. (The Pill changes the vaginal flora to make it more hospitable to this sexually transmitted disease, especially in younger women. See "Chlamydia" on page 494.)

Other conditions that make Pill use questionable are: gallbladder disease, mononucleosis, sickle cell anemia, and the presence of uterine fibroids (lumps of muscle tissue located in the outer wall of the uterus — see "Uterine Fibroids" on page 522). Anyone planning elective surgery within four to 12 weeks or major surgery requiring immobilization (see "Surgery" on page 95) should avoid using the Pill as should anyone having a long-leg cast or major injury to the lower leg because of possible circulation problems. Other women who should use the Pill with extreme caution are those with a history of epilepsy, depression (see "Depression" on page 49), varicose veins (see "Varicose Veins" on page 537), or anyone having very irregular periods or no periods (see "Amenorrhea" on page 411).

For years women past 40 were advised not to take the Pill because of their higher risk of heart attacks. In 1990, the Food and Drug Administration changed its Pill use guidelines to include nonsmoking, healthy women in this age group because of their perceived lower risk due to lower-dose Pills. However, there's no new research to show whether that judgment is correct.

If you already take the Pill, stop taking it and call your physician or clinic immediately if you have any of these problems: severe leg pain or swelling in the legs, bad headache, dizziness or fainting, blurred vision or loss of sight, chest pain or shortness of breath, coughing of blood, or abdominal pain — all of which could be symptoms of severe drug toxicity.

ADVANTAGES AND DISADVANTAGES

The typical U.S. Pill user is under the age of 25 (often a teenager), single, childless, and plans to have children in the future. Today many women take the Pill for an average of five years, which is longer than they once did.

The Pill affects every part of your body, from your hairline to your toes. Some women love the Pill and never have a complaint. For these women, the benefits easily outweigh the risks. Others are plagued by problems. The risk of side effects may be less with the low-dose Pill, which most women now take, but the likelihood and severity of side effects probably increase the longer the Pill is taken. The Pill may alter the absorption of certain vitamins and minerals (see the "Birth-Control Pill Diet" on page 32) including C, the B vitamins, zinc, and magnesium. These changes may play a part in causing side effects.

Advantages of the Pill are: high levels of effectiveness, freedom from having to do anything about birth control near the time of sex, lighter menstrual periods with less cramping and perhaps fewer symptoms of premenstrual syndrome (see "Premenstrual Syndrome" on page 408) and breast lumps (see "Breast Lumps" on page 227). There is also less risk of ovarian and endometrial cancers (at least with higher-dose Pills), and Pill use reduces the incidence of endometriosis for some women (see "Endometriosis" on page 329). In addition, there's some evidence that women who used the Pill for at least six years have denser bones past menopause.

Disadvantages of the Pill are the need to have the discipline to take a Pill at the same time of day each day, and its inability to prevent sexually transmitted diseases, much to the surprise of many teens. Other disadvantages are the chance of developing any one or more of the following side effects, most of which are reversible over time (spider veins may be an exception) or with effort (weight gain):

• Depression
• Headaches
• Weight gain
• Nausea (sometimes associated with increased motion sickness as well)
• Fatigue
• Diminished sex drive (even with low-dose Pills)
• Breakthrough bleeding (bleeding between periods)
• Menstrual abnormalities
• Depression of maximum performance for women athletes
• Uterine fibroids. Research is controversial and not conclusive, but the theory that the Pill causes uterine fibroids to form and grow is based on the belief that fibroids increase in size during pregnancy because of the extra estrogen produced during pregnancy, and perhaps in a pregnancy-mimicking way, the extra estrogen in the Pill user's body causes the same result
• Tender breasts
• Gum inflammation
• Chloasma, the facial "mask" associated with pregnancy
• Carpal tunnel syndrome, a painful condition of the wrist associated with Pill use, especially the high-dose version with its fluid-retention tendency (See "Carpal Tunnel Syndrome" on page 244.)

- Candidiasis, a yeast infection (See "Yeast Infections" on page 533.)
- Corneal swelling, which may make wearing contact lenses difficult
- Increased body hair (with mini-Pill or high-progestin Pill)
- Increase in blood pressure
- Higher chance of blood clots (Some researchers believe you can reduce your chance of developing blood clots, which occur in 20 out of every 10,000 Pill users, by exercising regularly. This Pill-induced risk for circulatory system problems stops when you quit taking it.)
- Higher cholesterol levels
- Visible vein changes, including darker, bluish veins and broken capillaries, or "spider" veins in the legs
- Gallbladder disease

It is important to know that it is not unusual to miss a period occasionally while taking the Pill correctly. It does not mean you are pregnant. However, if you've skipped some Pills during a cycle, you may be pregnant. If you get pregnant while taking the Pill, you may have a slightly increased risk for birth defects, as well as a twofold higher chance of twins.

While taking a low-dose Pill, I didn't menstruate one month and was afraid I was pregnant. Despite two negative home pregnancy tests and one negative birth-control clinic test, I wasn't convinced until my period came the next month. I wished they would have told me it wasn't unusual to skip a period once in a while.

The Pill made me depressed, so depressed I was suicidal. The psychiatrist I went to was the one who told me it was the Pill making me feel that way. I noticed a difference in how I felt within two weeks after stopping the Pill. I started on it when I was 16 and had taken it for six years without any problem until then. That was five years ago, and I've used the diaphragm ever since. But I tell you — I miss the Pill. It was so easy, so convenient. I felt free.

I loved the Pill, except it killed my sex drive. That didn't do me much good.

After winning our regional women's 10k road championships, I decided to quit taking the Pill. Well, my performance certainly did improve! . . . A couple months later, I started the Pill again and found it made me gain weight and caused me to run slower again. I stopped for the last time.

I took the low-dose Pill for two years and didn't realize how many side effects I had until I stopping taking it. When I did, I lost weight, my headaches and severe motion sickness were gone, as was my supersensitive stomach. I wasn't so tired, tense, and weepy anymore either. However, four years later, I still have bluish veins on my chest and legs (they started as soon as I went on the Pill) and probably will have them the rest of my life.

THE PILL AND CANCER

Concern about breast cancer and the Pill will continue for some time, especially as 80 percent of all U.S. women born between 1945 and 1964 have used it. After 30 years of use, the link between the Pill and breast cancer remains controversial and confusing. That's because breast cancer is mostly a postmenopausal disease of women in their 60s and 70s, and the majority of women who took the Pill in the 1960s are now in their 50s. (Cancers often remain undetected for 15 to 30 years after exposure to the disease trigger.)

Many studies, especially earlier ones, showed no link between Pill use and breast cancer. However, now that the original Pill takers are getting older, an equal number of studies have shown that the rate of breast cancer that occurs before age 45 (which is a small percentage of all women who have breast cancer) goes up with women who used the Pill at both a young age and who took it for five years, particularly before giving birth for the first time.

There are several arguments against a link between the Pill and breast cancer. Among them are:

• The factors that influence breast cancer are obviously not clearly understood.

• Yesterday's Pill-using women who appear to have a higher rate of breast cancer also took a higher-dose Pill than most women do today.

• Since it's believed that most side effects are dose related, a connection between Pill use in the 1960s and breast cancer doesn't necessarily hold true today, because the current dose of synthetic hormones in the Pill is less than it was in the 1960s.

• Since Pill-users are more likely to have frequent medical exams, they also may be more likely to have mammograms. These mammograms may indicate cancers that, without mammograms, wouldn't have shown up until the more common ages for breast cancer — past menopause. According to this argument, Pill-using women aren't getting more breast cancer, they are just getting their breast cancer detected earlier. However, a 1990 study showed that although in fact the incidence of breast cancer has increased, only a small portion of the increase was likely the result of increased screening. (See "Breast Cancer" on page 231.)

The relationship between Pill use and skin cancer (malignant melanoma) is unclear, but there is a definite link between cervical cancer (see "Cervical Cancer" on page 234) and the Pill, particularly after five years of Pill use, with the risk doubling with ten years of Pill use. (Women who take the Pill may, because of their more frequent medical exams, have more Pap smears and therefore a subsequent earlier diagnosis of cervical cancer.) There is also a threefold increased risk for noncancerous liver tumors and liver cancer although liver cancer is extremely rare in the United States.

WHY DOCTORS LOVE THE PILL . . . AND WOMEN OFTEN LEAVE IT

Some women who take the Pill quit within a year, according to U.S. government data. Many physicians believe women exaggerate their problems with the Pill, but most women report that they experienced one or more side effects, and many were downright miserable. Why this profound difference of opinion? Given the same set of facts, there are two points of view — consumer and physician.

The Physician View

• *Half of U.S. pregnancies are unplanned, so why not use one of the most effective birth-control methods?* The Pill *is* one of the most effective nonpermanent options. But not the only option.

• *Haven't the drug companies reduced Pill dosage to safer levels?* Safer, yes, but how safe is an individual matter.

• *Don't the Pill's good side effects outweigh its bad ones?* In addition to being an excellent contraceptive, the Pill often reduces menstrual cramps and blood loss, and if taken for five or more years, it reduces the risk of two cancers — ovarian and endometrial — and increases your bone mass.

The Consumer View

• *Sometimes the bad side effects outweigh the good.* According to many researchers, the Pill protects against some diseases while contributing to others, including, rarely, blood clots and perhaps cancer as discussed above. It's true that the woman most likely to have severe side effects with blood clots or high blood pressure smokes and is at least age 35, and physicians routinely warn these women away from taking the Pill. Only 12 percent of Pill-related deaths occurred among nonsmoking women under age 35. But doctors readily admit they cannot predict which women will experience side effects.

Aside from these serious side effects, the Pill much more commonly is also responsible for side effects often labeled "minor" discomforts by most physicians. But most practicing physicians have no personal experience with Pill side effects, because they are men. Maybe it's not major if it's not happening to you.

• *Women choose birth control based on how it affects them personally, not how it affects millions of other women.* Sometimes physicians defend the Pill's side effects by saying that you're more likely to die in a car wreck or from lung cancer than you are from the Pill. But women who quit the Pill are comparing it to other forms of birth control—not to ways to die. A woman's decision is as personal as her extra 10 to 20 pounds, her nausea, and her headaches. Women are so sure of their right to decide, two thirds of the time they quit the Pill without consulting their doctor or birth-control clinic. When a doctor recommends that a woman stop taking the Pill, it's usually for entirely different reasons—smoking or breastfeeding—than those reasons women give for quitting.

HOW TO USE THE PILL WISELY

The Pill may be the perfect contraceptive for you. But it's still a big-time, big-deal medication that you will take on a daily basis for many months or years. You can protect yourself and reduce your short-term and long-term risks and side effects by using the Pill wisely.

• *Understand the Pill risks and how to recognize them.* It's not realistic to expect your physician or clinic to anticipate how your particular body will react, nor to assume that they will describe contraindications and side effects in detail for you if you don't ask. Sometimes they don't tell you all the possible side effects, because they think then you won't take the Pill. (Or according to one physician survey, you'll make up symptoms.) How you will react, however, is very individual.

• *Ask for and read the patient insert description that comes with your brand of Pill.* It's up to you to know what the possible side effects are, and which are most relevant to you. Patient inserts can be confusing and conflicting, according to 1992 research, so be sure to ask questions when you don't understand the insert wording.

• *Take a Pill the same time every day to avoid having hormonal protection lapse, allowing ovulation.* In one large study, not only did a large number of women skip taking Pills every day, only 20 percent who took them every day took them at the same time every day.

• *Be aware of what medications or conditions can make the Pill lose its effectiveness. Then use other forms of contraception while using these drugs or during these conditions.* The following medications can affect Pill effectiveness in some women (that is, increase your chances of becoming pregnant while taking the Pill):

   ◦ Rifampin, an antituberculosis drug.

   ◦ Antibiotics, in particular, ampicillin, neomycin, sulfonamides, tetracycline, sulphonamides, penicillin V, chloramphenicol, nitrofurantoin, griseofulvin, metronidazole, and cephalosporins. In addition to pregnancy, these may permit breakthrough bleeding.

   ◦ Valium, benzodiazepines, and barbiturates.

   ◦ Anticonvulsants, such as phenytoin and primidone.

   ◦ Phenylbutazone, an anti-inflammatory drug.

   ◦ Some antimigraine preparations.

The following conditions that can affect Pill effectiveness are:

   ◦ Diarrhea or vomiting, because the hormone isn't properly absorbed.

   ◦ Traveling into many different time zones, which alters the time of day you take your Pill. Take a Pill every actual 24 hours, no matter what your watch says (or carry along an extra watch set to home time).

• *Know before you leave your medical office what you need to do if you miss taking a Pill or two.* Generally, the next step is to take the Pills you missed (instructions may be different if you missed three or more), *plus use another form of birth control for the rest of one cycle* (some studies show that most women don't do this), especially if the missed Pills were in the first half of the cycle. The procedure may vary a little depending on the particular brand and dose of Pill.

• *Get twice-yearly physicals including a Pap smear and, if you have more than one sex partner, a test for chlamydia.*

• *Take supplements to make up for those vitamins and minerals that are lost as a side effect of taking the Pill.*

• *Exercise regularly to counteract the risk of blood clots.*

If you decide to stop taking the Pill, know that there is no "grace" period when you can't conceive. If you don't want to get pregnant, start using another contraceptive immediately. There are women who are unable to conceive for a while after stopping the Pill, sometimes for a year or more, but they are an unpredictable minority.

I've taken the Pill since I was 17 and love it. When I was 19 I had toxic shock syndrome, so I can't use the diaphragm or the sponge. The Pill and I will stay together a long time.

I started using the Pill when I was in college, and my roommate and I shared one Pill prescription for awhile. Can you believe it? Amazingly, neither one of us got pregnant doing that. We were just lucky.

BARRIER CONTRACEPTIVES

WHAT THEY ARE

Barrier contraceptives are products that prevent sperm from entering the cervix (the neck of the uterus that protrudes into the vagina).

EFFECTIVENESS

The effectiveness rates of barrier contraceptives depend on the user's age, motivation, experience, frequency of intercourse, and the couple's fertility, in addition to the barrier product itself (see failure rates of contraceptives in chart on page 168). When used in combinations like condom/foam, condom/diaphragm, or condom/sponge, they are as effective as the Pill.

TYPES AVAILABLE

Barrier contraceptives work either by creating a physical barrier (condom, diaphragm, cervical cap) or by destroying sperm (spermicide in gel, foam, cream, or suppository form). Some products combine both approaches—like the TODAY sponge or the condom, diaphragm, or cervical cap when used with spermicide inside the devices. All of these methods will be discussed individually later in this section.

HOW TO DECIDE

Advantages are: negligible short-term side effects and no long-term consequences; some protection against sexually transmitted diseases, such as AIDS, herpes (condoms in particular), chlamydia, gonorrhea, and candidiasis (condom and TODAY sponge in particular); some protection against pelvic inflammatory disease (see "Pelvic Inflammatory Disease" on page 441), which may or may not be transmitted sexually, as well as from cervical cancer and communicable vaginal infections like trichomoniasis. (See "Vaginal Infections" on page 532.)

Disadvantages are: interference with spontaneity (less so with the cervical cap and diaphragm), and lower effectiveness rates (unless used in combinations). Barrier contraceptives are not recommended for women who are uneasy about touching their genitals, who have a partner who is not supportive, or who don't get the contraceptives out of the purse or drawer when they need to. Toxic shock syndrome is a rare side effect of the diaphragm and the TODAY sponge, but it can be avoided if users do not leave the devices in place longer than what is recommended. (See "Toxic Shock Syndrome" on page 506.)

Barrier contraceptives, both devices and spermicides, are apparently the oldest form of birth control, other than abstinence or withdrawal, and date back 5,000 years or more. Gumlike substances were used to block the cervix, including crocodile dung, opium, and beeswax. All apparently worked to some degree, and ingredients varied from culture to culture. Until the 1960s and the arrival of the Pill and the IUD, barriers were the only form of birth-control products available, because sterilization was seldom used. Because of the AIDS and sexually transmitted disease epidemics, condoms have regained some of the barriers' popularity and are the third most used form of birth control in the United States.

HOW TO USE BARRIER CONTRACEPTIVES WISELY

• *Be consistent and be correct,* whether you buy an over-the-counter method, like condoms or the TODAY sponge, or you have a prescription for a device. Women who never have unprotected sex and who follow the directions for their birth-control product to the letter are far less likely to have contraceptive failure.

• *If you are using a diaphragm or cervical cap, go to a health care provider who will carefully check the device for correct fit and patiently instruct you in its use.* A New York City study in the 1970s of more than 2,000 women, mostly unmarried and under age 30, showed diaphragms had a 97 to 98 percent effectiveness rate. In this study women were carefully fitted and counseled and asked to return within a week so the provider could answer questions and check the diaphragm fit. Clinic personnel involved in this study believed diaphragms were both safe and effective.

You may get more personalized help with barrier methods at a women's clinic where appointments may not be as rushed, and the staff is both experienced with barrier contraceptives and prepared to instruct you in detail over several visits. (See "Women's Health Centers" on page 598 in the Resource Directory.)

• *Change your barrier method to avoid losing interest and going without a contraceptive "just this once."* Barrier methods provide lots of alternatives.

I had the same gynecologist for years and we always got along fine, as long as I used the Pill and the IUD, that is. The last time I went in, I asked what he thought about condoms or the diaphragm, and he gave me a look like, "What are you doing here?"

You probably think I'm stupid, but I never felt comfortable putting in my diaphragm. I was never sure I was doing it right, so Max always put it in for me. After we got divorced, I worked up the nerve to go to a clinic and have someone take the time to show me how to do it myself.

Before I got married I always used a diaphragm with my lovers. But now my husband and I keep a drawerful of barrier contraceptives, and we take turns choosing which one to use. I have condoms in all colors, a box of TODAY sponges, my trusty diaphragm, even foam. Selecting the contraceptive is fun, not a chore.

MALE CONDOM

WHAT IT IS

A male condom (sometimes called a rubber) is a contraceptive sheath placed over an erect penis to collect semen. (See the female condom on page 197.)

EFFECTIVENESS

Condom effectiveness averages 84 percent with study results ranging from 77 percent to 98.1 percent. Some couples combine the use of condoms with other barriers, like contraceptive foam, to improve birth-control effectiveness.

TYPES AVAILABLE

Latex condoms made in the United States are more reliable than foreign-made condoms. U.S. condoms are available in different shapes and colors, with or without lubricants and/or spermicides. Some also have added ribs, bumps, and tips, which are mostly decorative, not functional. Condoms with spermicides are good for 18 months or two years (see expiration date on package) if stored away from heat and light. Although there is no conclusive research that indicates how often condoms actually break, government estimates are that about one in every 1,000 good-quality condoms may be defective during vaginal use though some manufacturer's research shows the breakage rate may be higher. Probably a greater problem than leakage is a condom that slips off during intercourse or withdrawal, or one that was not stored well.

HOW TO DECIDE

Advantages of condoms are: they are a reliable form of birth control, and they are the best protection against sexually transmitted diseases (STDs), such as AIDS, hepatitis B, chlamydia, gonorrhea, herpes, and genital ulcers as well as pelvic inflammatory disease (PID) and communicable vaginal infections, such as trichomoniasis and monilia. (See "Sexually Transmitted Diseases" on page 493, "Acquired Immune Deficiency Syndrome" on page 138, "Pelvic Inflammatory Disease" on page 441, and "Vaginal Infections" on page 532.)

Some couples use condoms for their disease prevention qualities while simultaneously using the Pill or another contraceptive for birth control. Condoms are available over the counter without a fitting or prescription, and are nonhormonal, noninvasive, and reversible. There is a shared responsibility because the male is the one who uses them.

Disadvantages are that condoms may interfere with spontaneity until you get accustomed to using them and incorporating them into sex play, and many men report condoms reduce sensation ("skin" condoms made from sheep intestines, which are thinner, may not do this as much, but skin condoms are not recommended as a prevention against HIV transmission because the virus can leak through).

The first condom dates back to at least 1350 B.C. Later, condoms were used for hundreds of years to prevent both sexually transmitted diseases and unwanted pregnancies, and at one point they were made from linen. Once hidden behind the pharmacist's counter, condoms weren't displayed on American store counters until 1975, and they used to be illegal in some states. Today condoms are the most used barrier contraceptive in the United States.

HOW TO USE A MALE CONDOM WITH PLEASURE

To use a condom, first examine it for possible flaws, and squeeze the reservoir end to keep out air. Use each condom only once, and have it put on before the penis enters the vagina. That's because the few drops of semen that are often discharged as the penis first becomes totally erect may contain enough sperm to fertilize an egg—and sperm deposited on the vaginal lips can reach the fallopian tubes, so pregnancy might occur even

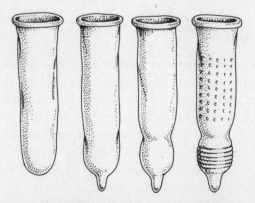

FOUR MALE CONDOM SAMPLES

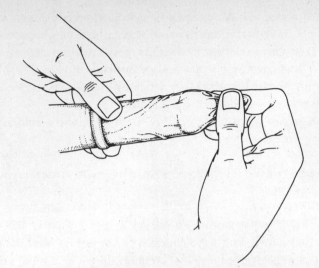

After squeezing the reservoir end, press the condom against the end of the penis and unroll with the other hand until it covers the length of the penis.

HOW TO PUT ON A MALE CONDOM

without intercourse. If in doubt about a condom's condition, throw it out and use another one.

To avoid breakage, leave a loose ½ inch at the tip of a condom, or use brands that have a built-in reservoir tip. Also, avoid "dry" intercourse. Use a water-soluble gel to lubricate your vagina if necessary (do not use an oil-based lubricant, such as petroleum jelly). In the unlikely event that a condom breaks or slips off during intercourse, inject spermicidal foam immediately. After intercourse, when the penis becomes flaccid, the condom should be held firmly in place until the penis is completely away from the vaginal area.

Although more couples are using condoms, many shy away from them. Condoms have been the butt of many a joke, and for centuries they have been associated with prostitutes, sailors, and extramarital sex. Condoms have always been excellent birth control, and they're now the next best thing to celibacy or a monogamous relationship in avoiding sexually transmitted diseases (STDs). It's easy to say "Use a condom," but it's quite another to do it.

Until the man in your life comes prepared with his own birth control, following are suggestions on how you can introduce men's condoms into your love life:

• *Buy them yourself.* Today most condoms in the United States are bought by women. You may find it difficult to buy your own condoms, carry one with you, and suggest a man use it. That may seem unwomanly or culturally unacceptable. Just because it's new and/or difficult, though, doesn't mean you can't do it. Maybe it just takes practice or a new perspective on who may pay the price if you don't use a condom.

• *Make them part of your love play.* Buy them in rainbow colors, and let them be fun — not a chore.

Be prepared for the following reasons why your partner might say he can't use a condom:

• *"I can't use a condom because I'll lose my erection."* That is a bona fide problem for some men, but if the condom is not put on until the penis is quite firm, it's not likely to cause a lost erection. In younger men, a condom may help an erection last longer. A solution is that you put the condom on him as part of love play.

• *"It's not romantic."* Tell him that unplanned pregnancies and unexpected diseases are definitely not romantic.

• *"I won't wear a condom because it's like taking a shower wearing a raincoat."* Research has shown that men who use condoms accept the sensation as the "natural" one. Assure him that he has more nerve endings than just those in his penis, and if he's sure he doesn't, are you sure you want to be with someone who focuses on his own body and not yours?

• *"Condoms hurt."* No, they don't. In spite of that, the biggest stumbling block to condom use in one large study of adolescents was the belief by more than one third that condoms are painful to use.

• *"I don't need a condom because I don't have a disease (and/or I've had a vasectomy)."* Unless you know your partner *very* well, you do not know if what he's saying is true. Besides, many people are carriers for STDs without knowing it because they don't have symptoms.

• *"I can't use condoms because they are too small (or too big)."* Currently in the United States, condoms come in two sizes, regular and extra-large.

It's not that I didn't think about contraception. I was nervous about AIDS. But the man had just come out of a year of meditating, hadn't he? It's hard enough to go to bed with a man for the first time in years without having to ask him to wear a condom.

I just come right out and say I have a dress code. If he doesn't wear a condom, I won't have sex.

FEMALE CONDOM

WHAT IT IS

A Reality female condom is a seven-inch-long lubricated polyurethane pouch that collects semen. (The lubricant is designed to duplicate the natural lubrication of the vagina during sexual excitement.) The condom has flexible rings at each end to hold it in place. The inner ring fits behind the pubic bone and is inserted like a diaphragm (but fits more loosely). The outer ring fits about one inch outside the body over the labia. This female condom resembles a small plastic bag and is stronger and lighter than a male condom.

The Reality condom is a brand name item and was conditionally approved in 1993 by the Food and Drug Administration. It became available in France and Switzerland in 1992. (See "Future Contraceptives" on page 224 for other female condoms.)

EFFECTIVENESS

Reality condom effectiveness averages about 74 percent in early studies.

HOW TO DECIDE

Advantages of the female condom are that it is a reliable form of birth control, and, if used properly, it appears to provide as good as or perhaps better protection than the male condom against STDs and communicable vaginal infections. Unlike the diaphragm, TODAY sponge, or cervical cap, the female condom also protects the entire vagina and labia from contact with semen. An erection is not needed to insert this female condom, nor does it have to be removed immediately after male ejaculation.

Female condom tear rates are reportedly less than 1 percent, and these condoms can be stored at room temperature for three years. These devices are available over the counter and are nonhormonal, noninvasive, and reversible. As with the male condom, some couples will use the female condom for its disease prevention while also using the Pill or another contraceptive for birth control. For women who like to use barrier contraceptives and alternate different methods with their partners, the female condom is a nice addition.

Disadvantages are that the female condom, like the male condom, may interfere with spontaneity until you get accustomed to using it and incorporating it into sex play. Some women find the outer ring that hangs outside of the body to be cumbersome. Women who don't like using tampons or other barrier contraceptives probably won't like the female condom either. There's been little report of loss of sensation for either partner, perhaps because the female condom is thinner than the male condom. The Reality condom costs $2 or more each, which is about four times more than the cost of one male condom.

HOW TO USE A FEMALE CONDOM

Pull apart the two sides of each individual package in the middle at the top to avoid damaging the condom. Be sure the lubrication is evenly spread by rubbing the outside of the pouch together. (If you find after using these condoms that you want more lubrication, add a drop of Reality lubricant which is probably available where you purchase the condoms. Avoid using other brands of lubrication.)

To use a female condom, first examine it for possible flaws. Use each condom only once, and insert it before the penis enters the vagina to avoid

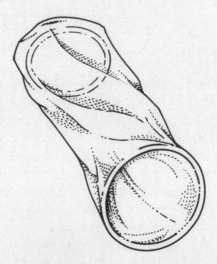

FEMALE CONDOM

HOLDING THE CONDOM

Hold the pouch with the open end hanging down. While holding the outside of the pouch, squeeze the inner ring with your thumb and middle finger.

INSERTING THE CONDOM

While still squeezing the condom with your three fingers, spread your vaginal lips with your other hand and insert the condom. This gets easier with practice.

POSITIONING THE CONDOM

With your index finger, push the inner ring and the pouch the rest of the way up into your vagina. Make sure the inner ring is up just past the pubic bone.

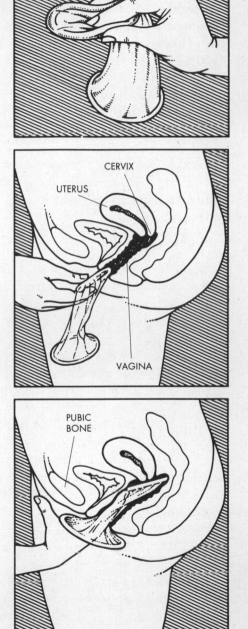

HOW TO INSERT A FEMALE CONDOM

both disease transmission and impregnation from the first drops of semen. (See additional instructions in the illustration of a female condom on pages 198 and 199.) After intercourse, squeeze and twist the outer ring to keep the sperm inside the pouch, and pull out gently. Do not flush the used condom down the toilet. Be conscientous about following the instructions. The FDA says the high failure rate is due to improper use of this condom.

DIAPHRAGM

WHAT IT IS

A diaphragm is a shallow rubber bowl several inches wide with a flexible rim. It snugly covers the upper vagina and cervix and remains in place by spring tension.

EFFECTIVENESS

Diaphragm effectiveness used without a condom averages 82 percent with studies ranging from 75 percent to 98 percent.

TYPES AVAILABLE

Diaphragms come in several sizes and types. It's generally recommended that you be fitted with the largest size your body can accommodate without your feeling it when it's inserted correctly.

HOW TO DECIDE

Advantages of the diaphragm are: it's nonhormonal, noninvasive, and reversible, and it offers some protection against sexually transmitted diseases. In fact, studies at an STD clinic showed the diaphragm and the TODAY sponge were more effective against gonorrhea, chlamydia, trichomoniasis, candidiasis, and bacterial vaginosis than was the use of the male condom. (They are not effective in preventing the transmission of the HIV virus, however.)

Disadvantages are: it may interfere with spontaneity until you get used to incorporating it into your love play; it requires a prescription; and women who have severely relaxed pelvic muscles (see "Uterine Prolapse" on page 527) or who have frequent urinary tract infections (see "Urinary Tract Infections" on page 515) are cautioned to use another form of birth control. There have also been reports suggesting that use of the diaphragm

DIAPHRAGM

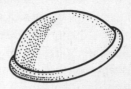

Inserting a Diaphragm

Positioning of diaphragm

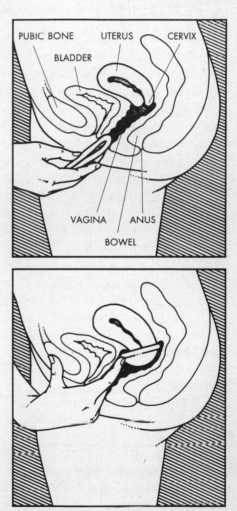

PUBIC BONE   UTERUS   CERVIX

BLADDER

VAGINA   ANUS

BOWEL

HOW TO INSERT A DIAPHRAGM

for more than one year affects the cervical mucus of some women, making it more difficult for them to conceive later.

Like other barriers, the diaphragm's historical roots are in ancient times. The modern version of the diaphragm was produced in Germany in the 1800s. The diaphragm then crossed the ocean to America with birth-control advocate Margaret Sanger. She provided diaphragms to women in the 1920s when birth control devices were still illegal in this country. Like other barrier contraceptives, diaphragms were more popular before the 1960s and the advent of the Pill.

HOW TO USE A DIAPHRAGM

To use a diaphragm, place a small amount of spermicide in the dome of the diaphragm. Spread the spermicide around the inner surface of the dome and rim. Get into a squatting or half-reclining position. Separate your vaginal lips with one hand while holding the diaphragm in your other hand. While squeezing the rim together, slide the diaphragm into your vagina and push it back as far as it will easily go. Use your forefinger to doublecheck the position of the diaphragm over your cervix.

You can insert the diaphragm, with contraceptive jelly, up to several hours before you have intercourse. Some women ask their partners to put it in as part of love play. Add new spermicide before each time you have sex, and leave the diaphragm in place for at least six hours after each time you have intercourse. To avoid the risk of TSS, don't leave the diaphragm in altogether for more than 24 hours.

To care for your diaphragm, wash it in warm water with a tiny amount of mild soap, rinse well, and dry with a towel. (Do not use talcum powder.) Store in its own container. Check for tears. Replace your diaphragm every two to three years or sooner if you have a baby, or gain or lose more than 10 pounds. Don't hesitate to get your diaphragm checked periodically for fit. Replace it immediately if the rubber changes around the rim or develops a hole. (To check for holes, fill the empty diaphragm with water.) Be aware that a diaphragm may move and have less contraceptive effect if you are on top during intercourse.

***

What can I tell you? My generation suffered from the conceit that the Pill was the only sophisticated contraceptive. If not the Pill, then withdrawal, a condom, or nothing—but never a diaphragm. Old-fashioned, cumbersome, messy, it totally deserved the disparaging nickname "midnight trampoline," or so we thought.

I quit taking the Pill after two years because I was tired of the headaches and tired of being tired. The people at the birth-control clinic were not happy when I switched to the diaphragm, but I love using it.

TODAY SPONGE

WHAT IT IS

The TODAY sponge is a 2¼ inch disposable disc, smaller than a diaphragm, shaped like a mushroom cap and made of polyurethane, embedded with spermicide (nonoxynol-9). It works three ways: it releases spermicide, absorbs semen, and blocks the cervix. This is a brand name item, so there is only one kind available.

EFFECTIVENESS

TODAY sponge effectiveness (used without a condom) averages 76 percent. The sponge works best for younger women who have not yet had children whether vaginally or by cesarean.

HOW TO DECIDE

Advantages are: it can be inserted unhurriedly hours before intercourse, thus providing a greater degree of sexual spontaneity, and it is available over the counter with no fitting and no prescription. It's also nonhormonal, noninvasive, and reversible, and is perhaps easier to insert than the diaphragm or cervical cap. It provides continuous protection for a 24-hour period (no matter how often you have sex within that 24-hour period), and also provides some protection against sexually transmitted diseases. In fact, studies at an STD clinic showed the TODAY sponge and the diaphragm were more effective against gonorrhea, chlamydia, trichomoniasis, candidiasis, and bacterial vaginosis than was the use of the condom. (They are not effective in preventing the transmission of the HIV virus, however.)

Disadvantages are: it has a higher pregnancy rate than the diaphragm, and it may be difficult for some women to remove. (If it is difficult for you to remove the sponge, reconsider using it.) In addition, it may cause a vaginal burning sensation, irritations and/or dryness from the spermicide that is used.

The TODAY sponge is not recommended for women who have had

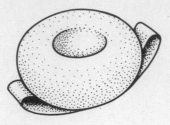

TODAY CONTRACEPTIVE SPONGE

toxic shock syndrome (see "Toxic Shock Syndrome" on page 506) or for women who have had children, as the contraceptive failure rate is higher with them.

Vaginal sponges (often sea sponges) have been in use for 5,000 years, and were first reported in ancient Egypt. The modern version of this old approach, the TODAY sponge, includes spermicide and was introduced in the United States in 1983. The spermicide in the sponge has been available for more than 20 years and is used in spermicidal creams, foams, and suppositories. However, the amount used in the TODAY sponge is about ten times greater than in other products when they are used alone.

How to Use the TODAY Sponge

To use the TODAY sponge, first wet the sponge to activate the spermicide, then insert it into your vagina, loop-side out for later removal. Leave it in place no more than 30 hours, or six hours past last intercourse. Avoid the TODAY sponge during menstruation or within six weeks after childbirth.

I love the sponge. I put it in in the morning and then I'm always prepared. It's easier than other barriers that have to be inserted closer to the time of sex, and it doesn't have the side effects I experienced with the Pill. My girlfriend told me the sponge is expensive. But I paid a lot for the Pill, so I'm not concerned.

CERVICAL CAP

WHAT IT IS

A cervical cap is a thimble-shaped rubber bowl that is inserted into the vagina and placed over the cervix to block sperm and is held in place by suction.

EFFECTIVENESS

Cervical cap effectiveness (when used without a condom) averages 82 percent; and study results range from 74 percent to 96.7 percent.

HOW TO DECIDE

Advantages of the cap are: it allows sexual spontaneity, since it can be left in for as long as 72 hours (twenty-four hours is considered the safest maximum to avoid toxic shock syndrome — TSS — though no reports of TSS have been associated with the cervical cap), and it does not require repeated applications of spermicide during that time.

It is nonhormonal, noninvasive, and reversible, and it may be more enjoyable for oral sex than other barrier methods, because there is practically no possibility of a spermicide taste. It also can be used by some women who cannot be fitted for a diaphragm, including women with severely relaxed pelvic muscles, and it will not usually be felt by you or your partner. It is not associated with urinary tract infections as is the diaphragm, and unlike the TODAY sponge, it can be used by women who have had children. It is economical because it seldom needs replacement and uses very little spermicide.

Disadvantages are: 15 to 20 percent of women cannot be fitted because one of the four currently available cap sizes does not match their anatomy, it requires a prescription, and occasionally there is a vaginal odor (this can usually be eliminated by removing the cap after 24 hours). In addition, a cervical cap is more difficult to insert than a diaphragm or sponge, and it is more easily dislodged.

Cervical caps are not recommended for women who have severe cervical laceration, infection of the cervix, inflammation of the ovaries and fallopian tubes, temporary vaginal infection (see "Vaginal Infections" on page 532), or an abnormal Pap smear (see "Pap Smear" on page 105). The Food and Drug Administration recommends that cap users get a Pap smear after three months of use and every year thereafter, because in a National

Institutes of Health study, 4 percent of cervical-cap users developed cervical tissue abnormalities in the first three months. If this happens to you,
choose another contraceptive.

Like other barriers, cervical caps are an ancient form of birth control.
The modern version appeared in the 1830s when a rubber cervical cap was
introduced in Germany. By the early 1900s, it was the most prescribed
contraceptive method in Europe among those few women who had access
to birth control. In this country cervical caps were first popular in the 1920s
and then that popularity, along with that of other barriers, diminished with
the advent of the Pill in the 1960s.

However, concern about IUD and Pill side effects created renewed
interest in the cervical cap in the 1970s. When use of the cervical cap was
resurrected in this country at that time, the FDA labeled it experimental, but
in 1988 it was approved by the U.S. government. (To find the best health
care provider for you to fit a cap, see "How to Use Barrier Contraceptives
Wisely" on page 191.)

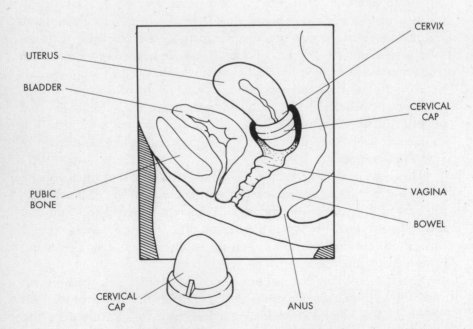

CORRECTLY POSITIONED CERVICAL CAP

How to Use a Cervical Cap

To use a cervical cap, fill it no more than one-third full of spermicide jelly or cream. Get into a squatting or half-reclining position. Separate your vaginal lips with one hand while holding the cap between your thumb and forefinger of the other hand. While squeezing the rim together, slide the cap into your vagina and push it as far back as it will go. Use your forefinger to press the rim around the cervix until the dome covers the opening. Avoid using a cervical cap during menstruation or if you have had toxic shock syndrome.

I've tried every birth-control method there is. I quit taking the Pill after gaining 15 pounds and didn't have a menstrual period for the next three years. While using the IUD, I developed a pelvic infection that kept me bedridden for weeks. This is my last chance. I won't get an abortion and I can't use those other things, so what's left?

Spermicide

What It Is

Spermicide is a chemical that destroys sperm on contact. It is packaged in aerosol foam, cream, jelly, and suppositories.

Effectiveness

Spermicide effectiveness (used without a condom or other barrier device) averages 70 percent, and study results range from 67 percent to 98.5 percent.

How to Decide

The advantages to spermicide are: it's available over the counter with no fitting and no prescription; it's nonhormonal, noninvasive, and reversible; it's perhaps easier to use than a diaphragm or a cervical cap; and it provides some protection against sexually transmitted diseases. Spermicide increases the effectiveness of barrier devices, as well as the effectiveness of other birth-control methods like IUD and natural family planning when used midcycle.

The disadvantages are: a higher pregnancy rate than for the diaphragm, TODAY sponge, and cervical cap; perhaps an unpleasant taste with oral sex; a 10- to 15-minute wait before sex when using suppositories (for example, Encare, Intercept, and Semicid); and occasionally no protection from an undissolved suppository. Some people may be allergic to the spermicide, resulting in itching or a burning sensation.

Although spermicides have been accused of causing birth defects in the offspring of women who used spermicides when they conceived, research since then has shown no link.

Two precursors of today's spermicides were highly acidic lemons and pomegranates used thousands of years ago. Today's acidic foams, jellies, creams, and suppositories (see "Future Contraceptives" on page 224) are usually made with Nonoxynol-9, the leading spermicidal ingredient. Spermicide preparations differ in strength. Diaphragm and cervical cap creams and jellies, for instance, are not as potent as forms intended to be used alone.

HOW TO USE SPERMICIDE

To use spermicide, insert the measured amount deep into the upper part of your vagina before sex. With a suppository, you need to wait 10 to 15 minutes to allow it to dissolve and foam. Check and be sure the suppository has dissolved. Do not douche for at least eight hours after sex. (Douching is a good thing to avoid in general. It increases your risk for both pelvic inflammatory disease and ectopic pregnancy.)

A t the age of 20 I started using foam, and 18 years later had a foam failure at age 38. What a shock! But foam did work for 18 years.

INTRAUTERINE DEVICE (IUD)

WHAT IT IS

An IUD is a small plastic or metal device that fits inside the uterus. No one is quite sure how an IUD functions, but it's believed that it prevents the sperm from fertilizing the egg. It may also be a uterine irritant, which prevents a fertilized egg from implanting on the uterine wall.

EFFECTIVENESS

Effectiveness of the IUD averages 96 percent.

TYPES AVAILABLE

Two IUDs are currently available in the United States. Progestasert, available since the late 1970s, is a T-shaped device which releases progesterone daily. This IUD needs to be replaced every 12 months. The newer IUD is the ParaGard Copper T380A, which became available in the United States in 1988, and can be left in for several years.

HOW TO DECIDE

Advantages of an IUD are: it's a highly reliable contraceptive, it allows for sexual spontaneity, and it's reversible.

Disadvantages are: many users have more menstrual cramps and lose more menstrual blood (which may cause anemia — see "Anemia" on page 158) than women who do not use an IUD; occasionally the device perforates the wall of the uterus; and some IUDs "travel" in the uterus or become embedded in the uterine wall and have to be removed surgically (this requires hospitalization).

In addition, Progestasert may increase the number of days of bleeding and spotting and is occasionally associated with serious hemorrhaging, although it may cause less menstrual cramping than the ParaGard Copper T380A. There may also be additional side effects caused by the contraceptive steroid released in the Progestasert device.

Other disadvantages of all IUDs are:

• *Pelvic inflammatory disease* (PID), which may occasionally lead to infertility and/or hysterectomy. This infection occurs somewhat more often in IUD users, especially those who are not monogamous, but not as often (two to five times greater risk) as with the earliest version of the IUD, the Dalkon Shield, which is no longer on the market.

It's believed that the increased risk for PID occurs when the IUD is inserted (rather than from contamination of the IUD string, which was the original theory). That's why a single dose of an antibiotic at the time of insertion is now recommended. With earlier versions of the IUD, the risk for PID increased the more years an IUD was in place. Today's IUDs, however, are not left in place for many years, and most infections will appear in the first four months of use, usually in the first 20 days. (See "Pelvic Inflammatory Disease" on page 441.)

• *Pregnancy.* When pregnancy occurs and an IUD is still in place, there's a 50 to 60 percent chance of a miscarriage (see "Miscarriage" on page 487). Over half of these miscarriages will occur in the second trimester of pregnancy when pregnancy loss is a more difficult experience both physically and emotionally. If the device is removed as soon as pregnancy is diagnosed, a miscarriage is less likely to occur. If you think you might be pregnant, contact your physician immediately.

• *Ectopic Pregnancy.* A tubal pregnancy occurs occasionally and is another reason a suspected pregnancy needs to be investigated immediately. Although ectopic pregnancies are rare, they are more likely to occur with the Progestasert rather than the copper IUD. (See "Ectopic Pregnancy" on page 488.)

• *Endometriosis.* For some women, an IUD will stimulate endometriosis, a usually painful disorder in which some of the tissue that usually lines the uterus grows in other parts of the body. (See "Endometriosis" on page 329.)

Women who have had PID, an ectopic pregnancy, tubal surgery, or currently have vaginitis (see "Vaginal Infections" on page 532) are advised not to use an IUD. The IUD is safest with a woman who has only one sex partner and who has already given birth.

The idea — a foreign body embedded in the uterus that tends to prevent pregnancy — has been known for thousands of years. But IUDs didn't become available in the United States until the late 1960s. In spite of the heavier menstrual flow and cramping which many women experienced, and the unexpected pregnancies that are a possibility with any birth control, IUDs were popular and considered care free among users. IUDs allowed sexual spontaneity with no attention paid to the device except checking the string.

Side-effect reports in the late 1970s changed that attitude for many women and physicians, however, and use of these devices declined through the 1980s. At least 325,000 women in more than 80 countries have filed claims against IUD manufacturers because of PID and infertility. These suits have resulted in U.S. manufacturers' reluctance to produce more IUDs beyond the two now available, although different types of IUDs are popularly used in 94 other countries.

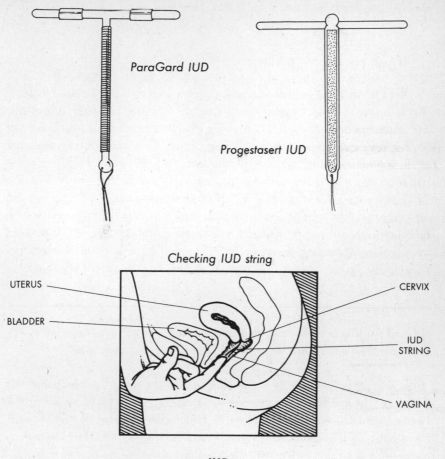

ParaGard IUD

Progestasert IUD

Checking IUD string

UTERUS

BLADDER

CERVIX

IUD
STRING

VAGINA

IUD

How an IUD Is Inserted

After a pelvic exam and depending on your history, perhaps a pregnancy test, you'll be given an oral antibiotic (to avoid infection) and a painkiller such as aspirin (to help ease the cramps caused by insertion of the IUD).

With a speculum holding open your vagina, your cervix and vagina are cleansed with an antiseptic solution. Next, an instrument called the tenaculum holds the cervix in place. An IUD is then folded into a slim plastic tube and inserted as close to the top of the uterus as possible. As the tube is slowly removed, the T-shaped arms of the IUD unfold within the broadest part of the uterus and the strings are drawn down through the cervix into the vagina.

HOW TO USE AN IUD

To use an IUD (which you and your partner will not be able to feel), check the two strings to see if they are in place before and after intercourse and after menstruation. IUDs may be expelled from your body without your knowing it. Expulsion most often occurs with intercourse, urination, or during menstruation. Although it's easier to insert an IUD during menstruation, the risk of expulsion is probably greater at that time.

Have your IUD checked if any of the following occurs: the strings can no longer be felt; your period is late, missed, unusually heavy (perhaps with blood clots), or you spot midcycle; you feel abdominal pain and/or have an increased temperature, fever, or chills; or you have a noticeable or foul vaginal discharge.

I loved the IUD and am sorry that most of them are no longer available. Yes, I know they don't work for everyone, but it was perfect for me.

I got an IUD in the early 1970s when it was all the rage. I got pregnant with it twice. The first time I miscarried at three months. When I told my doctor that I was sure the IUD was still inside of me, he told me not to worry. He said of course it was gone, I just hadn't noticed. I went to another doctor and asked him to x-ray my pelvis, but he said he wouldn't do it because pelvic x-rays of women are not safe. He, too, said surely the IUD was gone. While using foam, I got pregnant again three years later. This time the IUD came out at the end of a 20-week miscarriage, complete with massive PID.

NATURAL FAMILY PLANNING (NFP)

WHAT IT IS

Natural family planning (NFP) is a birth-control method that relies on periodic abstinence and a woman's awareness of her fertility pattern within the menstrual cycle.

EFFECTIVENESS

NFP effectiveness averages 81 percent (less for younger women or those with irregular menstrual cycles) and ranges from 65 percent to 98.5 percent for all women. As with other forms of birth control, reliability of this method improves with careful, consistent, and accurate following of instructions. (See "Fertility Awareness" on page 613 in Recommended Reading for information about using NFP during breastfeeding or when approaching menopause.)

HOW TO DECIDE

The advantages of NFP are: it's nonhormonal, noninvasive, and completely reversible, and except for the cost of a thermometer, it's free. Some women report pleasure in understanding their bodies better, and others find an increased awareness of and use of other forms of sexual play. It's also helpful for women who want to get pregnant and who want to know when they ovulate.

Disadvantages are: this method can be time-consuming; it requires a long period of abstinence; and it requires training and ongoing counseling if it is to be highly effective. Some women find the record keeping and body function monitoring tedious and distasteful. Some research has indicated a slightly higher rate of Down syndrome associated with pregnancies that occur despite NFP. The reason is that this method requires infrequent intercourse prior to ovulation, which may lead to fertilization with an "old" sperm. (See "Down Syndrome" on page 454.)

It has only been since the 1930s that there's been any certainty in understanding how to prevent conception through an awareness of a woman's period of fertility within a menstrual cycle. It was shown by scientists then in both Japan and Germany that the interval between ovulation and the next menstruation is usually 14 days, and the calendar, or rhythm, method began.

The rhythm method is based on the erroneous idea that women's menstrual cycles are regular and predictable. It is also based on a 28-day cycle from the beginning of one menstrual period to the beginning of the next. With rare exception, only Pill users have that regular a cycle. In a study of 30,000 women whose menstrual cycles for a year were evaluated, two thirds had cycles that varied by more than eight days. In other words, one month's period for one woman could be 25 days, and another cycle for the same woman could be 33 days or longer within the same year.

More information about ovulation was added in the 1970s with greater understanding of the role of cervical mucus. This led to the sympto-thermal method, or NFP. The most successful couples using this method have a high degree of motivation, limit sexual intercourse to the approximately 14 days prior to menstruation, and receive excellent information.

HOW TO USE NATURAL FAMILY PLANNING

NFP works best when it is taught by a well-informed teacher who is successfully experienced with this method. To use NFP, you check your basal (body at rest) temperature with a thermometer before rising in the morning, your cervical mucus, any midcycle spotting and pain (called Mittelschmerz), and changes in the cervix throughout your menstrual cycle to determine ovulation. You keep track of these changes on a chart. When your temperature rises one-half to one degree and remains elevated for three days, this signals that ovulation is taking place. It is considered safe to have intercourse after those three days.

Unsafe days are all those from the beginning of your menstrual period through the three days of elevated temperature, a period of time that averages two to three weeks, depending on the number of days in an individual woman's menstrual cycle. The safe days start on the first day after the three days of elevated temperature and continue until menstruation begins.

Some women use NFP by only checking their cervical mucus. However, this method is not reliable if you have a vaginal infection, use spermicides, or douche. (Douching is a good thing to avoid in general. It increases your risk for both pelvic inflammatory disease and ectopic pregnancy. See "Pelvic Inflammatory Disease" on page 441 and "Ectopic Pregnancy" on page 488.)

If you choose to combine NFP with a barrier contraceptive during your fertile period, use a condom. Spermicidal jellies and foams can alter the appearance of vaginal secretions, which will affect your daily cervical mucus checks.

_____

*N*FP really works for my husband and me. Neither one of us wanted to use anything chemical like the Pill or a barrier like condoms or diaphragms. We both seem to know a whole lot more about my body now that I keep track of fertility symptoms every day. When I went in for my first prenatal visit with our planned first child, I told the doctor exactly what day I got pregnant. He wasn't so positive, but I was.

*F*orget about getting information on natural fertility control from a doctor. Mine told me he didn't know much about it, and for me to contact the Couple to Couple League.

NORPLANT

WHAT IT IS

Norplant (also known as levonorgestrel) is a birth-control device that consists of six toothpick-size capsules made of silicone rubber which are implanted under the skin, where they release a hormone directly into the bloodstream. This hormone (progestin) is found in many birth-control Pills, but unlike the Pill, Norplant comes in only one dosage. It inhibits ovulation and makes cervical mucus thick and scanty (an inhospitable environment for sperm).

Norplant is implanted with a local anesthetic on the inside of the upper arm above the elbow, and most women report little or no pain with the insertion. Removal may be more difficult. As is true with any procedure, it's important to find a physician who has experience with it. As Norplant is new in the United States, you may have to search.

EFFECTIVENESS

Early research shows Norplant is 99.5 percent effective with a woman weighing less than 110 pounds and 91 percent effective with a 150-pound woman. (Reliability decreases because higher body weights dilute the hormonal effect.)

HOW TO DECIDE

Advantages of Norplant are: it's highly reliable, especially for small women; it's convenient; it allows for sexual spontaneity; it may be effective for as long as five years (according to the manufacturer); and it is reversible by removing all capsules. It can also be used by women who have side effects from the estrogen used in the Pill.

Disadvantages are: Norplant must be inserted and removed by health

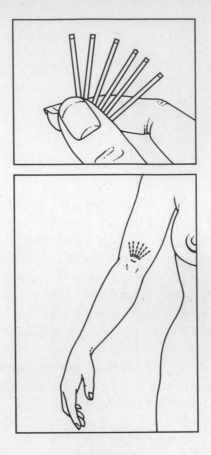

Norplant capsules

Location in arm

NORPLANT

care professionals, it may be visible (particularly in thin women), you cannot discontinue use on your own, it initially costs more ($200 – $500) than other contraceptives, and like the Pill, shouldn't be used during pregnancy.

Nearly all users report irregular menstrual bleeding, including prolonged menstrual periods, spotting between periods, or no periods (see "Amenorrhea" on page 411) for several months. Headaches, breast tenderness, mood changes, dizziness, weight gain, skin rashes, enlarged ovaries, and other side effects occur less often.

As with the Pill, Norplant should not be used by smokers or women who have acute liver disease or liver tumors, breast cancer, unexplained vaginal bleeding, or blood clots in the legs, lungs, or eyes.

The list of side effects to the Pill grew as 50 million women in the United States alone since the 1960s used oral contraceptives and reported their experiences. Millions of women worldwide haven't used Norplant yet (the number is closer to one and a half million), so all side effects are probably not known yet. However, many will likely be related to the side effects of the Pill. In fact, women who have specific side effects from the use of progestin in the Pill (such as the minipill) may have similar reactions to Norplant as well. (See side effects of the Pill on page 184.)

Norplant became available in the United States in 1991. It was originally manufactured and sold in Finland and is now available in at least 23 countries.

DEPO-PROVERA

WHAT IT IS

Depo-Provera is a synthetic hormone that is injected into your body, usually in the buttocks or arm, in a physician's office or clinic to provide contraceptive protection by inhibiting ovulation for 90 days. (It can also be taken in tablet form for other purposes.) It's believed this drug prevents the release of eggs and thickens the mucus lining the entrance to the uterus so that sperm cannot enter.

EFFECTIVENESS

Its effectiveness averages 99.6 percent.

HOW TO DECIDE

Advantages are: it's highly effective and convenient.

Disadvantage are: it can cause irregular menstrual cycles, abdominal discomfort, weight gain, hair loss, fatigue, headaches, skin problems, decreased libido, depression, among other side effects. Many women are unable to conceive for six to 12 months after the last shot wears off. And, in addition, infants exposed in utero to Depo-Provera through method failure are twice as likely to have low birth weight.

Depo-Provera has been turned down twice by the Food and Drug Administration since 1967 because of potential hazards to users, but it was approved for birth control in 1992. Currently, it's used in 90 other countries as a contraceptive.

MORNING-AFTER BIRTH CONTROL

WHAT IT IS

"Morning after" birth control is the name given to birth-control methods that are used within a few days of unprotected sex to prevent implantation of a fertilized egg within the uterus.

TYPES AVAILABLE

The Food and Drug Administration has not approved any method for morning-after birth control, but there are several methods that are used. They can only be obtained through a physician or clinic, and should be used only if their benefits outweigh the risks for you.

Several Birth-Control Pills

You will most likely be told to take two birth-control Pills at least within 72 hours of sex, and two more Pills 12 hours later. (Timing is essential.) Not every Pill brand works, so it's best not to try this on your own. Get good advice. Over the years, both the brands and the hormone-dose strength of recommended Pills for morning-after birth control have changed. Be sure to thoroughly discuss this possibility with a physician or clinic personnel so that you understand not only the procedure for taking Pills for this purpose, but also danger signs of their use. Those include severe abdominal pain, severe chest pain, severe headache, vision or speech problems, or severe leg pain.

Half of women who try this will experience nausea or vomiting with birth-control Pills. If you weren't pregnant to start with, or if you were pregnant and the Pills successfully prevented implantation, you'll menstruate within two to three weeks. This is one-time birth-control use. Be sure to use other birth control later on a continual basis. If you don't menstruate, and you are indeed pregnant and have used morning-after Pills, there may be potential side effects for your baby from this high-dose use of the Pill. (Once again see side effects of the Pill on page 184.)

Because of the Pill's common side effects of vomiting and nausea, two other drugs with fewer side effects have been suggested for morning-after use. One is Danazol, a drug commonly used for endometriosis, and the other is RU486, the controversial drug used to cause an abortion within the first few weeks of pregnancy. (See "RU486" below and "Danazol" on page 332.)

IUD Insertion

An IUD should be inserted within five to seven days of unprotected sex to prevent a fertilized egg from implanting. You'll want to consider all the advantages and disadvantages of IUD use before using this approach. (See "Intrauterine Device" on page 208.)

Menstrual Extraction

Menstrual extraction is performed by inserting a plastic tube (cannula) into the cervix and gently withdrawing the endometrial lining of the uterus by suction, using a syringe. This procedure was developed by feminists in the 1970s not as birth control, but as a way to remove menstrual blood. Although not originally intended as a do-it-yourself abortion, menstrual extraction can be performed before a woman knows she's pregnant, or up to two weeks past a missed period. It's inexpensive, easy, and requires no anesthetic.

However, infection is a possibility, and there is no research on either safety or effectiveness of this procedure. Also, if a woman is pregnant, menstrual extraction doesn't always work, so the pregnancy may continue. The most likely facility to offer menstrual extraction is a clinic staffed with women who are interested in self-help healthcare methods. (See "Women's Health Centers" on page 598 in the Resource Directory for help in locating a clinic near you. See also "Menstrual Extraction" on page 613 in Recommended Reading.)

RU486

In addition to its "morning-after" capability, RU486 can be taken as an abortion drug for three days within 49 days after the last menstrual period. It softens the cervix and blocks the effect of progesterone, which is needed for implanting and maintaining a fertilized egg. It is usually used with prostaglandin to increase the strength of the contractions. A miscarriage with bleeding comparable to a heavy menstrual period results more than 99 percent of the time. RU486 is not recommended for use by smokers or women who have heart problems or diabetes or in those who are in poor health, especially if they are past the age of 35.

This drug is available in France, the United Kingdom, and Sweden. China also has its own version of RU486. By 1993, RU486 was not available in the United States.

EFFECTIVENESS

The number of U.S. women who use these methods and their effectiveness for morning-after contraception is unknown. To begin with, no one knows how many of the women who use these methods were really pregnant. Pregnancy tests don't work that early. It's a given that none of these methods are 100 percent effective, though 1992 research that included women's ovulation history as a measure of pregnancy risk showed that both the Pill and RU486 were very effective.

HOW TO DECIDE

Maybe you've had a barrier contraceptive fail (broken condom, dislodged diaphragm), or you forgot to take several Pills, or you just didn't use any birth control. Or maybe you were forced to have sex when you didn't want to and were unprepared. (Estimates are that a U.S. woman has perhaps as high as a 25 percent chance of being raped in her lifetime.) In any case, you definitely don't want to be pregnant.

What are your options? You can do nothing, and probably your period will come just as it always does. Estimates vary anywhere from 1 to 30 percent as to what your chances are for conceiving with one unprotected midcycle intercourse. Your chances for conceiving are higher if you're in your teens or early 20s. Another option is to wait and see if you are pregnant and deal with that situation then. However, if you don't want to wait, there is morning-after birth control.

---

*A*fter I reported the rape, the police were very helpful and suggested that I immediately talk to the rape counseling people. And I did. After listening to my story, they told me that one of my options was to take these birth-control Pills, so that I wouldn't have to also deal with an unexpected pregnancy. After thinking about it, I decided to do it. The counselor was wonderful and told me how I would feel and what the warning signs were that meant I should call her immediately if they happened. She also told me that I might throw up. I'm glad she told me, because I did throw up.

I had sex once when I thought it was my fertile time and I hadn't used any birth control. I worked at a medical clinic, so I knew about morning-after Pills. The doctor warned me that taking these Pills could make me throw up and feel lousy for a few days, but they didn't. Frankly, I don't think I would have noticed. I was just so relieved not to be pregnant.

WITHDRAWAL (COITUS INTERRUPTUS)

WHAT IT IS

Withdrawal is the removal of the penis from the woman's vagina and vaginal lips before male orgasm. To be successful, withdrawal must occur before the first few drops of semen are discharged as the penis becomes totally erect, since they may contain enough sperm to fertilize an egg.

EFFECTIVENESS

The effectiveness of withdrawal averages 76 percent (less with younger couples).

HOW TO DECIDE

Advantages are: it's free, always available, no prescription or office exam needed, no storage, and no planning required except during intercourse.

Disadvantages are: it interrupts lovemaking, resulting in sexual dissatisfaction for many, and it has a high rate of failure. The man needs to be especially aware of his orgasmic timing which may be particularly difficult for younger men and can be anxiety-provoking.

Withdrawal has been used as a form of birth control since prehistoric times, and nearly 20 percent of U.S. couples use it the first time they have sex. The true extent of its use tends to be underreported in published survey findings, some researchers claim, especially if couples also use more effective methods. The most likely couples to be successful are those in which the male is a master-timer, the couple is experienced with withdrawal, and they are motivated to use it consistently.

Like barrier contraceptive methods, reliance on withdrawal was reduced with the advent of the Pill in the 1960s. But despite its built-in frustration and unreliability, withdrawal is still commonly used by millions of people in many parts of the world where contraception is not readily available. For example, in the former U.S.S.R., withdrawal is the third most common method of birth control. Perhaps not coincidentally, abortion is the first.

I think withdrawal is the most anxiety-ridden experience I've ever had. Instead of enjoying myself, I spent the time asking myself, "Will he or won't he?" You can keep Latin lovers. I'll stick with American men.

DOUCHING

WHAT IT IS

Douching as birth control is quickly flushing out the vagina after intercourse to wash away and/or destroy sperm.

EFFECTIVENESS

Its effectiveness averages 60 percent. The only birth-control method with a higher failure rate than that is using none.

HOW TO DECIDE

The only advantages are: it's nonhormonal, noninvasive, and reversible.

The biggest disadvantage is that it usually doesn't work. Sperm can complete their journey within seconds. A douche may merely hasten them, but it has other disadvantages, too. Douching about once a week (practiced by one third of young U.S. women) is associated with increased risk for both pelvic inflammatory disease and ectopic or tubal pregnancy.

In spite of douching's high failure rate as birth control, it's been used as a contraceptive for centuries and is still used in many parts of the world, including in the United States. In this country, as well as others in the developed world, folklore claims that many a teenager, who's as fertile as she will ever be in her life, has shaken up a bottle of cola and squirted it up her vagina in hopes of a contraceptive effect. Following up on this claim, in 1985 researchers at Harvard Medical School reported that as a contraceptive, Coke is not it.

We went into the bathroom at a party, and one of the other girls showed us how to shake up a Coke and use it for birth control. You get it real fizzy, then squirt it "up there." I thought I'd die laughing, but we all did it because we needed to. It wasn't so funny later when one of the girls turned up pregnant.

BREASTFEEDING AS CONTRACEPTIVE

HOW BREASTFEEDING WORKS

Breastfeeding inhibits ovulation and delays menstruation, creating, for some women, a period of sterility.

To use this method to maximum effectiveness, you need to breastfeed with frequent suckling around the clock. Your child should receive no other food, either liquid or solid. Breastfeeding may be more effective as a contraception in non-Western cultures where babies are carried on their mothers' bodies and are allowed to suckle as much as they want. (For more information on breastfeeding as child spacing, see "Breastfeeding" on page 614 in Recommended Reading and contact La Leche League listed under "Breastfeeding" on page 561 in the Resource Directory.)

EFFECTIVENESS

Effectiveness of breastfeeding as a contraceptive is 93 percent to 97 percent, but only until you menstruate the first time after childbirth.

HOW TO DECIDE

Advantages are: it's nonhormonal, noninvasive, and eventually reversible.

The disadvantage is that breastfeeding is useful only as a short-term contraceptive for nearly all U.S. women, because most breastfeeding women in this country wean their babies from the breast by three months. Some breastfeeding mothers do not menstruate for nine to 12 months, and occasionally for 18 or 24 months, after the baby is born. For these mothers, breastfeeding can be a natural form of child spacing. Other mothers menstruate when their babies are three months old, in spite of giving the babies nothing but breast milk. And 3 to 7 percent of breastfeeding women never have a period before they conceive again.

*B*reastfeeding was wonderful child spacing for me. My kids were two and three years apart, and during those years I didn't have to deal with other birth control. Of course, I breastfed my three children for nearly two years each, and I'm sure most mothers aren't interested in doing that.

I asked a doctor if I could conceive while breastfeeding, and he said there was probably only one chance in a million of my getting pregnant without having a period first. Little did I know then how little he knew. I got pregnant a few months later while breastfeeding without a period. My two kids are 20 months apart.

FUTURE CONTRACEPTIVES

Research and development funding of new contraceptives in the United States has declined, in part on account of IUD lawsuits and family planning politics. In spite of that, there are new products and updated versions of old ones in the offing.

What's often underestimated with contraceptives of the future is side effects. That's because it's not until millions of women use products that a true measure can be made of consequences. However, it's likely that the side effects of the future birth-control products listed below will be similar to those of the current contraceptives using the same chemicals or techniques. The following products and procedures are still experimental and some of them may never be available in the United States.

• *Skin implants—hers and his.* Copronor is an implant that is absorbed into the body and prevents pregnancy for 18 months, while another implant, Uniplant, provides birth control for 12 months. A 90-day biodegradable capsule that would be implanted into a man's arm that works by reducing sperm count is being studied as well.

• *Female condoms.* The Women's Choice Female Condomme is a sheath like the Reality condom that is inserted tampon fashion with a reusable plastic applicator. The Unisex Condom is in essence a latex panty which is held in place with thin latex straps that fit much like a bikini. It has a built-in rolled pouch that fits over the vagina and which is partly pushed into the vagina before intercourse. Manufacturers say it can be worn by both women and men.

• *Made-to-order cervical cap.* This is a cervical cap designed for a woman's own cervix. It would come with a built-in, one-way flow for menstrual blood and could be left in place indefinitely.

• *Disposable diaphragm.* "Once" is a use-once and throw-away diaphragm that comes in four sizes with its own premeasured spermicidal gel. Similar in design and expense to the TODAY sponge, each Once will cost $1 to $2.

• *Female sterilization without surgery.* A new, simpler method could be performed in a doctor's office under local anesthesia rather than general anesthesia, which always has more risk. Instead of making a small incision in the abdomen, a physician would use a special probe fitted with a flexible light which would be inserted through the cervical canal. This would allow the physician to see and block off the opening of each fallopian tube.

• *Reversible vasectomy.* A shug, which consists of two silicone plugs held together by a nylon suture, is a device designed to block sperm transport. It is surgically implanted and can be removed later. (See "Breast Implants" on page 302 for side effects of silicone.)

• *Nasal spray.* A synthetic hormone that mimics the secretions of the pituitary gland is sniffed once a day to inhibit ovulation. Reports on side effects are mixed. Although dosage may be difficult to regulate, researchers in Scotland and Sweden report good results. But that sniff currently costs $400 per month.

• *Vaginal ring.* Developed by the World Health Organization, this product is a combination of diaphragm and Pill. It's a circular ring, which contains chemicals used in the Pill, and it is inserted into the vagina, just like a diaphragm. Like the Progestasert IUD, hormones leak out through the plastic and are absorbed into the body. This ring can be left in for three weeks and taken out the fourth. The chemical dosage is lower than that in the Pill, so the ring may have fewer side effects as a result.

• *Once-a-year shots — hers and his.* Research is going on in several countries to develop contraceptive vaccines that would cause the body to reject any pregnancy that forms. A woman would get a single injection once a year or so, rather than taking a Pill every day. Theoretically, there would be fewer side effects than those associated with the Pill. Another version of this is a monthly shot for the same purpose. The World Health Organization is sponsoring research on a male vaccine, potentially reversible, that blocks sperm from fertilizing eggs.

• *Arm-patch birth control.* Similar to the transdermal patch used for estrogen replacement therapy (see "Estrogen Replacement Therapy" on page 337), this contraceptive patch would slowly release hormones through the skin and into the circulatory system and would be changed every seven days.

• *Male pill.* One version of the male Pill, which has been researched in China, uses a cottonseed derivative, gossypol. It causes sperm count to drop below impregnating levels and renders remaining sperm nearly immobile. Fertility returns in about three months. A major side effect is permanent sterility in as many as 20 percent of men who take it.

• *Male 90-day shot.* Tests in several countries began in 1987 for a contraceptive using a synthetic version of testosterone. Another version is a high-dosage Pill using testosterone to suppress sperm production.

• *Male plug.* This is a polyurethane gel plug that is inserted into the sperm duct to reduce the sperm count to almost zero. The plug is removable and is being tested in China.

BLADDER INFECTION: *see* Urinary Tract Infections (UTIs)

Breast Lumps

What They Are

Breast lumps (erroneously also known as fibrocystic breast disease) are those that contain one or more harmless, often painful, pockets of fluid. They are not cancerous. Most women have noncancerous breast lumps at some time during their years of menstrual cycles. They are a more intense version of the breast tenderness that many women feel premenstrually from their teen years.

A less common kind of noncancerous breast lump is fibroadenoma. This kind of lump is smooth, round, solid and movable. It nearly always occurs to women younger than 25, and may well require a biopsy and surgical removal, as these lumps don't go away on their own. They are not, however, considered a precursor to cancer.

Signs and Symptoms

Symptoms of breast lumps vary from mild to severe and include: tenderness (perhaps pain) in one or both breasts, especially near the arms; breast

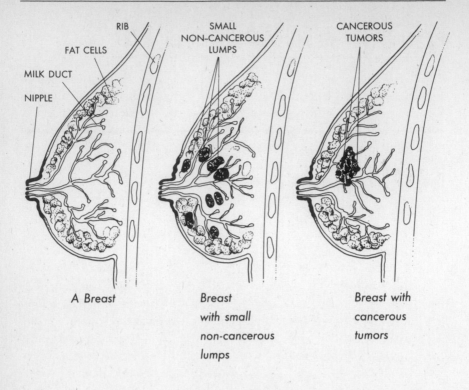

RIB
FAT CELLS
MILK DUCT
NIPPLE

SMALL
NON-CANCEROUS
LUMPS

CANCEROUS
TUMORS

A Breast

*Breast
with small
non-cancerous
lumps*

*Breast with
cancerous
tumors*

BREAST LUMPS

fullness; and lumps that come before a menstrual period and go away a day or two after it starts.

MAKING THE DIAGNOSIS

If there's some doubt about whether a breast lump is benign, depending on its location and how it feels, an ultrasound can be taken to discover whether this lump is hollow (suggesting a harmless lump) or solid. Another option is a needle aspiration: A needle is inserted into the lump and fluid removed. This is performed in your doctor's office. Often this will make the fluid disappear altogether. Biopsy, in which a sample of breast tissue is removed and examined under a microscope, is the most thorough option, because it provides the most reliable answers.

The cause of breast lumps is unknown, but they are not a disease and they do follow the pattern of normal hormonal fluctuations.

PREVENTIVE MEASURES YOU CAN TAKE

The following guidelines may help you reduce or eliminate breast lumps and are in any case healthful steps to take. Research findings on some of these suggestions are mixed. If the addition or subtraction of any of these approaches is going to work for you, you'll probably notice some improvement after several months. With this caveat in mind:

• *Reduce dietary fat* (some say to 25 percent or less of your food intake). Dietary fat, it's believed, triggers the secretion of lump-producing hormones. (See "How to Find Fat in Your Food" on page 29.)

• *Avoid caffeine* in coffee, tea, chocolate, colas, and in many over-the-counter drugs.

• *Breastfeed* your babies for at least several months each. This often reduces or eliminates the problem. (See "Feeding Your Baby" on page 292.)

• *Increase your intake of vitamins E, A, B₆, evening primrose oil, and the mineral selenium or take supplements.* (See books by Fuchs, Gaby, and Hendler on page 604 in "Food" section of Recommended Reading for specific dosages.)

• *Eat more fiber and maintain a normal weight* to help your body process the fats you do eat. (See discussion of fiber on page 28 and chart of recommended weights on page 429.)

• *Restrict excess salt.*

• *Exercise* to stimulate circulation to your breasts. (See "Exercise" on page 41.)

TREATMENT OPTIONS

Breast lumps usually stop altogether after menopause, unless you take estrogen replacement therapy, and may subside if you breastfeed for at least several months or take a low-dose birth-control Pill. It's believed that the consistently low hormone levels of the Pill are a deterrent to breast lumps. (See "The Pill" on page 181.)

In addition to the use of the Pill, these lumps may subside if you take Danazol, a synthetic form of the male hormone androgen. This drug, which costs about $200 per month, may eliminate severe breast lumpiness and pain, but possible side effects are the elimination of your menstrual periods, weight gain, facial hair, and rarely, voice deepening. There are other drugs (gestrinone, tamoxifen, and bromocriptine) used to eliminate severe breast lumps, but Danazol is the most common.

How to Avoid Anxiety over Breast Lumps

The biggest problem with harmless breast lumps is the anxiety they cause. Symptoms of benign breast disease and cancer can be the same. Here are suggestions on how to reduce or avoid cancer anxiety:

• *Remember that 80 to 90 percent of all breast lumps are noncancerous.*
• *Know the difference between noncancerous and cancerous lumps.* That knowledge may give you more assurance. Harmless lumps are tender, soft, and fluid filled, and they tend to be most painful before your period. Cancerous lumps are often (although not always) painless, hard, and not affected by the menstrual cycle. (See Love's book on page 613 in Recommended Reading for a thorough discussion of cancerous and noncancerous breast lumps.)
• *Go to your health care provider and get an opinion* if you think you have a suspicious lump. And while you're there, have her describe to you what you should look for in breast lumps. Not going and trying to push your worry into your subconscious makes your anxiety bloom. Take someone with you who will be supportive of you and who will take notes on what's said. (You may be too upset to listen accurately.) Also, if a friend comes with you, you're more likely to keep the appointment.

I was scared to death, because I was positive my time had come. My doctor performed a needle aspiration on my breast lump, and the wait for the results was agonizing. When she told me I didn't have cancer, I was very grateful to her.

Breastfeeding: *see* Childbirth

Bulimia: *see* Eating Disorders

Cancer

What It Is

Cancer is a group of more than 100 diseases, each of which causes cells to grow and divide in an abnormal way.

Following is a list of the seven most common cancers, listed in order of overall prevalence for U.S. women.

Breast Cancer

This is the most frequently diagnosed cancer in women, and the second leading cause of cancer death. Symptoms are: breast lump (usually painless), skin dimpling, persistent skin irritation, bloody nipple discharge, and/or persistent pain or tenderness. Although breast cancer's cause(s) are not clear, known risk factors (which account for only one fourth of diagnosed breast cancers) are: family history (though this risk decreases with age), late childbearing, x-rays of the breast, exposure to the pesticide DDT, and use of diethylstilbestrol (DES). Other contributing factors, but still controversial with mixed research findings, are: a high-fat diet, early menarche (age of first menstruation), alcohol use, obesity, teen smoking, and use of the Pill

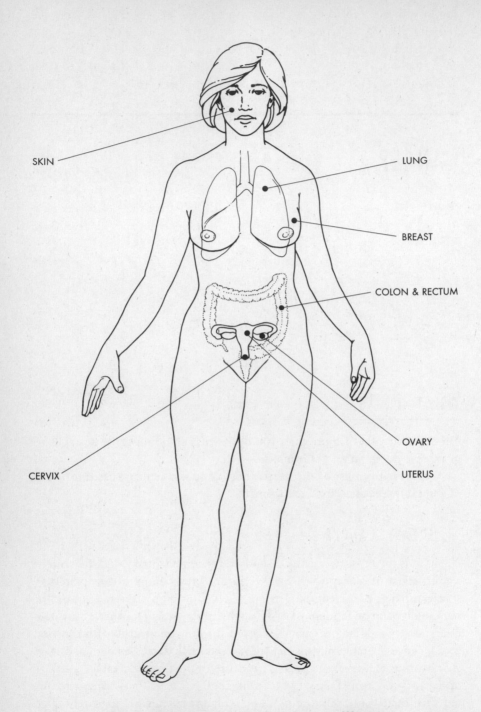

SKIN

LUNG

BREAST

COLON & RECTUM

OVARY

UTERUS

CERVIX

THE 7 MOST COMMON CANCER SITES IN WOMEN

and/or estrogen replacement therapy. (See "The Pill and Cancer" on page 186 and "Estrogen Replacement Therapy" on page 337.)

Screening methods are self-exam, mammograms (see "Mammogram" on page 100), and fine-needle aspiration (withdrawal of specimen cells). Traditional treatments are: surgery (lumpectomy and mastectomy), radiation, chemotherapy, and the drug tamoxifen.

LUNG CANCER

This is the leading cause of cancer death for women. Symptoms are: persistent cough, sputum streaked with blood, hoarseness, shortness of breath, chest pain, recurring pneumonia or bronchitis, fever, weakness, weight loss, difficulty swallowing, arm and shoulder pain, and one drooping eyelid. Risk factors for lung cancer are: cigarette smoking, sidestream smoke, occupational and environmental exposures, and diet low in vitamin A. Traditional treatments are: surgery, radiation, and chemotherapy.

COLON AND RECTAL CANCER

This is the leading cancer for women who are past the age of 75. Symptoms are: rectal bleeding, blood in the stool, diarrhea, increasing constipation, bloating, bladder symptoms, lower back or abdominal pain, unexplained anemia, and skin tags (small flaps of flesh on your face, neck, or elsewhere). Risk factors for colon and rectum cancers are: polyps in colon or rectum; inflammatory bowel diseases; high-fat, high-protein, low-fiber diet; and a family history. A possible risk factor is alcohol consumption. Screening methods are digital rectal exam, sigmoidoscopy, and home test kits. Traditional treatments are surgery, drugs, and occasionally chemotherapy, for advanced disease.

UTERINE (ENDOMETRIAL) CANCER

Symptoms are: postmenopausal bleeding or other unusual vaginal bleeding. Risk factors for uterine cancer are: menstrual problems, infertility or no full-term pregnancies, family history, obesity (particularly in upper body), diabetes, heart disease, estrogen replacement therapy (ERT) after menopause, and irregular ovulation. This cancer is screened with a pelvic exam and endometrial biopsy, a sometimes uncomfortable (or painful) office procedure in which a small piece of tissue from your uterine lining is removed for laboratory analysis. Traditional treatments are: drugs, surgery, and chemotherapy.

OVARIAN CANCER

Symptoms are: chronic abdominal pain, indigestion, postmenopausal vaginal bleeding, difficult or frequent urination, back pain, weight gain, nausea, and vomiting. Risk factors for ovarian cancer are: family history of breast or ovarian cancer (especially sister-sister or mother-daughter links), childlessness (the more children you have, the lower your risk), personal history of breast or colorectal cancer, history of menstrual problems or infertility, history of therapeutic radiation to the pelvis or trunk, history of regular use of talcum powder on underwear, sanitary napkins, or diaphragms, and perhaps use of fertility drugs. This cancer is usually screened with a pelvic exam and ultrasound. Traditional treatments are: surgery, chemotherapy, occasionally radiation, and the drug Taxol.

CERVICAL CANCER

Symptoms are: unusual vaginal discharge, urinary complaints, pain in lower pelvis, constipation, and bleeding with intercourse. Risks for cervical cancer are: teen sex, more than three sex partners, herpes or genital warts, dysplasia (deformed cells, which, if left untreated, may lead to cervical cancer), and smoking. Another risk factor for cervical cancer is having a mother who took DES during pregnancy. (See "Herpes" on page 494, "Genital Warts" on page 495, and "Diethylstilbestrol" on page 309.) Vaginal douching more than once a week is a risk factor for cervical cancer, and it has other disadvantages, too. It's associated with increased risk for pelvic inflammatory disease and ectopic pregnancy. Cervical cancer is screened with a Pap smear (see "Pap Smear" on page 105). Traditional treatments are: surgery (often laser), cryosurgery (which uses a liquid freezing agent), the newer loop electrosurgical excision procedure (LEEP), radiation, and chemotherapy.

SKIN CANCER

The most serious (often fatal) skin cancer and also the least common is melanoma. The common skin cancers, which are many times more prevalent, are easily treated by surgical removal by your physician. Melanoma's rate of occurrence is increasing faster than that of all other cancers, and it's now the No. 1 cancer for women ages 25 to 29, due in part to a depleted ozone layer (that part of the atmosphere that blocks out many dangerous ultraviolet rays).

Symptoms are: change in appearance of a mole (it may itch, be painful or bleed easily, grow darker, thicker or larger) or an irregularly shaped mole.

Risk factors for skin cancer are: overexposure to the sun, especially week-end sunbathers who periodically get sunburns, and those who have a history of many blistering sunburns in the teen years (80 percent of average lifetime sun exposure occurs before age 20); light complexion, especially with freckles; ease of burning and inability to tan; family history of melanoma; and living in the Southwest, particularly Arizona and Colorado. Screening methods for skin cancer, including melanoma, are self-exams and examinations by a physician. Traditional treatment is surgery.

PREVENTIVE MEASURES YOU CAN TAKE

In spite of the unsupported fear that "everything causes cancer" and the continuing mystery about who will get cancer and when, you can take preventive steps to reduce your risk for these seven cancers common to women. The following steps will enhance your health in other ways, too.

• *Stop smoking*, no matter what your age or how long you've smoked. (And don't spend time with other people who smoke.) Estimates are that smoking causes about one third of U.S. cancer deaths. Lungs that have early, precancerous changes will often return to normal when the person stops smoking. Stopping smoking may also reduce your risk for cancers of the breast and the cervix. (See "Suggestions for Users of Recreational Drugs" on page 40.)

• *Eat high-fiber foods* (vegetables, fruits, and whole grains, in that order), *foods rich in vitamin A* (carrots, sweet potatoes, apricots and spinach), and *cabbage-family vegetables* (broccoli, cauliflower, cabbage, and kale). This reduces your risk for colon cancer. (See "The Anti–Breast Cancer and Healthy Heart Diet" on page 28.)

• *Reduce fat in your diet* (use less fat and oil in cooking; eat lean meat, fish, and low-fat dairy products). This reduces your risk for cancer of the colon and perhaps of the breast. (See "How to Find Fat in Your Food" on page 29.)

• *Maintain a normal weight.* This will reduce your risk for cancers of the uterus and colon.

• *Exercise regularly.* You'll reduce your risk for cancer of the breast, cervix, colon, uterus, and ovary. Less active women have cancer two-and-one-half times more frequently than women who begin regular exercise during their teens and maintain it later. (See "Exercise" on page 41.)

• *Breastfeed your babies.* Studies indicate that nursing reduces your risk for the kind of breast cancer that occurs before menopause. (See "Feeding Your Baby" on page 292.) Research provides a cancer-deterrent number that ranges from four months to at least a total of 12 to 18 months of breastfeeding for all of your babies combined. (Your risk for breast, ovarian, and endometrial cancers reduces as well with multiple full-term pregnancies, particularly four or more.)

• *Reduce your exposure to hazardous materials*, such as asbestos, polyvinyl chloride, and the pesticide DDT.

• *Protect yourself from the sun* and you'll be less likely to get melanoma. Use sunscreens and hats, and avoid office worker's weekend sunburn. (See "Skin Health" on page 59.)

• *Choose cosmetic surgery wisely.* Implants to enlarge your breasts will reduce the accuracy of mammogram screening for early breast cancer. (See "Mammogram" on page 100.)

• *Avoid x-rays* of all kinds, including dental. (See "Dental Health" on page 61.)

• *Use barrier contraceptives.* These help reduce your risk of cervical cancer, which is associated with the viruses that cause herpes and genital warts. (See "Barrier Contraceptives" on page 190.)

• *Be aware of the controversy over estrogen replacement therapy (ERT).* Research findings are mixed. Earlier research suggested that ERT protected a woman from breast cancer. Other, more recent research, however, suggests that ERT use may double the breast cancer risk, and ERT that includes progestin increases the risk for breast cancer fourfold. ERT also increases the risk of endometrial cancer.

• *Consider the use of fertility drugs carefully.* These drugs stimulate the ovaries to overproduce eggs, which may or may not be the connection to the increase in ovarian cancer by users of these drugs in early 1990s research.

TREATMENT OPTIONS

TRADITIONAL CANCER TREATMENTS

• *Chemotherapy.* The intent of this combination of chemicals (drugs) is to kill cancer cells or stop them from growing, to relieve pain, or to destroy tiny tumors that have traveled from the original site that was removed by surgery.

• *Surgery.* This procedure removes cancerous tissue, reconstructs body parts after cancer removal (for example, breast reconstruction after mastectomy), and/or relieves symptoms.

• *Radiation.* This treatment uses high-energy x-rays to kill cancer cells. Radiation can be delivered by a beam directed at the tumor by a machine or intravenously by injection.

If you are treated for cancer, you may have any combination of these three methods. None of these treatments is 100 percent effective — that is, none is guaranteed to cure everyone completely and permanently. However, many people are able to live a reasonably normal life for months or many years after these treatments, depending on the type of cancer and the extent of its growth.

All of these therapies damage the body to some degree. Chemotherapy often results in at least temporary hair loss and low levels of hemoglobin, the oxygen-carrying cells in the blood, leaving you vulnerable to infections. Cancer surgery can sometimes cause a deformity, and radiation causes nausea, vomiting, and an increased risk for other cancers. Furthermore, there are no absolute guidelines for treatment of certain cancers, such as cancer of the breast. Often what is recommended depends on where you live.

(See "Cancer" on page 555 in the Resource Directory for organizations to call for the most up-to-date information on effective treatments. See also Dollinger on page 614 in Recommended Reading for detailed information about traditional cancer treatments.)

A NOTE ABOUT LUMPECTOMIES VERSUS MASTECTOMIES

Research continues to show that lumpectomy (removal of the lump) plus radiation is as effective in the treatment and cure of most cases of breast cancer as a mastectomy (complete removal of the breast with perhaps lymph glands from underneath the arm).

Many doctors would rather do the mastectomy, however. They may feel more secure ("for sure I'll get it all") or just more at home with an operation that is more familiar. Or it may be that a mastectomy is the preferred treatment in their part of the United States. However, women who have had a mastectomy often feel regret, whereas most women who have had a lumpectomy do not. If you want a lumpectomy and it is appropriate for your kind of breast cancer, find a surgeon both experienced and comfortable with this procedure.

COMBINING CONVENTIONAL AND ALTERNATIVE CANCER THERAPIES

Since all cancer treatments have mixed results and not all women prefer the same therapies, an unknown number of women who have cancer experiment with a variety of treatments. They may work with several health care providers at the same time, while using both conventional and alterna-

LUMPECTOMY

Lumpectomy removes only cancerous tissue

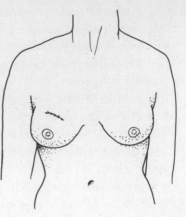

SIMPLE MASTECTOMY

Simple mastectomy removes breast and sometimes portion of underarm lymph nodes. (See the "Immune System" illustration on page 10 for view of lymph nodes.)

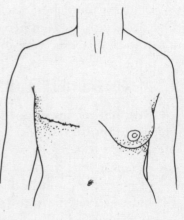

RADICAL MASTECTOMY

Radical mastectomy removes breast, chest muscles, and chest and underarm lymph nodes.

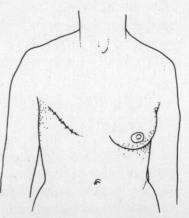

tive options. As with other difficult-to-treat diseases, the woman who is most likely to combine therapies believes she has the right to do this, acts with confidence and persistence, and can pay medical fees, either from insurance or personal income.

Acupuncture may relieve the pain of the cancer itself and the nausea of traditional treatment, and it may also strengthen organs and enhance healing. Visualization or guided imagery has been known to boost the immune system, and meditation is used for pain relief. (See "Acupuncture" on page 82, "The Immune System" on page 9, and "Meditation" on page 59. See also "Alternative Medicine" on page 609 and *Unconventional Cancer Treatments* on page 614 in Recommended Reading for a comprehensive U.S. government review.)

I rely on deep spiritual faith, believing it the ultimate source of all healing. After having provided myself with the best medical care available, I also successfully used visual imagery, meditation, and other life-affirming, stress-reducing techniques that enhance the immune system. After all, God helps those who help themselves.

HOW TO GET THE BEST CANCER TREATMENT FOR YOU

Since there are no absolutes in cancer treatment, your personal preferences are important. Try to choose a treatment you believe in wholeheartedly, since this may boost your chances of successful treatment.

• *Expect to be overwhelmed when you're given a diagnosis of cancer.* Nearly everyone is, that's normal. It's also quite usual to feel hopeless and helpless, but with the support of friends and family and a review of your options, that will probably pass.

• *Get a second opinion* because of the variety of treatment options available and to avoid an inaccurate diagnosis or inadequate treatment. According to government research, most cancer patients do not get up-to-date treatments. In addition, the "gospel" of correct treatment changes, and good physicians give conflicting advice. (See "Second Opinion" on page 95 and also "Second Surgical Opinion Program" on page 596 in the Resource Directory.)

• *Call the National Cancer Institute (NCI) Hot Line* (see NCI in "Cancer" on page 556 in the Resource Directory). They can answer your questions about any cancer and send you printed information. They offer information about where to obtain second opinions, direct you to locations of clinical trials, and access the P.D.Q. (Physician's Data Query) computerized data base, which describes the latest cancer treatments. (See other toll-free listings in the same section.)

• *Don't rush into treatment, unless that's your style.* Many women think that the quicker they do something, the better everything will be. But cancer doesn't always grow that quickly unless it has reached a critical mass. Breast cancer, for instance, is usually slow growing and may go undetected for 10 to 20 years. You have several weeks to think through what your options are, if you want to do that. Specialists say that if you wait much longer than a month to decide what to do, however, you may feel worse on account of anxiety.

• *Choose a doctor whose style and gender is what you want.* After you've gotten at least a second opinion, you'll need to choose a physician to guide your treatment. Some women want a woman doctor. If that's you, find one. Some women prefer a doctor who is reserved, others want a doctor to be openly friendly. Find a doctor you like, because you'll be spending a lot of time with this person, and her attitude can affect how you feel. (See "Choosing the People" on page 86.)

• *Know your own style and do what you want.* Some women, especially older women, prefer to let a doctor make their medical decisions. If that's the way you like it, it's okay for you to say no to your children or to your friends who want you to try something else. On the other hand, some women want a doctor who will explain all options in detail so they can make up their own minds. When it's your cancer, you choose.

• *Prepare yourself for cancer treatments.* Preparation may help the treatment go better and speed your recovery. (See "Surgery" on page 95.)

• *Talk with other women who have had cancer,* especially the same kind that you have. They can tell you about recovery and what's helpful and what's not.

• *Choose a doctor who is very experienced in dealing with your kind of cancer.*

I became intimately acquainted with the physical manifestations of fear. There are several of them. There's the blocked feeling in your windpipe and throat that threatens to choke off your breath. There's the sudden weakness in the legs that causes you to stumble, walking up the steps.

My husband and I are professional people and we are accustomed to making decisions. But when we got the diagnosis back, we were frozen. We didn't know anything. We were like helpless babies.

Until I was diagnosed, I had no idea what the treatment options and survival rates were, and I was forced to make important decisions quickly and under great pressure from a physician who wanted me to accept his choices.

I knew that breast cancer was a real possibility for me because my mother and sisters all had it, and I was beginning to get suspicious lumps. I had more time to investigate options than most women, because I was thinking ahead. I read a great deal about breast cancer, and researched the procedure that I thought best for me. I talked to a number of physicians, but in the end, I decided. I was the one in tune with my problem.

My sister-in-law discovered that she had cancer with a mammogram, had a biopsy and a lumpectomy — all within 48 hours. Now all she has left is radiation therapy. That's how I would want to do it — fast, get it over with. I wouldn't want time to think about it and worry about how I have cancer. Once it's cut out, cancer no longer exists.

A friend knew that she had a good chance of having breast cancer, so that when her doctor told her the bad news, she was not totally shocked. She took two weeks to sort through her options, and her whole family helped. She called the cancer information 800 number to get information about breast cancer, as well as the names of specialists and treatment centers. Her children investigated alternative therapies, and her husband always went with her to interviews.

I switched doctors because I like working with people who are nice, informal, and relaxed — and happy to see me. It took some looking to find this person, but I feel better already.

When I discovered that I might have ovarian cancer, I asked my young doctor, whom I liked a lot, how many of these particular operations she had performed. When she said dozens, I decided to find someone who had performed hundreds. I found that person and she had more options for me.

WHICH WOMEN WITH CANCER HAVE THE BEST OUTCOME?

Some women have better cancer survival rates than others. Here are some factors that contribute to cancer survival:

• *Race.* More white women survive cancer than women of other races who have cancer, but this is due to socioeconomic differences, not racial differences. (See Chapter 5 on page 113.) However, Latina women are statistically the least likely to have cancer.

• *Support from others.* Women who have family, friends, and therapy groups to help them often recover sooner. Even knowing that, we may feel reluctant to ask for help. Many of our friends may want to help, but don't know what to do. Ask them to do specific things: spend time with you, take over projects, or whatever. Another option is to meet with other women like yourself in self-help groups or group therapy.

• *Diet.* Research shows that an especially nutritious diet, plus vitamin and mineral supplements, will speed your recovery.

I learned I could handle a lot with the help of my family and friends. Someone was with me all the time I was in the hospital. We made arrangements with the hospital to bring in an extra bed at night.

I wished people would have called me during the months I was getting cancer treatment. My mother taught us not to call people when they were sick, but I have to say I found out that wasn't right — not right at all. My husband needed support, too. It would have been nice for someone to have asked him how he was feeling. Now when I hear about someone being sick, I call that person.

CANCERPHOBIA

At current rates, four out of five women will never have cancer. Yet only AIDS has more women fearful than cancer, and less than 1 percent of all U.S. women have been diagnosed with AIDS. Cancer is not the leading killer of women, heart disease is. Yet heart disease doesn't seem to cause the same amount of angst. That may be because heart disease statistics have not been converted into the one-in-nine risk that we see associated with breast cancer. That statistic is a theoretical quantification of what would happen if all women lived to be 110, and as such it is misleading. We are not all equally likely to get breast cancer (or heart disease, or AIDS). Most women who have breast cancer are in their 60s and 70s. The highest possible risk of getting breast cancer in any given year is rarely greater than 1 percent, and your chances of dying from breast cancer are even less.

Cancerphobia, which has existed since ancient times, is fueled by the mystery of breast cancer in particular. Most women who have breast cancer do not have known risk factors, which contributes to our feeling of powerlessness over this disease. However, nearly 90 percent of women will never have breast cancer. Moreover, cancer is increasingly something women are living with. More than half and perhaps as many as three fourths of all women who have been treated for breast cancer are cured.

A 20-year-old student of mine came to me in a panic because she was worried that a mammogram she was scheduled to have would show that she had cancer. When I attempted to reassure her that breast cancer was unlikely in a 20-year-old, she was quite sure it could happen to her because it happened to Reagan's wife, didn't it?

Carpal Tunnel Syndrome (CTS)

What It Is

Carpal tunnel syndrome (CTS) is a painful condition in the wrist and forearm. It is caused by swelling of the connective tissue, which is in the shape of a tunnel surrounding the carpals (wrist bones) resulting in the compression of the median nerve at the wrist. (See the musculoskeletal illustration on page 16 for the location of the carpals.)

Signs and Symptoms

Symptoms of CTS may be mild or severe. They are: intermittent numbness; tingling or pins-and-needles sensations in thumb, index, and middle finger; pain that can radiate to elbow, upper arm, and shoulder; burning sensation in the fingers; and weakness of the thumb. Symptoms are often worse at night. Some women with these symptoms do not have CTS and may have, instead, one of many other conditions, including pinched nerves in the neck.

MAKING THE DIAGNOSIS

The presence of CTS in the early stages can be evaluated by physical examination, performed by an experienced physician, along with an apparatus that uses an electrical stimulus to detect inflamed or irritated nerves.

Thumb muscle deterioration can be confirmed by an electromyogram test, which measures the electrical activity in muscles, or can be diagnosed with ultrasound (see "Ultrasound" on page 476) or magnetic resonance imaging (MRI).

CAUSES

According to most experts, repetitive wrist flexing and grasping motions — five in particular — cause the nerve damage that results in carpal tunnel syndrome. This condition and other repetitive motion traumas are the fastest-growing U.S. occupational hazard.

Carpal tunnel syndrome is more common in women, especially those who are pregnant, who have edema, or who have a history of premenstrual bloating (see "Pregnancy" on page 447 and "Premenstrual Syndrome" on page 408).

Some research has also shown a link between CTS and women who have a history of gynecologic surgery, particularly hysterectomy and perhaps oophorectomy (removal of the ovaries). Natural menopause is not associated with an increased risk for CTS. (See "Hysterectomy and Oophorectomy" on page 354.)

CTS shows up most often among assembly-line workers, those who use vibrating equipment, and grocery store checkout clerks, particularly those using electronic scanners. It's estimated that as many as one in ten Americans will develop CTS, but in some studies, a majority of clerks who use electronic scanners report CTS symptoms. That's because they may be checking up to 600 items per hour, or perform 10 of these repetitious movements per minute.

CTS also affects people who work for long periods of time at the keyboards of typewriters or video display terminals, as well as people who repeat the same actions with their hands — for example, butchers, musicians, packers, cooks, housewives, and carpenters. It may also be related to repeated use of the wrist in racquetball and handball. (See "Carpal Tunnel Syndrome" on page 614 in Recommended Reading.)

I had to change jobs when I became pregnant because my wrist bothered me too much. Instead of checking groceries, I worked in the office, and the pain went away in several weeks.

PREVENTIVE MEASURES YOU CAN TAKE

• *Change jobs if your CTS is caused by repetitive motion.* Of course, that's not always possible. Try changing the way you do the repetitive motion to avoid putting pressure on the median nerve of the wrist.

• *Ask a physical therapist to show you the correct position in which to perform a motion to avoid CTS.* Some women make sure their wrist is straight, not twisted. But if you're not sure, a physical therapist can show you as well as help you evaluate your posture and demonstrate helpful hand-and-wrist exercises.

• *Rest more*, thereby reducing the frequency of the motion. If your onset occurs during the last trimester of pregnancy, CTS is likely to disappear after you have given birth.

• *Take vitamin B_6*, a vitamin necessary for the health of the carpal tunnel. Although this solution doesn't work for everyone, in some studies as many as 30 to 40 percent of those women who try vitamin B_6 recover, especially if their hand muscles have not lost strength yet. Some women with CTS, especially those whose blood originally showed a deficiency in B_6, are relieved within two to six weeks. (See books by Gaby and Colbon on page 604 in "Food" section of Recommended Reading for information on the careful use of this vitamin.)

TREATMENT OPTIONS

A wrist splint, which allows the fingers to move but holds the wrist still, is sometimes used to minimize pressure on the nerves. Sometimes this solves the problem in a day or two, and other times it doesn't work at all. Anti-inflammatory drugs or injections of cortisone into the wrist to reduce swelling are also used. A possible risk of this approach is the danger of the needle being inserted incorrectly, causing damage to the wrist. Drug side effects are also possible. This therapy works best when symptoms have been short term. In a British study, postmenopausal women had CTS symptoms relieved by taking estrogen replacement therapy (see "Estrogen Replacement Therapy" on page 337).

Surgery is sometimes used as a last resort to free the pinched nerve, relieving pressure. This is an option that will work only once. About 5 percent of people with CTS might require it after all other options have been exhausted. After surgery, the hand will be bandaged for two weeks with limited movement for the following four to six weeks. Surgery usually improves hand and wrist function, although a possible after-effect is lingering fingertip numbness. Also, according to one 1991 study, about one third of people who had CTS surgery reported significant scar pain and weakness two years after surgery.

Childbirth

Vaginal Birth

What It Is

During vaginal childbirth, a baby is born through the mother's birth canal, or vagina. "Natural" childbirth usually refers to a vaginal birth that occurs without drugs. (See "Cesarean Birth" on page 267.)

Following is a description of the five phases of labor; questions to ask prospective birth attendants and birth place employees in your search for a good and safe birth; a description of common hospital procedures; the old and new ways of knowing your due date; information about babies that come early or late; and a topic about which most women can't know too much — suggestions on how to get pain relief.

The Five Phases of Labor

Labor is divided into five phases. You may or may not experience them all, and you may or may not experience them in the usual way.

Part 1 is the latent phase, the least intense and the longest. At the end of this phase, the cervix is opened to the width of three to four centimeters (at 10 centimeters the cervix is dilated enough for the baby to totally emerge). Sensations may be mild contractions, menstrual-like cramps, indigestion, and/or diarrhea. Walk around, eat lightly, urinate often, relax, and make yourself comfortable.

Part 2 is the active phase, more intense and more brief than the latent phase. At the end of this phase, the cervix is opened to about six to seven centimeters. Sensations are stronger, with more frequent contractions and less time in between. You may now experience "bloody show," a pink, mucous discharge (although this may appear before labor begins), increasing backache, and fatigue, as well as the spontaneous rupture of the membranes (this, too, can occur at any time). Most of you will be in the hospital or birth center by now. Walk, if possible, or change position frequently, and relax between contractions.

Part 3 is transition, the most intense phase, where your body completely opens the birth canal in preparation for pushing. Contractions are very strong, seemingly continuous. On average, it takes from 15 minutes to an hour for the cervix to dilate the last three centimeters. During transition you may feel rectal or lower back pressure; you may also feel warm and sweaty or chilled and shaky; you may experience trembling, nausea, and/or vomiting. You may also feel crabby and especially vulnerable. Use breathing techniques that are helpful. Don't push unless you know you're through transition. Be patient, you're almost there.

Part 4 is pushing out the baby, which can take minutes or hours. Your cervix has now dilated to 10 centimeters. Many women feel an overwhelming urge to push, though some don't (especially those who have an epidural, a type of spinal anesthesia). Get into an upright position if you can, and push when you feel the urge. Pant or blow when you're told by your birth attendant to stop pushing. You may feel a stretching, stinging sensation in the vagina when the head crowns and a slippery, wet feeling as the baby emerges.

Part 5 is the delivery of the placenta (the afterbirth). After the baby has been born, mild contractions for up to 30 minutes will occur and the placenta will emerge.

Labor and vaginal childbirth can last from a few hours (especially when the woman hasn't noticed painless contractions early on) to many hours, sometimes days. The belief that every labor should conform to the one-centimeter-an-hour rule (that is, the cervix should dilate at a rate of 1 centimeter per hour, especially during active labor) is like saying all women should be five feet, four inches tall, because that's a U.S. average, too.

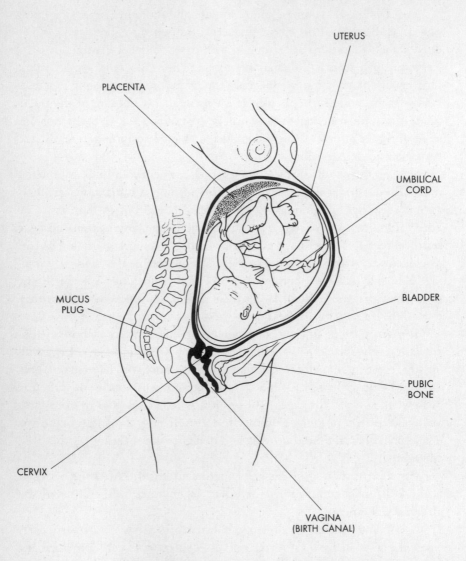

UTERUS

PLACENTA

UMBILICAL
CORD

MUCUS
PLUG

BLADDER

PUBIC
BONE

CERVIX

VAGINA
(BIRTH CANAL)

Full-Term Pregnancy

CHOOSING A BIRTH ATTENDANT AND BIRTH LOCATION

Before giving birth, you will want to give some thought to where you'd like your baby to be born and whom you'd like to have on hand. These choices are interconnected—for example, your favorite obstetrician may deliver babies only at a certain hospital, or you may feel strongly that you want several family members present, but your local hospital may have a policy against this. Or your medical insurance policy may make up your mind for you.

The question of what women want in birth, ignored through the late 1950s, has evolved into a featured position in today's hospital commercials. Words and phrases like, "homelike," "your choice," and "come talk to us about your birth plan" are common. In the United States you have the choice of two kinds of doctor (obstetrician or family practice doctor) or two kinds of midwife (certified nurse midwife or direct-entry midwife) for a birth attendant.

Following are the four choices that you have for a birth place:

1. *Traditional hospital birth.* You will labor in one room and give birth in another—the delivery room. The atmosphere is stainless steel and bright lights, with equipment out in the open and all the people probably in green gowns, except perhaps you.

2. *Hospital birth room (or private labor, birth, and recovery room).* You will labor and give birth in one room, usually in a special birthing bed. The bright lights are recessed, and most equipment is covered except for the electronic fetal monitor (see "Electronic Fetal Monitor" on page 484), and wallpaper instead of paint probably covers the walls. Be warned that the room you want may already be occupied when you show up at the hospital, unless all of the rooms on the maternity floor are like this. This room provides a typical doctor's version of a home birth and has taken the place of the once-popular in-hospital birth centers.

3. *Freestanding birth center.* This is a certified nurse-midwife's version of a home birth. Here the bed is often a regular double bed, and the rooms really do look homelike because they are often in converted homes. Drugs for pain relief are rare, and transfer to hospitals for births is possible but unusual.

4. *Home.* Here everything is familiar, and all arrangements are up to you. Most home births are attended by direct-entry midwives, although a few take place with either nurse-midwives or doctors, or more rarely with only the mate present.

Although U.S. women have more birthing choices than women in the rest of the world, more than 98 percent occur in choice Nos. 1 or 2. Doctors, mostly obstetricians, assist at nearly all U.S. births, with midwives helping an estimated 4 percent of the time (usually in a hospital or free-standing birth center). However, the number of practicing midwives is increasing each year.

Research comparing the safety of these four options is incomplete, but the studies that have been done show that births at out-of-hospital birth centers and home births (when women are well-nourished and have had prenatal care) are as safe as hospital births. A study in 1989 of 84 U.S. freestanding birth centers showed high satisfaction for these new mothers, and a cesarean rate that was half (less than 5 percent) that of hospital cesarean rates for low-risk populations. (See "Midwifery" on page 615 in Recommended Reading.) The United States ranks 22nd among nations for infant mortality, according to most researchers. Nearly all of the countries that have better outcomes for babies, which includes Japan and all of western Europe, have midwives assisting women at most births.

Healthy babies can be born and good experiences can be had in all four places. The best place for you to give birth is where *you* feel safest and most comfortable. Around the world all countries have their own childbirth culture that is perceived as adequate, effective, and safe — whatever it is. That's true in the United States as well.

Your best way to a healthy baby and satisfactory birth experience are a good prenatal diet (see "The Pregnancy Diet" on page 34), waiting until you're well along in labor before you go to the hospital, and having a labor companion (a woman-friend or doula) with you in addition to your mate. Some women worry that their mates will be insulted if a woman comes with them during the labor. Experience shows, however, that both the laboring woman and her mate usually benefit with the calm help of another person who is there just for them. In fact, women who have a doula with them (with or without a mate) have shorter labors, less use of epidural anesthesia, and fewer cesareans. (See "Bring a Friend" on page 93.)

Many of you will be limited in your choice of birth attendant by your medical insurance, but you can still research your options. When you're choosing a birth attendant, make an appointment just for an interview, not an exam. (Some health care providers charge for these interviews, others don't.) Decide in advance what is important to you. Following are some questions to help you clarify which issues matter most to you, as well as questions to ask of any prospective birth attendant (in addition to whatever questions you have about costs):

Questions to Ask Physicians

• *What happens most of the time in the hospital to the women whose births you attend?* Do most of them give birth in the traditional unit or in the birth rooms? Do most of them have a variety of labor procedures performed on them (see "The Ten Most Common Hospital Childbirth Procedures" on page 256)? If so, which ones? What do you think is the safest way for me to give birth? (The answers to these questions will give you a general idea of what you can expect from this person.) Instead of trying to persuade a doctor to do things your way, try to find a doctor who thinks as you do. Many women mistakenly believe that physicians will alter their usual care just for them. That's not common, no matter what you may be told. Doctors believe that their "usual" care is best. Why else would they do it?

• *How close are your prenatal appointments?* The closer they are, the more you'll wait.

• *What is your recommendation about prenatal testing?* Which test(s) do you use? What is your experience with these tests? (See "How to Make the Best Use of Prenatal Testing" on page 464.)

• *How many babies do you help birth each month?* More than 30 suggests this person won't have much time for you, whereas fewer than 10 suggests someone with individual time for each pregnant woman.

• *How many of those births are you there for, and how many are covered by your colleagues?* Women report more satisfaction when their favorite midwife or physician is there for the birth, but most obstetricians who are in group practices are present for only about half of the births of their patients. (This is far less likely to happen with midwives.) To avoid potential unhappiness over this, arrange to meet others in the practice who might be "on call" for you, and decide for yourself ahead of time who among them you would prefer if your physician is not there. If you don't like one of the colleagues, find out if there is a way to get around using this person. (For more information about finding "Dr. Right," see "Choosing the People" on page 86. Also see "Childbirth" on page 615 in Recommended Reading.)

Questions to Ask Hospitals

When most women choose a doctor, often little thought is given to the hospital. However, that's where most of you will spend the bulk of your labor, all of your birth, and the first day or two of postpartum recovery. And more than 90 percent of your time will be spent with hospital nurses, not the birth attendant you chose, unless that person is a midwife.

Following are questions to ask as you shop for a hospital or out-of-hospital birth center. For those of you who are assigned to a particular hospital because of the requirements of your medical insurance, the answers to the following questions will still be helpful to you because you'll know more about what to expect and will have time to plan to find ways to meet your particular needs.

• *What are the rules for the use of your labor/birth room?* Is the use first come, first served? Will I have to move to another room for recovery? Do I have to be at a certain point in my labor to be checked in? If so, how many centimeters and where will I be assigned before that?

• *Who can be present at the birth besides my mate?* A friend? My other children? Who can be there if I have a cesarean? (See "How to Have the Safest and Most Satisfying Cesarean Birth" on page 279.)

• *Does your hospital have its own childbirth education classes?* Some women complain that hospital-taught classes only tell you what you're going to get, not what your other options are. If you want to know more, seek out independent childbirth educators and compare curriculums. If you want to know about nondrug labor pain relief (a popular issue), find a teacher who is also trained as a midwife. (See "Childbirth Education" on page 562 in the Resource Directory.)

• *What is the nurse-patient ratio?* Many hospitals are short-staffed, and maternity floors are no exception. Birth centers usually have a low ratio of laboring women to nurses, and some traditional hospital units do as well. But many hospitals may have one nurse responsible for as many as five or six women in labor. In addition to calling and asking what the ratio is for the hospital you're considering, notice when you take the hospital tour if the nurses are watching the fetal monitor screens at a central nurses' station. If they are, they're not likely to have much circulating time to spend with you.

• *What are the required labor procedures at your hospital?* All U.S. hospitals have routine procedures that will vary somewhat from doctor to doctor. Some hospitals and physicians are very flexible and agreeable to most requests, but many are not. U.S. government hospital records in 1989 showed that whether women are considered at low risk or high risk for labor problems, they will all have about the same amount of intervention during labor as well as the same rate of cesarean birth. In the end, you'll get what most women get at that facility.

• *What kind of breastfeeding help do you offer?* Women who receive help with breastfeeding in the hospital report fewer problems and more nursing success then and later. "Helpful" help generally comes from staff lactation consultants or doctors and nurses who have themselves successfully breastfed or who have specialized knowledge. Many staff lactation consultants work part-time, however, so they may not be working when you're in the hospital. (See "Breastfeeding" on page 561 in the Resource Directory for referrals.)

• *When will my baby be separated from me?* What is your usual routine for rooming-in?

If you choose a birthing center, find out if there is a home visit follow-up program after you and your baby return home.

Questions to Ask Midwives

Midwives (meaning "with woman") are women who are trained to assist at normal, uncomplicated births. One kind of midwife is a *certified nurse-midwife* (CNM), who is a registered nurse with several more years of training in caring for pregnant and laboring women. Certified nurse-midwives must meet the requirements of the American College of Nurse-Midwives (ACNM). (See "American College of Nurse-Midwives" on page 564 in the Resource Directory.) Most work in hospitals, clinics, and birthing centers.

Direct-entry (formerly known as *lay*) *midwives*, who often have less classroom training than CNMs, receive their training from special midwifery schools in the United States and Europe, by apprenticing with experienced midwives, or through a combination of both. Some have backgrounds as nurses, and most attend home births, and some also go with laboring women to hospitals as labor assistants. (See *"Midwifery and the Law"* on page 565 in the Resource Directory to find out the legality of direct-entry midwives in your states.)

Certified nurse-midwives (CNMs) and some direct-entry midwives have more experience than typical physicians in helping women through their entire labor and birth because midwives are trained to be with women for the whole process. And they usually are extremely well versed and helpful with breastfeeding.

Midwives manage the health care of normal pregnant women, including health education, nutrition, and regular monthly check-ups, and will refer you to a physician if they suspect a problem beyond their knowledge. Most CNMs work for a physician, whom you may see at least once during the course of your pregnancy. Many direct-entry midwives also have a backup physician who you might see once during the pregnancy, or who will be with you if you need to go to the hospital. Many midwives work in pairs for labor, so that usually two of them will attend your birth.

• *How long have you been a midwife?*
• *How many births have you attended as the primary midwife?*

- *What is your training, and where did you get it?*
- *How soon will you meet me when I'm in labor?*
- *Will you stay with me during all of labor?*
- *What complications have you seen and how did you manage them?*
- *How do you monitor labor?* Do you use a fetoscope or ultrasound? Do you take blood pressure? How do you check my dilation and the position of the baby?
- *Does your fee include prenatal checks and lab tests?* If so, which ones? What is your opinion about prenatal testing? (See "Prenatal Testing" on page 461.)
- *How many of your home-birth or out-of-hospital birth-center clients transfer to the hospital?* For what reasons?
- *What could come up that would rule out a birth-center birth or a home birth?*
- *What kind of equipment do you bring to a home birth?*
- *What is your episiotomy rate?* How would you help me avoid an episiotomy (surgical cut between the vagina and the anus to widen the opening of the vagina)? Do you encourage the use of perineal massage? Will you show my partner and me how to do it?
- *What kind of childbirth education classes do you recommend?* For what reasons?
- *Who is your back-up if you are unavailable for my birth?* Midwives, particularly direct-entry midwives, rarely miss their client's births.
- *How many home visits will you make after the baby is born?* Midwives at some birth centers and virtually all midwives who attend home births will check you and your baby at home at least once or twice.

Questions to Ask Yourself

- *How do I feel with this person? Do I trust her?*
- *Is this person respectful of my needs?*
- *How prompt and dependable will she be with appointments?*
- *How thoroughly does she answer my questions?*
- *Of all the prospective birth attendants I've interviewed, who makes me feel the safest?*

THE TEN MOST COMMON HOSPITAL CHILDBIRTH PROCEDURES

If you envision a natural childbirth with a minimum of medical interventions, be aware that the following procedures are common during hospital birth. This list is organized in the order in which these procedures usually occur.

1. Shave of pubic area

2. Enema (Both shaves and enemas are not as common as they once were, but they still occur.)

3. Supine position on a bed

4. Amniotomy (breaking of the bag of waters if it hasn't broken already)

5. Electronic fetal monitor (EFM), either external or internal

6. IV (intravenous attachment in your arm for fluids)

7. Pitocin (the synthetic version of oxytocin, the hormone that starts labor naturally) to start or speed up labor. A newer induction drug is prostaglandin gel.

8. Drugs for pain relief

9. Episiotomy

10. Vacuum extractor or forceps to help remove the baby from your body

Most women have many of these procedures. None of them is 100 percent safe, and most are not helpful, as reported in worldwide research. Some women choose some of these procedures voluntarily. On other occasions they are performed because the hospital staff is accustomed to them (shave, enema, supine position on a bed), for convenience (amniotomy, IV, Pitocin or prostaglandin gel, electronic fetal monitor, episiotomy), or out of fear of malpractice (electronic fetal monitor). Some women ask for pain relief medication, but some women report that they were given drugs for pain relief without their knowledge — usually in an IV along with Pitocin. (See Korte and Scaer on page 615 in Recommended Reading for more information about these procedures.)

You have the right at all times to refuse treatment of any kind from health care providers, although many women are unaware of that right. (See "Your Legal Rights" on page 94, and "Court-Ordered Cesareans" on page 272.) Discuss these procedures with your birth attendant in advance, so that when they're used on you, you'll know they were in your best interests, and were not just a matter of routine.

I f you're having difficulty deciding who the right birth attendant is for you, or where you should have your baby, then someone else will decide for you. Whoever that someone is — your partner, your doctor, the person speaking in the hospital ad — choose them well. Because if you're like most other women, your choice of birth attendant and place of birth will influence your birth experience and satisfaction more than any other factor. *Find the person who has the most experience with what you want.* That's true whether you want a high-tech pregnancy and birth, or whether you're looking for a midwife with years of home-birth experience.

WHEN WILL LABOR BEGIN?

Knowing the age and size of the baby is considered essential for the prenatal tests — amniocentesis and chorionic villus sampling, scheduled cesareans, the management of premature labor, and the birth of babies who have diabetic mothers. It is of less importance for normal, full-term pregnancies of women who go into spontaneous labor and give birth vaginally. There are two methods for determining your due date, and neither one is 100 percent accurate. In fact, only 5 percent of babies are born on their estimated due date.

Determining Your Baby's Due Date

The new way: ultrasound. When an ultrasound scan (see "Ultrasound" on page 476) is used at the most reliable time for gestational dating (14 to 17 weeks), there is an allowance for a two-week error in the estimate, or seven days before or after the estimated due date. Ultrasound performed after 30 weeks has an error factor of plus or minus three and one-half weeks. In addition, the accuracy of ultrasound to determine the weight of a fetus is often wrong by at least 10 percent, and that error increases with the very largest and the very smallest babies. In spite of these ranges of errors, ultrasound is considered the "gold standard" for establishing due dates.

The old way: last menstrual date and monthly physical exams. Your due date is figured by adding two weeks to the date your last menstrual period started, plus nine months. Some women don't remember the date their last menstrual period started, or they may not menstruate regularly. Occasionally, some women get pregnant while breastfeeding without menstruating at all between pregnancies. But even if you know your last menstrual date, the formula often gives an inaccurate due date. That's because many of the calendar wheels used in health care offices are incorrect; it's a formula based on a 28-day menstrual cycle. It's likely that not many women besides Pill users have that regular a cycle. Two thirds of U.S. women have cycles that not only average more than 30 days, but will vary by eight days in the same woman over the course of a year.

A longer-than-28-day menstrual cycle is probably the reason why most women find that if labor is allowed to happen on its own with no interference, they will still be pregnant, not in labor, on their due date. This is because the calculated date is wrong, not because their body or their baby is late.

I *currently am about three months pregnant. On my first visit to the doctor, I explained that my menstrual cycles are long (approximately 38 days), but he still figured my due date in terms of the conventional 28-day cycle. The doctor now tells me that the size of the fetus is somewhat small (since he assumes the date of conception is about two weeks after my last period), and he wants me to have an ultrasound test after I'm four months pregnant. I assume I ovulated about 10 days late, since my cycle is 10 days longer. When I told him how far along I thought I was, he agreed that was the size the fetus was, but he still wanted me to have the ultrasound.*

Premature Rupture of the Membranes

Premature rupture of the membranes — that is, when a woman's water breaks before her due date — is often associated with premature labor and low-birth-weight babies (those that weigh less than five and one-half pounds). In the past, depending on how far along the pregnancy was, the usual treatment following premature rupture of the membranes was to induce labor or perform a cesarean if the mother didn't go into labor within 24 hours. The reason for this was fear of infection developing in the uterus.

A newer and safer option is not to induce labor and to wait until it starts on its own. If the mother is hygienic and no vaginal exams are performed, the rate of infection does not increase. Waiting also reduces the number of cesareans and the incidence of respiratory disease in the babies.

Premature Babies

These are the 10 percent of U.S. babies who are born before 37 weeks, and who often are also of low birth weight. Premature births are usually unexpected and traumatic and 30 percent of the time start with the premature rupture of membranes. No cause is known for most premature births, but of known causes, some are induced labors (responsible for 25 percent of premature births), giving birth to two or more babies, poor diet (including a deficiency in the mineral zinc), smoking, infections, alcohol abuse, placenta previa (when the placenta gets between the baby and the birth canal), and having a planned cesarean (before labor starts).

Other reasons are use of infertility technology, especially in vitro; untreated sexually transmitted diseases; pelvic inflammatory disease; untreated urinary tract infections; drugs, including cocaine; and being a DES-daughter.

Solutions for preventing or delaying premature births have had mixed results. In France, the rate of premature births dropped by more than one third in one decade due to the offering of more frequent prenatal appointments to low-risk women and paid work leave for these pregnant women when necessary. As for stopping premature labor once it's started (up to 48 hours or more), a common solution in the United States has been the use of drugs, including ritodrine. It's been used for decades, but it came under fire in 1992 for being both ineffective and risky. In addition, units that monitor fetal movement, which women wear around their abdomens at home, have been found to be ineffective in the United States as well in preventing premature birth. (See "In Vitro Fertilization" on page 373, "Sexually Transmitted Diseases" on page 493, "Pelvic Inflammatory Disease" on page 441, "Urinary Tract Infections" on page 515, "Pregnancy and Recreational Drugs" on page 451, and "Diethylstilbestrol" on page 309. See also "Premature Birth" on page 615 in Recommended Reading and on page 569 in the Resource Directory.)

Postdate Babies

These are infants that are born two weeks past due (or 42 weeks' gestation). No one knows how many babies are truly overdue, as there is no exact method for determining due dates and not all babies have exact nine-month gestations, nor is there a list of universally accepted postdate symptoms (though doctors and midwives usually have their own personal lists). This inconclusiveness keeps the treatment of allegedly postdate babies controversial. Research, however, shows that interfering with a pregnancy because it's "overdue" does not apparently improve the outcome of the baby. In spite of that, a primary reason for labor induction (which occasionally leads to a cesarean) is the so-called postdate baby.

HOME REMEDIES TO SPEED UP A SLOWED LABOR

Some labors are naturally slower than others. Some labors are too slow. When many hours have passed and the mother is especially fatigued, or when there's concern about fetal distress, it's a good idea to see if anything can be done to hasten the birth. (However, be aware that research shows that fetal distress as determined by an electronic fetal monitor is often an inconclusive diagnosis of questionable accuracy, unless it's confirmed by a fetal scalp test — and sometimes those are wrong, too, or the readings are misinterpreted.)

Home remedies are:

• *Stay upright as much as possible.*

• *Walk if you can.* If you're already at the hospital, ask your partner and your labor companion to help arrange for you to walk despite your possible attachment to an electronic fetal monitor.

• *Sit or stand in warm water.* Have someone help you stand in the shower or sit in the tub, so that your contractions might become more efficient.

• *Squat.* Squatting, especially during the pushing stage, shortens labor because the birth process is aided by gravity. In the centuries-old supported-squat position, someone stands behind the mother and holds her up under her arms to allow her knees to bend and relax.

• *Use nipple stimulation.* For years midwives have suggested nipple stimulation as a way to speed up a slowed labor. This is because oxytocin, the hormone that is released during labor, is also released during breast stimulation and orgasm. (See "Sex" on page 45.) Nipple stimulation is now also suggested in some hospitals. If you want to try it, you may want to forgo the electric breast pump (it can be very uncomfortable if you're in labor) you may be offered by the staff. Instead, have your mate close the door, ask everyone else to leave, and work it out between the two of you.

• *Have an orgasm.* If massaging the clitoris during labor feels good, it will reduce the pain and speed up labor.

Often a too-slow birth is helped along by the security of being with people you are comfortable with. That's usually your partner and your labor companion. Some labors slow when women get to the hospital, and that's often caused by the insecurity of being with strangers in a strange place. Labor, like making love, seems to work best in privacy.

When Pam's labor slowed and she wanted to move around, we arranged with the nurses for her to get up. They disconnected her fetal monitor strap, her husband supported her while she walked, and I followed carefully dragging the IV stand which was on wheels. We were quite a parade in the hall, but it worked.

Home Remedies to Reduce Your Pain During Labor

Pleasure and pain are not opposites. They can occur simultaneously. For example, imagine the feelings of the long-distance runner as she comes in at the end of her 26th mile, or the cyclist after a 100-mile road race. Both experience the pain and exertion while feeling the pleasure of released morphine-like endorphins (body chemicals) which cause the euphoria, known as "runner's high."

Labor is the most exhausting thing that most women ever do. And, like a 100-mile bike race, labor hurts. The pain comes from several sources. One is the uterine muscle contractions themselves having to get strong enough to move the baby down into the birth canal. Another source of the pain is the pressure exerted by the baby's head widening the path to get through. Many women describe it as the worst pain they've ever experienced. (In one large survey, only 2 percent of mothers reported painless births.) Women who use drugs report that drugs do not relieve all of the pain either. Women who give birth without anesthesia may suffer more pain, but studies show they can also experience more pleasure.

Some women experience an endorphin high, sometimes called a birth orgasm as the baby's body comes out (if forceps or a vacuum extractor are not used) when they give birth without drugs, especially those that block sensation during pushing (such as an epidural). If you expect to feel pleasure, this expectation may be self-fulfilling, so think positive. Just remember, though, you'll feel the pain, too. And that's okay. Birth is one big sensation.

To increase your pleasure and reduce your pain by working with it for as long as you can during labor:

• *Encourage your supporters to be natural tranquilizers.* In conclusive research, laboring women who had a labor companion with them and no epidural reported pain that was no different in intensity than that of laboring women who had epidurals and no woman friend with them. Ask your partner, your labor companion and your midwife (your doctor will probably not be there until you're ready to give birth) to give you help in deeds (holding, stroking, hand squeezing) and words. Ask for positive reinforcement ("You're doing great!"; "You're almost there!") only. Labors and laboring women thrive on words that are encouraging.

• *Get in a position that feels good.* For some women, that's sitting, or lying on their side, or standing, or walking, or moving into a supported squat (someone supporting you under your arms so that you don't have to hold yourself up), or getting on the bed or floor on all fours, or trying all of these. Experienced birth attendants know that you'll find your best pain-reducing position.

• *Take warm water baths or showers.* They not only can speed up a labor, but they can take the edge off of the pain. Water makes it easier for you to reduce your inhibitions and allow labor to happen. Warm washcloths, electric heating pads, space heaters, and warm socks are also helpful for some women.

• *Find out if you like cold temperatures, too.* Cold cloths on the lower back or perineum relieve pain sometimes as well. Try ice, fanning, and open windows.

• *Have someone give you a foot and ankle massage.* An accupressure point just behind the ankle bone is particularly helpful. (See Stillerman on page 620 in Recommended Reading for specific labor-massage instructions.)

• *Get a backrub.* Tell your helpers where it feels best to apply pressure. Strong force applied to a spot on the lower back during contractions using the "heel" of the hand is often helpful.

• *Plan for acupuncture and/or acupressure.* Specific points (see the "Acupuncture" illustration on page 83) are especially helpful during labor. You'll need an acupuncturist to apply the needles, but your supporters can apply the acupressure (needleless acupuncture) themselves. (See "Acupressure" on page 56).

• *Practice perineal massage to reduce your risk for either a tear or an episiotomy.* Get comfortable, and have your partner press oiled fingers back and forth across the bottom part of your vagina for about five minutes each day of your last month of pregnancy. This massage makes your skin more elastic. Whether you avoid an episiotomy, however, also depends on the skill of your birth attendant. Midwives are accustomed to catching babies without episiotomies, and they know how to support the perineum between contractions. Physicians, however, are accustomed to either giving an episiotomy or allowing the perineum to tear.

• *Listen to relaxing, soothing music,* whether with earphones and a tape recorder with cassettes or a radio in the room. This isn't for every woman, but those who like it find that it can shorten labor.

• *Use visualization to reduce the pain.* Midwives often encourage women to visualize each contraction pulling the baby down and out through the body. Practice meditation during your pregnancy so that you don't have to learn how to do it when you're in labor. (See "Meditation" on page 59.)

• *Have a helper use therapeutic touch.* This is a no-touch method of healing that involves holding one's hand several inches away from the other person's body. It may be helpful, particularly for those women who are distracted by someone touching them. (See "Therapeutic Touch" on page 56.)

• *Wear your own clothes during labor if you want to.* There's no binding rule that states that you have to wear a hospital gown, although a nurse may say that.

• *Bring a favorite thing or two from home*, like a family photo, pillow, or even a favorite scent — such as fresh lilacs in the spring — to make your room more like home for you. (See Lieberman under "Childbirth" on page 615 in Recommended Reading for more pain-relieving suggestions.)

N*o one told me about the pleasure of birth. All I ever heard about was the pain. Luckily, the baby crowned before they could give me the epidural, so I felt that pleasure as I pushed out my son. You can imagine my astonishment!*

M*y friend who was with my husband and me was great. She seemed to know when a massage or a wet cloth on my forehead would help. She certainly knew a lot more than my husband and me. And I'll always be grateful to her for encouraging me to get up and move around. It seemed so impossible, but she said she would help. Once I spent 10 minutes on my feet, I was ready to push.*

T*he midwives used acupressure points and massage for pain relief. At best it really helped the pain, and at worst it felt good.*

DRUGS DURING LABOR

However, if the pain is making your birth experience a nightmare for any of a number of good reasons, drugs are an option. Many laboring women go into the hospital expecting not to use any drugs, especially those 85 percent of women who have attended childbirth education classes. However, most receive at least one drug, while those who have a cesarean average many more. Other pregnant women swear by the drug approach and discuss their options early on with their physician.

So that you don't have to depend on the advice of strangers at the last minute while you're in labor, here are some suggestions on drug use:

• *Know your drug options in advance.* Generally speaking, there are medications for early labor (one to five centimeters) and medications for established labor (six to 10 centimeters). Early labor painkillers are usually tranquilizers, but sometimes sedatives and narcotics are used as well to promote sleep and reduce anxiety. The most popular medication in the United States (sometimes used by more than 80 percent of all laboring women in some hospitals) for an established vaginal labor (and cesarean birth) is epidural anesthesia which is usually administered by an anesthesiologist. With this procedure, anesthesia is injected into the lower spine and numbs the body from your waist to your toes. An epidural (done correctly) provides excellent pain relief, doesn't affect your alertness, will sometimes speed your labor, and usually affects your baby less than comparable drugs.

• *Be aware of the general consequences of drug use.* Drugs used in labor affect both your baby and you to varying degrees, depending on the type of drug used, the dosage, and you and your baby's individual biochemical response.

◦ *Effects on your baby.* Each drug has its potentially mild to severe effects on the baby, including the possibility of fluctuating heart rate during labor and, after birth, slower motor and sensory responses, breathing difficulty, limpness, interference with sucking, and intense irritability.

Your use of drugs might affect your baby a lot or a little, and side effects can either last a short time or a while. Both tranquilizers and epidurals can cause depression and lower Apgar scores (a quick evaluation of a newborn's condition, including appearance, pulse, reflex, muscle tone, and respiration), and epidurals can cause low blood pressure and a high body temperature in your baby.

No drugs during labor are considered totally safe for the baby because all drugs cross the placenta. Not only are babies' bodies more sensitive than ours, their brain development is not complete at birth. Furthermore, some of the most commonly used drugs have not been approved for use in labor by the FDA. Generally, it's best for your baby if you use the fewest drugs as late in labor as possible.

◦ *Effects on you.* Drugs used in early labor can cause depression in you, too, along with drowsiness, nausea, and vomiting. Although doctors consider epidurals to be safer than other forms of analgesia, they still have their side effects, including: longer labors, particularly the pushing stage, greater likelihood of the use of forceps or a vacuum extractor (many women can't feel enough to push out the baby themselves), greater likelihood of Pitocin to speed up a slowed labor, a cesarean (sometimes labor stops altogether or drug effects on the baby cause a dangerously low fetal heartbeat), confinement to bed, constant electronic fetal monitoring for the duration of your labor, and frequent blood pressure monitoring (because of increased risk for low blood pressure).

An unknown number of women have epidurals — even during cesareans — that do not take, a phenomenon called an anesthesia window. Usually this results in one side of the body with full sensation and the other side with no feeling. After birth, headaches, backaches (some persisting for a year), nausea, vomiting, shivering, and difficulty in urination are common. (See Enkin on page 615 in Recommended Reading for more information about obstetric drugs.)

• *Discuss drugs in advance with your birth attendant.* Don't wait until you're in labor to ask what her usual recommendations are. (See "Do Your Homework About Prescription Drugs" on page 74 for questions to ask.) Ask if the women she helps in labor usually have drugs. If they do, find out what kind of drugs are administered and when. You'll then have some sense of what you can expect. (Remember, what happens to you in labor will be just about the same as what happens to all the other women she helps in labor.)

• *Think about what you'll do for pain relief before labor ever starts.* If you know you want drugs and you want them as soon as possible, tell your doctor and the hospital nurses. If you want to avoid drugs altogether or for as long as possible, plan on using the home remedies mentioned above to reduce pain from the very beginning. Have people with you who know how to do these things (massage, acupressure, and so on).

Perhaps most important of all, plan to have your baby at a place where nondrug methods of pain relief are encouraged. Either work with a midwife or go to a hospital where nurses are trained to use a fetoscope. (See an illustration of a fetoscope on page 478, and a discussion of fetoscopes on page 484 under "Electronic Fetal Monitors.") If nurses don't use a fetoscope to listen to your baby's heartbeat, they will use an EFM and it will then be very difficult for you to change positions, much less move around.

• *Find out how far along you are.* When you're in labor, ask the nurse or your doctor to examine you. If you're going to be at 10 centimeters in a few contractions, you may want to forgo any medication now because you're almost there. Once you're through transition (10 centimeters), you're ready to push and most of the pain will be behind you and the exhilaration of the birth just ahead.

Should you worry about your baby and feel bad if you end up using drugs during labor? No. When we're in labor, we all do the best we can in our circumstances. And that's all any baby would expect.

---

*I*t seems it ought to be quite enough to have gotten pregnant, lived through nine months without killing the hundreds of people who volunteer precise instruc-

tions on how to be a parent, and produce a healthy baby; but no, there is more. You must get through labor without drugs.

CESAREAN BIRTH

WHAT IT IS

A cesarean birth is a major operation in which the baby is lifted out through a surgical incision in the mother's lower abdominal wall and uterus. Cesarean births accounted for 23.5 percent of U.S. births in 1991.

Before a cesarean, your pubic hair will be shaved, and you may be given an enema. Next you will have a catheter inserted into your bladder, and you will be anesthetized by either an epidural, spinal, or general anesthesia, although the epidural is used most of the time. The first incision is through the thick layer of tissue that holds the organs of your abdomen in place. Then the second incision, the one in your uterus, is made. At this point, the membranes surrounding your baby will bulge and rupture. Your baby will be born in about ten minutes after the procedure began, but another half hour or so will be spent stitching you back together. The length of your hospital stay will vary from five to nine days. (See "Surgery" on page 95.)

CAUSES

Cesareans are usually performed for a combination of reasons. They can include a previous cesarean, a slowed labor, a distressed baby, placental problems, maternal hypertension, or pre-eclampsia, a serious condition in which a woman has hypertension, as well as fluid retention and protein in her urine. She may also have headaches, nausea, or vomiting. But the reasons for your cesarean can also have nothing to do with your body or your baby. They can include the misinterpretation of the electronic fetal monitor, your choice of doctor and hospital, your doctor's fear of malpractice, your age, educational level, and insurance coverage — reasons that are fighting words to many physicians, but supported by a large body of research nonetheless.

No discussion of cesareans today is complete without mentioning "unnecessary" cesareans. The issue is controversial because in 1970, when these operations were considered last-resort medicine, the cesarean rate was 5.5 percent. Today it's nearly 25 percent, and babies are no better off. Infants in 21 other countries are more likely to survive than are infants here, and all of these countries have considerably lower cesarean rates. More babies survive in Japan per capita than anywhere else, and the cesarean rate there is 7 percent. Public health researchers say fewer babies die in the developed world today not because of more cesareans, but rather on account of better birth control, legal abortion, blood banks, prenatal care, and clean water supply, among other reasons.

Since all hospital records will indicate a valid medical reason for each cesarean, who decides and how do you know when your cesarean is unnecessary? It's confusing. Decisions for cesareans are usually grey, not black and white, but here's what some experts say. The American College of Obstetricians and Gynecologists states that 12 to 16 percent is a reasonable cesarean rate, the U.S. government prefers 15 percent, the World Health Organization says 10 to 15 percent, and some researchers claim that less than 10 percent is the ideal.

Of all cesarean births, 95 percent are attributed to the following causes:

• *Previous cesarean.* More U.S. cesareans occur for this reason than any other. Although most women are physically able to have a vaginal birth after a cesarean (VBAC), only 24 percent do in the U.S., although the rate is much higher in Europe. (See "Vaginal Birth After Cesarean" on page 285.)

• *Dystocia.* This is a catchall label for ineffective or prolonged labor, or a too-small pelvis or too-large baby. The rate of labor will vary from woman to woman, pregnancy to pregnancy. Labor can be speeded up by drugs, like prostaglandin gel or Pitocin, which is the synthetic version of oxytocin, the hormone that starts labor naturally, and slowed down by many other drugs, including epidurals. Some women find that their labors slow up because they feel inhibited by the unfamiliar surroundings of a hospital, or they are intimidated by nurses or doctors.

Cephalopelvic disproportion (CPD) — when the pelvis is too narrow to permit passage of the baby — is considered rare, and it is usually the result of severe childhood malnutrition. However, some researchers claim that women of short stature (less than five feet) are at a greater risk for CPD, especially if they are pregnant with large babies. Others claim that giving a woman that label is a self-fulfilling prophecy. What it may mean for you if you are around five feet tall and had a cesarean is that the reason listed for your cesarean, appropriately or not, is CPD. Since the average birth weight has increased only 2 ounces during the past 20 years, we do know that larger babies are not the real reason for a climbing cesarean rate.

• *Fetal distress.* Usually this is the label given an abnormal heart rate as indicated by an electronic fetal monitor (EFM). Some researchers believe that fetal distress — that is, changes in the baby's heart rate — is normal and necessary for the baby as she or he gets ready to come into the world. The problem for doctors is knowing the difference between normal fetal stress and abnormal fetal distress. Despite the EFM's use as the standard of care for evaluating this problem, there are no universal specific guidelines for knowing the difference, or when deciding the difference, what to do next. Since interpreting EFMs is more of an art than a science, the deciding factor is your doctor's experience.

• *Breech birth.* This is a buttocks- or feet-first presentation instead of the usual head-first birth position of the baby. Today about 80 percent of breech babies (which account for 3 percent of all births) are born by cesarean. Vaginal delivery of a breech baby can be tricky because the head is last to come out, but some research shows the method of delivery makes no difference on the baby's outcome.

I had a breech baby by c-section. He was my fifth child. All my other children were normal deliveries. That's why my doctor wanted to do another c-section with No. 6. He said I could die, the baby could die, or I could lose my uterus.

I thought my labor was going along just fine. It was hard work and it hurt, but I knew I was going to have my baby soon. Then the nurse came in and said that I was too slow, and that they would have to give me something to speed up the labor. That didn't seem to work, so many hours later, much to my disappointment, I had a cesarean.

My labor was going along fine until the nurse asked me if I wanted an epidural for pain. That sounded good to me. But shortly after they gave it to me, my labor stopped. My doctor told me that I would have to have a cesarean.

I had labored for many hours and got tired of hearing the nurse complain about how slow I was. Finally, my labor stopped. My husband saved the day, though. He told my doctor that we didn't want that nurse in our room again. Soon another nurse came who was very helpful. I gave birth several hours later without any more interference.

I had two cesareans for CPD: The x-rays showed an "absolutely contracted pelvis" and my obstetrician told me that "a five-pound baby couldn't maneuver that pelvis" and asked if I'd had rickets as a child. I am five feet, one inch and wear a size five shoe and size three dress. I delivered by elective section first a six pound, 10 ounce daughter and later by section a six pound, 12 ounce

daughter. From there I went on to have a VBAC; my son was seven pounds. . . .
Now, I just had another son this past February at home. He was nine pounds,
which is almost DOUBLE the weight I was told I could deliver.

The remaining 5 percent of cesarean births are due to:

• *Premature birth.* Some research shows that premature babies, especially
the very-low-birth-weight babies, are more likely to survive if they are born
by cesarean. Other research indicates that the method of delivery doesn't
matter.

• *Chronic problems in the mother such as diabetes, cardiac disease, and hypertension.*
These medical conditions do not always require a cesarean, and some would
argue that if you have a high-risk pregnancy with chronic problems, the last
thing you need is major surgery.

• *Genital herpes.* (See "A Note About Herpes and Cesarean Births" on
page 499 for the reasons.)

• *Uterine fibroids* occasionally cause the uterus to contract less effectively,
though many women give birth vaginally despite these. (See "Uterine
Fibroids" on page 522.)

• *Toxemia* often results in a very sick mother, and the baby needs to be
born quickly to avoid any fetal consequences.

• *Placenta previa* is a placenta that blocks the birth canal and often results
in hemorrhage.

• *Placenta abruptio* is a placenta that partially or completely detaches from
the uterine wall before the baby is born, thus depriving the baby of oxygen
and other nutrients.

• *Prolapsed cord* is an umbilical cord that hangs down into the vagina,
impairing blood flow to the baby.

• *Babies who are small for their gestational age* often are delivered by cesarean.
However, research shows that the outcome is the same for these babies
whether they're born by cesarean or vaginally.

Who has a cesarean is often an issue of extremes. The oldest and
youngest women have the most cesareans, as do those with the least and
most prenatal care. The cesarean rate for women who are 35 and older is
33 percent; for teenagers age 15 to 19, it's 18 percent, but increasing faster
than the rate for most other age groups. Women who have private insurance have a cesarean rate twice as high as women without insurance and
those who do not pay at all.

When women are middle or upper class, regardless of whether they're at low or high risk, they have more cesareans, especially with their first-born babies. Women in the lowest economic classes are more likely to go to public clinics where they also have a higher rate of cesareans, particularly women who have had many pregnancies or who qualify for Medicaid.

Women who go to doctors or hospitals with high cesarean rates are also more likely to have a cesarean. Some doctors are quicker to suggest that you may need a cesarean, either during labor or even before labor begins if you've been labeled "overdue."

The same is true in hospitals. Nurses in high–cesarean rate hospitals are quick to move into a "let's get ready for a cesarean" mode, especially if your labor has been induced, and you have "failed." ("Failed induction" is what is written on the hospital record.)

Cesareans are also more convenient than vaginal births. In the United States, most cesareans occur on weekdays, and the fewest occur on Sundays and holidays and between the hours of midnight and 8 A.M. Doctors generally spend less time with you, too, if you have a cesarean, and, according to a national insurance survey, they usually make more than a third as much money.

Some critics say cesareans are what doctors learn to do best in their training, rather than staying by the side of laboring women for many hours. Although there are admirable exceptions, many women in the United States report that they do not see their obstetricians until their labors are well advanced, and then only periodically. These doctors may be in the hospital at the time or in contact with the nurses' station by beeper, but they are not necessarily beside the laboring women.

The good news is that the U.S. cesarean rate has been stable for six years, putting a halt to its previous steady annual increase. Researchers who follow the relation between study results and practice claim that peer pressure in a community — what colleagues say and do — has more influence on the cesarean rate than any other factor.

---

*M*y friend had warned me to get a midwife and avoid obstetricians. But I told her that my Ob was the right person for me. After all, he agreed to my birth plan, didn't hassle me too much about genetic testing, and he even wore Birkenstock sandals. However, I was 41 weeks when I went into labor, and all of a sudden he started talking about doing a cesarean. I said I didn't want one, but after I labored to nine centimeters, he convinced my husband that I needed one.

I couldn't wait to see the baby and went to the hospital at the first sign of labor. Because my labor was slow then, they decided to give me some Pitocin to *speed it up. All that did was make everything more painful. The nurses didn't help by telling my husband that I didn't do well with induction. Many hours later, I had a cesarean.*

COURT-ORDERED CESAREANS

The controversy over the rights of an unborn fetus versus the wishes of a pregnant woman has resulted in several dozen women in at least 11 states being forced to have cesareans without their consent in teaching hospitals. When these mothers didn't agree that their babies were in jeopardy, the attending physicians all sought and received court orders, usually within six hours, to proceed with the cesareans.

None of the pregnant women was asked for her side of the story by the judge. Most of these low-income women were African-American, Asian, or Latina, almost half were single, and about one fourth did not speak English as a primary language.

In all reported cases of fetal distress in court-ordered cesareans, as determined by electronic fetal monitor readings, none of the babies showed signs of any impairment after they were born, even though at least some damage to the babies had been expected. In some reported cases in which doctors failed to obtain court orders for cesareans, women went on to have successful vaginal births. The American College of Obstetricians and Gynecologists says, "Resort to the courts is almost never justified." In spite of that statement, and information that shows the court-ordered cesareans have not saved lives, research reported in leading U.S. medical journals in the 1980s shows that about half of surveyed obstetricians said it's okay to have court-ordered cesareans.

To avoid being subjected to a forced hospital procedure of any kind, *do not be alone in a hospital*, especially if you are pregnant. Vulnerability is so intense during labor that most women can be talked into almost anything. Choose a health care provider who respects your opinions and who discusses options with you. (See "Be Aware of Your Doctor's Malpractice Fears" on page 76.)

ADVANTAGES OF A CESAREAN BIRTH

In dire circumstances, a cesarean might save your baby's life, or prevent your child from being damaged, especially when there are problems with the placenta or you have severe toxemia. Emergency cesarean deliveries can be lifesaving to both mother and baby.

Some think cesarean-born babies look prettier at birth, because they usually do not have the temporary head-molding that vaginally born babies sometimes have. However, because some cesareans occur when the baby is well into the birth canal, some cesarean-born babies have the temporary molding as well.

A cesarean can give instant relief from the pain of labor, if the medication given is both accurate and effective. (However, postoperative pain for most women lasts longer and far exceeds the pain from an episiotomy that some women experience who have vaginal births.)

If you plan a cesarean, you will have the convenience of scheduling the birth and planning arrangements for other family members.

Some believe that cesarean delivery guarantees a "maidenlike" vagina, so-named since it is theoretically unstressed because the baby didn't come through it. This is apparently a key reason for cesareans in Latin countries where the cesarean rate is 31 percent in Brazil; 27 percent in Mexico City; and 27 percent in parts of Puerto Rico. Vaginal birth should not be avoided for this reason, since the strength of a woman's perineal muscles (those of the vagina and the surrounding area) is related to her body structure and perineal-tightening exercises, not necessarily to damage from childbirth. (See "Kegel Exercises" on page 47.)

DISADVANTAGES OF A CESAREAN BIRTH

A disadvantage of a cesarean for the baby is a greater chance of being premature. Babies born by cesarean, on average, have lower birth weights and have completed fewer weeks of gestation than vaginally born babies. These babies account for the greater part of admissions to high-risk nurseries. Some of these babies were born before their due dates because of medical emergencies that threatened their safety or the safety of their mothers. However, others were probably born too soon because of miscalculated due dates or overeager doctors.

Another possible disadvantage of cesarean birth is respiratory distress syndrome (or hyaline membrane disease), a condition in which the baby's lungs are not strong enough to get sufficient oxygen to body tissues. This is more likely to happen with cesarean-born babies, especially those where the mother did not experience any labor and the cesarean was performed with general anesthesia.

Another disadvantage for the baby is the lack of stimulation from not being born through the birth canal. Many doctors believe babies are better off without the stress of labor, since they think the vagina is a source of danger to the infant's head. But others believe it is ridiculous to think that the natural way for babies to be born could be treacherous.

Researchers explain that the stress hormones, catecholamines, are secreted by the infant's adrenal glands and released in the baby during labor to prepare the infant to survive outside the womb. The infant's lungs are cleared in preparation for normal breathing, and a rich supply of blood goes to the heart and brain. These hormones also dilate the pupils of infant eyes in preparation for bonding.

Babies born by cesarean often have lower Apgar scores and other side effects of anesthesia. (See "Drugs During Labor" on page 264.) They also stay in the hospital longer with their mothers and both baby and mother are at least theoretically exposed to more hospital-caused infections. For many of the mothers of these cesarean-born infants, there is a lingering notion that there's something wrong with their baby just because she or he was born by cesarean.

Disadvantages of a cesarean for you are the pain of a major operation, including that from the healing of the incision, adhesions, and gas pains. Occasionally, anesthesia is administered incorrectly and doesn't relieve the pain of surgery. Another disadvantage for you are the side-effects from the drugs which are used immediately before, during, and after a cesarean. Little research has been done on the effect of their combined use, but some believe that the depression and psychological disturbance some women feel for many months after a cesarean may be heightened and/or caused by this combination.

Your risk for an infection after a vaginal birth is 2 to 4 percent. Your risk for an infection after a cesarean in the United States is considerably higher. Among the most common infections after a cesarean is endometritis, an infection of the lining of the uterus, which causes fever and abdominal tenderness. This occurs to one third of women who've had cesareans, depending on the physician's skill, the choice of hospital, and whether you were sick before you went into labor. The risk is higher for insulin-dependent diabetic women, and the infection rate is lower (but not absent) with women who receive antibiotics immediately before or after the cesarean and with women who had a planned cesarean, since the membranes are intact at the time of the operation.

Women at greatest risk for endometritis are teenagers and others who are poor, probably because most receive less-than-ideal treatment and little or no prenatal care; women whose membranes ruptured six hours prior to the operation; women who were connected to an internal fetal monitor; and women who had seven or more vaginal exams during labor by health care providers.

Other common infections are wound infections. The women who are most likely to have these are those who had their membranes ruptured prior to the operation, those who were connected to an internal fetal monitor, and those who are obese, because of the difficulty in stitching together the layers of the abdomen. Other possible surgical consequences are abscess, peritonitis, and gangrene. In addition, as with any other major abdominal operation, there is a risk for hemorrhage, often requiring blood transfusions. Most women lose two units (nearly two pints) of blood during a cesarean, but don't require transfusions. Other possible surgical consequences are a temporary paralysis of the bladder and bowel and/or a surgical item left in your body, which requires follow-up surgery.

Difficulty with breastfeeding is another disadvantage of a cesarean. (See "Breastfeeding" on page 614 in Recommended Reading and on page 560 in the Resource Directory.) Difficulty in movement, which is typical after a cesarean, is also an inconvenience.

Occasionally a sick baby has to be moved to a separate facility away from the mother. Usually this is due to complications that develop during pregnancy or childbirth, but it may also be a consequence of the cesarean itself.

Another disadvantage of having a cesarean is that it delays your contact with your baby, too. This may be especially true if you have general anesthesia.

Your recovery after a cesarean is slower than recovery following vaginal birth. This is due to the combination of major abdominal surgery and the normal changes in your body after childbirth, as well as the 24-hour demands of an infant who allows you little time for recuperation unless you have help. Your return to physical exercise will ordinarily also be slower than it is for women who give birth vaginally because of the extra fatigue from the operation and the need to avoid stress on the cesarean scar.

Only one third of women who have cesareans, as opposed to three fourths of women who have vaginal births, feel they've regained their physical energy in six weeks. This is particularly true if there were complications for either mother or baby. If you return to work before you've recovered, you may feel under par for months.

A lack of confidence about mothering skills is not unusual with women who had cesareans for vague reasons. This sense of inadequacy may be due, in part, to the mother's preoccupation with trying to understand what happened to her. She may not be paying as much attention to her newborn, which may also be a result of delayed contact with her baby at birth. These feelings may not linger for some women, but for others, they may. Women who have had difficult births, including cesareans, are more likely to report that their child shows behavior problems.

Some women after a cesarean feel a sense of failure and guilt, and the disappointment of unmet expectations. This may be especially true if the reason given for your cesarean was "maternal fatigue" or "inadequate labor." You also may be made to feel inadequate by others who make thoughtless or unkind remarks. When you need the most support, when you would benefit from praise and offers of help, your friends may make the worst comments. This is especially true if you've been part of the "natural childbirth" culture, those women who expect to have unmedicated births.

Fear of disfigurement, which many people feel after surgery of any kind that leaves a visible mark on the body, may trouble you, too. (Women who give birth vaginally may feel this way, also, if they have stretch marks.)

My doctor was positive that my baby was due now. I was positive that I still had a few weeks to go based on my calculation of when I last menstruated. But he insisted that ultrasound and the stress tests showed that I was ready. So I had a cesarean because my first child was born that way. When my new daughter was born, she was a few weeks premature and ended up spending a week in the high-risk nursery. Easy to say now, but I should have said no to the surgery.

Every time my baby has a bad day, I find myself thinking back to my cesarean and wondering if it messed him up somehow.

My doctor told me I'd experience some discomfort if I had a cesarean. He said it wasn't much worse than giving birth vaginally. He couldn't have been more wrong. After my vaginal birth, the only pain I had was from an episiotomy for a week or so, and that wasn't terrible. The pain after my cesarean is terrible, and it goes on and on.

I never took drugs, not even aspirin, before I got pregnant. After my cesarean, I felt emotionally unstable for months. My doctor said that was due to childbirth, so I thought it was a bad case of baby blues, but now I wonder. I've read about drug reactions and many of the symptoms sound like what I had.

The pain was so great that I couldn't bear the thought of having anyone touch me, much less a baby sucking on my breast. A helpful nurse convinced me that if I took some pain medication, I would be okay. And she was right.

Breastfeeding became impossible. It was too hard to pump my breasts after the cesarean; I hurt all over. I was worried about my sick baby, too, who had been transferred to Children's Hospital.

I wanted to hold my baby for a long time when they brought her in the first time, but it hurt too much. I knew we would get better acquainted later.

J ust saying that all that matters is a healthy baby . . . and attempting to "pretty up" the cesarean as an ordinary birth is ridiculous. It's major surgery — and it's horrible to have surgery and then have to take care of a baby at the same time. Women are truly heroic to do this.

I was tired and hungry because I'd been sick the day before. I was exhausted from the labor and wanted it to be over. When my doctor came in, she told me I needed a cesarean. She said I wasn't strong enough to go through labor. It was a relief at the time to have the cesarean, but later I felt awkward around some of my relatives because they were strong enough to have vaginal births.

I t's terrible being a childbirth educator and having a cesarean. When my friends found out, what they were anxious to tell me is not "Congratulations" or "How can I help you?" The messages that they gave me were: "Too bad you couldn't have waited a little longer," and "If you had only done this or that, maybe it would have been a vaginal birth."

Cesareans are associated with certain long-term disadvantages, in addition to the immediate challenges of surgery. These include:

• *Greater risk of death as a result of complications.* The ultimate disadvantage of a cesarean is the risk of maternal death. In a 1988 study, 46 percent of women of all ages who died in childbirth had had cesareans. Although only nine women in 100,000 die as a result of childbirth in the United States (this rate may be underestimated due to incomplete and/or conflicting reporting from individual states), you are twice as likely to die when you have a repeat cesarean and four times as likely if you have a primary cesarean. Many of these deaths are from side effects of anesthesia. Although some cesareans are due to medical complications that place the mother at a greater risk of death, not all of the cesarean-related deaths can be attributed to medical emergencies. Only some cesareans are performed because the mother and/or the baby were sick.

• *Injuries to urinary tract, bladder, or bowel.* These injuries and urinary incontinence may not be apparent at the time of the cesarean, but will show up weeks or months later. There is always the possibility of damage to internal organs, or scar tissue that may cause problems later, after abdominal surgery of any kind. These injuries are more likely after a repeat cesarean.

- *Repeat cesareans for most women.*
- *Depression* (see "Cesarean Depression" on page 281.)
- *Hysterectomy.* Occasionally, problems caused by a cesarean are severe enough to require this operation (see "Hysterectomy and Oophorectomy" on page 354).
- *Placenta previa.* Women who have cesareans have a higher risk of having placenta previa (when the placenta gets between the baby and the birth canal) in subsequent pregnancies.

HOW TO AVOID AN UNNECESSARY CESAREAN

Here are suggestions to help you improve your chances of avoiding an unnecessary operation:

- *Choose a midwife.*
- *Or choose a physician who has a low cesarean rate* and who helps women birth at a hospital that also has a low cesarean rate. Once you are in labor, you are generally committed to the style of childbirth your doctor or midwife ordinarily practices. And don't expect to discuss your disagreements in a rational and calm way. It's probably impossible to be calm and rational after many hours of labor.
- *Don't choose an obstetrician who has just been sued for not performing a cesarean.* Many doctors who have been sued for that reason readily admit that they increase their cesarean rate after that. (You can find out who has been sued at your county courthouse.)
- *Go to the hospital only after you're well established in labor.*
- *Keep upright and mobile* as much as possible during labor.
- *Educate yourself about nondrug solutions to pain relief.* (See "Home Remedies to Reduce Your Pain During Labor" on page 262.)
- *Be realistic about birth plans.* Having your doctor agree to and sign your birth plan is often recommended as an effective way to get the birth you want. And sometimes it is. However, the caveat with birth plans is that they go out the window as soon as you or your baby are perceived to be in danger. Then your doctor's judgment takes over. Few laboring women or their mates are likely to argue about their birth plan when they are told their child is in trouble.

Books and classes usually don't prevent cesareans either. Millions of low-risk women who read many books and went to childbirth preparation classes have had cesareans during the last few years.

- *Have a labor companion (a woman friend) with you* in addition to your partner. In 1991 research, the rate of cesareans was cut in half when a labor companion stayed with a birthing woman. (See Klaus on page 615 in Recommended Reading.)

---

*A*n obstetrician who was sued a few years ago was stunned. After that, he said he did too many cesareans for a while, and wishes he hadn't. Now his rate is about like everyone else's, but he has a lingering feeling that the next lawsuit could be just around the corner.

*M*y birth plan was two pages long, and it had been signed by my doctor and the nursing supervisor. But it became garbage when I was told that my baby was in distress and I needed a cesarean.

I had planned on moving around during my labor, but my doctor told me I needed a fetal monitor and had to stay in bed. I had expected to eat and drink lightly, but he told me I couldn't because I needed an IV and Pitocin when my labor slowed down. The only person who seemed surprised at what happened during my labor was me. My doctor and the nurses all acted like my labor was very typical.

I spent nine months in my first pregnancy doing all the right things, everything from exercising, and reading all the right books, to practicing relaxation and eating well. I labored on my back for 18 hours with tubes and wires in me, and ended up with a cesarean I never expected, or thought necessary. But what could I do?

HOW TO HAVE THE SAFEST AND MOST SATISFYING CESAREAN BIRTH

Some women welcome a cesarean, others are left shocked and dazed by it. Whether your cesarean was welcomed or not, learn what you can from the experience and move on. Own your cesarean. Make it yours, not something that was done to you and left you powerless. Your baby, whether planned or unplanned, born vaginally or by cesarean, breastfed or bottle-fed, wants and deserves the best care you can give. Some guidelines:

• *Have someone there just for you.* Cesarean birth is much more satisfactory if you have a partner with you. Your helper can hold your baby after she or he is born, and tell you everything that happened during the time that you were in the operating room, which is something you'll want to know. Women need to discuss their childbirth experience in great detail. If you can't do that, you may feel there's a piece of the experience that's missing.

• *Take childbirth classes that help you understand what to expect* in the event that you have a cesarean.

• *Choose a physician and hospital — for a planned cesarean — that are prepared to perform surgery when you go into labor.* Some physicians would rather schedule your cesarean at a convenient time for them, whether this means slowing down your labor until they can accommodate you or scheduling your cesarean before you've had a chance to go into labor.

• *Have every step of the cesarean and the preparation for it explained to you.* People who are prepared for any kind of surgery experience less anxiety, recover sooner, and return home in fewer days. Your helper can ask questions for you if explanations are not volunteered. Some preparations — for example, the enema, pubic shave, and/or catheter — may be negotiable. Ask that your arms not be strapped down. (See "Surgery" on page 596 and "Cesarean Birth" on page 558 in the Resource Directory.)

• *Arrange for regional anesthesia.* Women report having better cesarean experiences when they are awake, and your baby will be in better condition with regional anesthesia, too. In addition, the need for drugs will be reduced, you'll lose less blood, and you are likely to be less depressed. Ideally, you should have an anesthesiologist who has experience in giving regional anesthesia for cesareans. Sometimes you may be told that, for your particular problem, general anesthesia is best, but usually the choice of anesthesia is optional. Or you may be told that the anesthesiologist on duty prefers general anesthesia. In this case, request another anesthesiologist who is both experienced and comfortable with using regional anesthesia for a cesarean.

• *Consider listening to the music of your choice on headphones during the operation.* Your headphones can be removed before the baby is pulled out, and replaced later while they're stitching you, if the baby is no longer in the operating room with you.

• *Ask to hold your baby as soon as possible, and have the baby examined near you so that you're not separated unnecessarily.*

• *Arrange to nurse your baby as soon as possible*, if you're planning to breastfeed.

• *Have help when you get home.* That's a good idea for any new mother, but especially for you. You're recovering from major surgery and you also have the responsibility of a newborn. (If you feel up to keeping the baby in your hospital room with you, be sure to have a helper with you at all times the baby is present.)

I did everything I could to have the best birth possible. . . . The day I had waited so long for finally arrived and I was able to use all my knowledge and positive energy to work for my "dream" birth. I had a 30-hour labor (contractions two to three minutes apart). I squatted, I walked, I ate, I drank, I used a hot tub, I laughed, I cried. I did what I wanted to do. I also had a cesarean. Am I disappointed I didn't have a VBAC? Of course. But did I have a good birth experience? Yes! I was thrilled with this birth. . . . I planned for every possibility, I hoped, I dreamed, and I did everything I could do to birth my son. I had choices this time and all the decisions were mine. [Unlike my first c-section] I have NO regrets.

My husband was there in the operating room and a day or two later I asked him to write down everything that happened to me and especially to our son, up to when I came to. Those papers are precious to me and help me feel more a part of the birth.

I went into labor before my scheduled day and was given medication to slow labor until the morning when it was more convenient for the surgical staff.

My sister came to the hospital after I had my cesarean to give me a "lovebath" of help and affection.

CESAREAN DEPRESSION

Cesarean depression is very common, and yet it is seldom discussed in medical circles. Many women experience a sense of failure and disappointment for six months or so after having a cesarean, especially an unexpected one. In fact, women who have emergency cesareans experience a sixfold higher incidence of depression. These negative feelings may last many months, even years. The women with longer lasting depression frequently have nightmares and anxiety dreams that go on for many months.

Some women accept the memory of the cesarean and put it into perspective with the rest of their lives only after personal therapy or association with a cesarean support group. But we can't always expect a neat-and-tidy ending. None of us probably ever totally resolves the major disappointments in our lives, no matter what our particular list of disappointments might be, whether important love affairs or failed marriages, career reversals, lost babies, or for some women, unexpected cesareans.

Some therapists have compared the depth of some women's depression after a cesarean to the stress disorder associated with some Vietnam veterans — post-traumatic stress disorder (PTSD). In addition to nightmares, other symptoms of PTSD are jumpiness and sleeping difficulties. Although considered rare, PTSD is not limited to veterans or women who are depressed after a cesarean. Children exposed to violence, women who have been raped, battered wives, and victims of terrorists may also share some of these symptoms.

These groups also may share a lack of appreciation and understanding from others. Some women who have had cesareans are asked why they didn't try harder. Women who have been raped are often told that they "asked" for it. And many Vietnam veterans have been told that what happened to them didn't matter, because it was a worthless war. This lack of support at critical times can make hurtful events worse.

The women who are most likely to experience cesarean depression are those who:

• *Expected "natural childbirth."*
• *May have had inadequate help and support during the cesarean and/or after the surgery.*
• *May have had general anesthesia, or a combination of drugs that may have caused unpleasant side effects.*
• *Felt coerced into the surgery by the hospital staff and/or by their partner.*
• *Felt that the cesarean was mostly an operation and not a giving-birth experience.*
• *Expected to breastfeed, but found that the cesarean made this difficult.*
• *May have experienced complications after surgery or a difficult convalescence.*

Many women who experience cesarean depression found that others, including family members and some of the hospital nurses, expected them to bounce right back immediately after surgery. And that didn't happen. No one expects a woman or man who has just had major abdominal surgery, like removal of a gall bladder, for instance, to start taking care of a newborn within days.

Stress on the marriage also contributes to cesarean depression. Many women find that their marriage was intensely troubled by the aftermath of the cesarean. Infants usually don't enhance marriages, and their emotional and physical demands are great. Women who have had cesareans are less able to handle the challenges an infant presents because they are physically weakened and may be emotionally distressed as well.

On the other hand, the women who are *least* likely to experience cesarean depression are those who:

- *Want above all a healthy baby*, not a good birth experience.
- *Trust their doctor's judgment and feel their cesarean was necessary.*
- *Planned their cesarean*, or knew from the beginning that it was a distinct possibility for medical reasons.
- *Are not believers in the "natural childbirth" style of birth* and welcome the pain relief of anesthesia.
- *May have had other major events in life not go according to plan either*, and have learned to adapt.

If you think you are experiencing cesarean depression, talk to someone about it, whether friends, family, or especially other women who have had cesareans. Or contact a therapist who is both understanding of, and experienced with, women who have had cesarean depression. (See "Finding a Therapist" on page 607 in Recommended Reading.) You'll avoid the side effects of keeping your feelings bottled up, and you'll know that you're not alone.

Contact and/or join a cesarean support group. (See the cesarean organizations mentioned earlier in the Resource Directory.) They'll provide you with information and emotional support. They also give you an opportunity to help others, which will help you resolve your own cesarean experience. Some women receive emotional relief after just one meeting.

I had my first child three-and-a-half years ago by cesarean. . . . I have a few friends who have also had cesareans but I find it hard to talk to them about my feelings. They seem to have done so much better at putting it all behind them. For me, it has changed my life and made me feel awful about myself. Why couldn't I have a normal birth? What was wrong with my body that I didn't dilate after all that labor? I wonder if I am abnormal to still get upset about having a cesarean. Even now I sometimes cry when I think about it. Shouldn't I be over this by now? My husband doesn't really know how much this still bothers me. He hates to talk about it and prefers to minimize it.

I had nightmares for a full nine months. They still recur occasionally. I have incredible feelings of anger, frustration, disappointment, helplessness, and bitterness — and the intensity and depth of these feelings frighten me.

I went into the hospital in early labor wondering if I would remember all the different breathing techniques I learned for pain relief, never dreaming that none of that mattered and what I should have done was take a cesarean class.

Recovery from my first cesarean was so much easier than it was after my second one two years later. The first time my husband and my sister lavished attention on me for weeks, and I didn't have to do any physical work. After the second cesarean, no one was there for me. My husband was busy with his job, and my sister was busy with the two-year-old. Everything was harder the second time, and I now had two children, not just one.

My obstetrician told me that it was more important for the anesthesiologist to feel comfortable than it was for me to be awake during my cesarean. So I had general anesthesia to please the doctors. I was so mad. When I finally became conscious, I didn't care about anything—certainly not my baby.

I was upset that I found out about the decision for surgery incidentally when the nurse came in to prep me. I wanted to say no, but I was afraid they would put me to sleep and do the surgery anyway. Especially since the anesthesiologist had said if I didn't cooperate they would put me under with general anesthesia.

I didn't want the cesarean and said no. But my husband was insistent. He said I couldn't jeopardize his baby. I was furious then and still am.

It has been almost two years since my son was cut from me in a procedure that was not a birth. . . . First our son was taken to the nursery and kept from us for seven hours for no apparent reason. My husband, who went home to change and get my pillows, was told by a nurse over the phone to stay away from me so that I could rest—did they really think that I would rest after having my child and husband taken from me?

I told myself, well, at least I'll breastfeed. But that didn't happen either. Nothing was working right. The nurses either would not help me or didn't have time to help me with breastfeeding; my baby was under bilirubin lights; and my mother kept telling me my baby was better off on formula.

My friends have all had vaginal births, and though they were tired for a few weeks, their fatigue didn't drag on like mine. Instead of getting mad at them for not understanding, I explained to them how I felt and why, and asked them to help me with specific chores. They were great once they understood what I needed.

My husband complained when I felt wiped out for months, but he didn't offer to help.

*S*ix months after my cesarean, my husband and I were in marriage counseling. I can look back now and understand that much of the friction was caused because of how terrible I felt physically until the baby was a year old. I don't plan on having any more children, but if I ever did, I would also plan on household help for the first year.

I wouldn't have a baby any other way but a cesarean. Most of my friends have cesareans and it seems to me that that's the best way these days. I think childbirth is safer, and I know my doctor thinks babies turn out better when they're born by cesarean.

I didn't realize how much buried emotion I still had about my cesarean until a friend took me with her to a group meeting that was just for women who had had cesareans. All of us had so many similar feelings. It was great to know that I wasn't alone or somehow inadequate.

*N*ow that I'm part of this cesarean support group, I feel like I can help other mothers achieve what I didn't with my first birth. And that's become very important to me.

Vaginal Birth After Cesarean (VBAC)

Although it's acknowledged that 50 to 80 percent of births after cesareans could be VBACs, and even though some doctors have success rates of 85 to 90 percent, currently in the United States only 24 percent of births following a cesarean are vaginal. This varies geographically, with VBACs occurring twice as often in the West as they do in the South. In Europe, however, VBACs have always been standard practice because European doctors and midwives believe that the reason for the cesarean is rarely present in the next pregnancy.

For many years in the United States, women rarely had VBACs because physicians were concerned that the cesarean scar would rupture, and the mother would die. In fact, uterine scars rarely rupture, even after multiple cesareans, and the consequences are not as severe as once feared. Ruptured scars occur just 0.5 percent to 1 percent of the time. Most women in their subsequent pregnancies after a cesarean feel some pain around the scar in mid- and late pregnancy, but that apparently has no effect on the ability of the uterus to stay intact.

Not every woman wants a VBAC, nor can every woman physically have one. It's as important to have the option of a scheduled cesarean as it is to have the option of VBAC.

Although the overall number of VBACs has increased, including those of women with multiple cesareans and women having twins and triplets, the number who wish to have a VBAC in the United States is far greater than the number who successfully do so. There are several reasons for that. Women may change their minds about the VBAC, or the situation may truly require another cesarean. But what's most influential are the helpers who are with these women and where they are (hospital, birth center or home) during the labor and birth.

Here's a description of the woman most likely to have a successful VBAC:

• *She wants a VBAC and, more importantly, believes that it's possible for her to have one.* A good positive attitude does not guarantee a VBAC, but lingering fears and doubts make VBAC less likely.

• *She has a supporter or two with her during labor, whether partner or labor companion who believe it's possible for her to have a VBAC.* During labor, it's hard to keep anything in perspective. This is why committed helpers are so important during a VBAC attempt.

• *She avoids naysayers during her pregnancy and labor, so that she doesn't pick up their worries, and she associates with friends who believe she can have a VBAC.* Since VBACs are not common in our culture, most people have negative programming about them, whether they know anything about them or not.

• *She has a doctor or midwife who also believes VBAC is a good option for her.* Midwives and physicians who are successful and enthusiastic about VBACs believe your labor is like that of any other woman giving birth vaginally. They do not hover and ask how your scar is feeling, nor do they keep reminding you that the operating room is prepared in case you need another cesarean. They don't say you can have a "trial" of labor, and then tell you that it's over after a few hours. You may have to travel to find a health care provider both enthusiastic and experienced with VBACs, but they are available.

• *She is having her baby at a place where VBAC is acceptable and welcomed, and if it's at a hospital, the nursing staff has experience and confidence in VBACs.* Ask what a doctor's or a hospital's VBAC success rate is. That matters more than whether or not they say they'll let you try for a VBAC. Ask if they require a second opinion before a second cesarean is performed. (Second opinions reduce the number of cesareans — see "Second Opinions" on page 95.)

• *She has a low transverse uterine scar, not an abdominal scar, which may be vertical.*

• *Her previous cesarean was due to one of the four reasons for 95 percent of all cesareans: previous cesarean; dystocia (difficult labor) or prolonged labor (including pelvis too small or baby too big); fetal distress; and breech birth.* These conditions are least likely to have an effect on subsequent births. However, women who have chronic problems like diabetes or heart disease may continue to have the same problems that initially caused a cesarean, resulting in subsequent cesareans.

If you're interested in having a VBAC, get in touch with the people in your area who are committed to VBACs. Some childbirth instructors offer special courses to VBAC-to-be parents to help dispel their fears and to provide them with all the encouraging statistics that are available. People feel strongly about VBAC; once you start making inquiries, you will be able to find the support you need.

---

*M*y husband and others worried that I was setting myself up for a big disappointment (planning a VBAC after two cesareans). A safe, healthy delivery for both baby and myself was my first priority. If I ended up with a c-section, I would be disappointed, but I'd know I'd given it my best shot. It would definitely be better than scheduling the birth.

I am happy to say that the birth of my second child was one of the most beautiful experiences I have ever had. . . . Eighteen hours after my water broke, my daughter was born vaginally and given directly to me. I was totally overwhelmed at the whole thing. Here I was told I could never do it, and yet I did. The experience was unbelievable.

*T*his time I really wanted a VBAC, so I surrounded myself with my cheerleaders. I told them to leave their worries at home and bring nothing but praise for me.

I didn't tell my mom my plans for a VBAC this time, because she worried through my first pregnancy. She always expected the worst would happen to me. This time I didn't tell her I was pregnant until I was in maternity clothes. And now when she asks about this pregnancy, I'm very vague.

I changed doctors with this pregnancy, because I knew I'd never have a VBAC with him. He was always worried. When I told him that I wanted a VBAC, he told me that my scar might rupture and I might die. When I said that I had read that rarely happens, he said, that's true, but it still might happen to me.

My doctor promised a trial of labor, but he didn't tell me that I could labor only four hours and if I didn't have my baby by then, I would need another cesarean. Who has a baby in just four hours?

I am through with persuasion, pleading, and groveling to get what I want—a VBAC. I've found a midwife in a hospital practice 75 miles from here who trained in Europe and thinks I can easily have a VBAC. A 150-mile round trip is a small price to pay to get what I want.

My doctor was willing for me to have a trial of labor, but he admitted he was nervous about it. The nurses at the hospital were most discouraging though. They told my husband that trial of labor never works and it's bad for the baby.

I wanted a VBAC so bad that I didn't go into the hospital until I was nine centimeters. The nurses and my doctor were so anxious about the baby and angry with me that my labor stopped. And I had another cesarean. I unintentionally got pregnant again, but this time I gave birth at home with a lay midwife. I finally did it!

THE BIRTH CYCLE AND EMOTION

Pregnancy, childbirth, and breastfeeding may generate more emotions than any other part of your life. The memory of the increased emotion of these months stays for years. Some women feel energized and reinforced by giving birth. Others feel let down.

It's a rare woman who can't give you details about certain parts of her births. That's because when you're pregnant, your whole life is changing. If it's your first baby, your whole way of being will be different. Your body is changing, that's obvious, but also your thoughts, your feelings, your outlook on life. You're not just having a baby, you're bringing another being into the world. And given the emotional swings of pregnancy, it's not surprising that today you say to yourself, "I don't want to do this" and tomorrow you believe you're contributing to society.

It's natural to feel the emotion of fear at times during childbirth. However, fear can cause you to make mistakes, be anxious, and sometimes act hostile. The fear of a threatened cesarean can actually create stalled labors, "difficult" births, and fetal "distress."

Women who are past 35 tend to be apprehensive because of the erroneous belief that these women are "elderly" and prone to problems. Another group that often worries is single mothers, who comprise 28 percent of all new mothers.

If your pregnancy is becoming more of a worry than a pleasure, you might want to consider spending time with people who think pregnancy and childbirth are wonderful events. That may be your family or friends or established pregnancy and childbirth groups. (See "Childbirth Organizations" on page 563 in the Resource Directory.) That also includes the person you choose to be your health care provider.

I really treasure that first look into her eyes, and the thrill of her calming at my voice was indescribable. It was the first time in my life that I felt valuable and necessary, and my life with her since has reinforced my sense of me.

My mom had natural childbirth with all of us. Every year on our birthdays, she would get out the photo albums and we would "ooh!" and "aah!" over our birth photos. She always said that birth was wonderful, and all of us would think so, too. I was surprised when I got pregnant to hear all the worries that my pregnant friends had. Their worries started to worry me, so I decided to see less of my friends and more of my mom and my sisters.

CHILDBIRTH PAST 35

Many women who give birth past age 35 are healthy, well-educated, working professionals, which is the profile of women at any age who are most likely to have a safe pregnancy and healthy baby.

Healthy, nonsmoking 35- or 40-year-old pregnant women who do not have chronic diseases like diabetes or hypertension can give birth with as much ease as younger women. This is a controversial finding which is contrary to popular belief. If you do have a chronic health problem, that doesn't guarantee difficulties with your pregnancy and birth. It does mean that you and your birth attendant will need to pay more attention to certain aspects of your prenatal care.

Older mothers have a higher cesarean rate — one in three versus nearly one in four for younger women — but this may be in part due to some health professionals' outdated ideas. Although M.D.s can't be blamed for all the problems that some older pregnant women experience, researchers in 1990 could not find a specific physical reason for the higher cesarean rate and speculated that it was due to "conservative treatment" of women over the age of 35.

Although statistics show that older mothers are more likely to have a low-birth-weight baby, the size of a newborn baby is related more to the mother's education and economic status than to her age. Women who are poor and who have had little or no prenatal care are the most likely to have low-birth-weight babies, and that happens more commonly to these women as they grow older, especially past age 40.

Birth defects are a concern for all mothers-to-be, but there is only one defect associated with older moms and that's Down syndrome. Your chances of having a baby with Down syndrome do increase with age, but the statistics are very different at 35 than at 45. In a group of 378 pregnant women who are 35 years old, 377 will not give birth to a baby with Down syndrome. The chance for a Down baby continues to increase with age with the risk one in 106 at age 40, one in 30 at age 45, and one in 11 at age 49. (See "Down Syndrome" on page 454 and "Risk for Birth Defects by Mother's Age" on page 456.)

Having a baby at 35 or 40 isn't new; what's new is the trend for so many women to have first-borns at an older age. Until the 1970s, women having babies in their 30s or 40s were usually pregnant with child Nos. 5 or 6. Their general health cannot be compared to that of many of today's past-35 women who are having baby Nos. 1 or 2. Right now only 8 percent of all U.S. babies are born to past-35 mothers, but this group of pregnant women, whether married or single, has more than doubled in size in a decade and is the fastest-growing group of new mothers in the United States. This is not just a U.S. phenomenon; it's happening in some other Western nations, too.

If you are older, your first challenge is to get pregnant. The ability for women to conceive decreases after their 20s. Estimates are one in nine women aged 35 – 39, and one in five women aged 40 – 44 are infertile (see "Infertility" on page 364). Similarly, over-40 men are not as likely to impregnate women as are younger men. Once you've successfully gotten pregnant, you may feel more confident once you're past the point of miscarriage (usually the first trimester). Many studies show that older women miscarry at twice the rate of younger women. But some studies do not distinguish between healthy women with their first or second pregnancy and those women who have a history of chronic health problems, repeated pregnancy loss, and/or infertility (see "Miscarriage" on page 487).

Older mothers also have a higher mortality rate. Although the rate of women 35 or older who die after childbirth has dropped nearly 50 percent in recent years, women in this age group are three times more likely to die in childbirth than younger women. This is in part due to the higher rate of cesareans — major abdominal surgery with heightened risks primarily due to anesthesia, hemorrhage, and infection.

White women past age 35, however, have the same mortality rate as women in their 20s. It's African-American women who are past 35 who are more likely to die, especially as a result of ectopic (or tubal) pregnancies. (Although these pregnancies end in the first trimester, the data is included in childbirth mortality statistics.) This is not due to their race, but rather the mother's education and the size of her wallet. Lack of education and lack of income are both associated with too-little or too-late prenatal care.

As an older mother, your biggest challenge is to have a worry-free pregnancy. That's because if you're planning on a normal and uneventful pregnancy and birth, which is the ideal attitude at any age, you can't ordinarily expect a lot of positive support. Instead, you are likely to hear concern and horror stories from a variety of kibitzers, including family, friends, co-workers, and many doctors and nurses.

Your enemy is unfounded fear, not your body. New research shows that anxiety — both your own and that exhibited by your partner, family, friends, or especially health providers — can actually cause slowed labors. In this way, fears become self-fulfilling.

To avoid the side effects, both physical and psychological, of inappropriate worry (and its companion, stress) on your pregnancy and impending birth:

- *Surround yourself with true supporters, not naysayers.*
- *Educate your mate, family, and friends if you need to.*
- *Find a birth attendant, whether physician or midwife, who mirrors your philosophy about pregnancy.*
- *Do what you can to avoid an unnecessary cesarean* (see "How to Avoid an Unnecessary Cesarean" on page 278).

I changed doctors because the one that I was going to was always worrying aloud about all the things that could go wrong with my labor because I was 42. I decided that between him and my mother I needed some relief.

When I became pregnant and looked obviously older than 35, people always assumed that I was having my third or fourth child. They were speechless and concerned when I nonchalantly told them that I was pregnant with my first child. . . . Although today's trend is toward delayed parenting, 45 years old was pushing the norm. Others were so concerned about my age that this clouded the congratulations and attention I had expected as a first-time mother-to-be. . . . Our healthy and alert son Jason was born full-term.

During my pregnancy I had to reassure my obstetrician that everything was fine. Just because I was 38 didn't mean I would have a problem. After my labor started, I blew down the highway, blew while they slipped me into their little gown, and blew as I climbed onto the labor bed. About four pushes later, we had a new son. The doctor allowed the cord to stop pulsing, and all procedures on the baby were delayed until he went to the nursery when we were ready. I don't think I came down for three weeks!

I was in labor for 17 hours and it wasn't going anywhere. . . . My doctor and I were worried because of my age (37). She had told me that older women tend to have longer labors. I'd done a lot of reading that said it was safe, but I had nagging fears. I agreed to the cesarean. I'd rather be safe than sorry.

I had my baby at home with my husband, two special friends, and my midwife. They all knew I could have a normal birth and weren't freaked because of my age. I never told my parents that I planned on having the baby at home because they were upset enough that I was pregnant at 41. I figured that what they didn't know wouldn't hurt them, and besides, I didn't want to listen to their worries. I didn't need that. No black clouds for me, thank you.

FEEDING YOUR BABY

Most women today breastfeed newborns, but by the time those babies are three months old, most are bottle-fed. There are advantages to both methods. The best method for you is the one you prefer.

BREAST OR BOTTLE? HOW TO DECIDE?

Breast milk contains over 100 ingredients that are not found in cow's milk and cannot be duplicated. Moreover, breast milk is individualized to each baby. (The milk at two weeks is different from the milk at two months or two years.) Mother's milk is more digestible than cow's milk, and is less likely to cause the baby to become overweight. Your baby will not be allergic to your milk, although occasionally a baby is allergic to something the mother ate.

Mother's milk is cheaper than formula and is more convenient, provided the mother is the primary caregiver. (If you are away from your baby, however, you can express milk and refrigerate or freeze it — as many working mothers do.) Your baby is not likely to become constipated or have diarrhea and is less likely to get sick, because immunities are passed from the mother's colostrum, the yellowish fluid the mother has in the early days, and from the later milk. This immune system boost is a boon to any mother and baby, but especially the mother who works away from home whose child is in daycare. Even if you can breastfeed only for a few weeks, you'll be passing this immunity along to your infant. In addition, at least six months of breastfeeding reduces your baby's risk for developing certain allergies later on.

Breastfeeding decreases your risk for breast lumps, ovarian cancer, and early-onset (before age 45) breast cancer if you breastfeed for several months or more. (It may also reduce your risk for the more common breast cancer that occurs after menopause.) It also reduces your risk for ovarian cancer. Breastfeeding also shrinks your uterus back to its prepregnant size sooner, and the flow of lochia, that red-brown discharge you have after birth, decreases sooner as well. Breastfeeding also suppresses ovulation and menstruation for some months, usually depending on how often you breastfeed every day. Nursing may contribute to child spacing, but it's not a reliable method of birth control by itself unless you plan to have about eight or more children. (See "Breastfeeding as Contraceptive" on page 223.)

Every mother, whether breastfeeding or bottle-feeding, can get reinforcement from her senses, from the sight, smells, feel, and sounds of her baby. But the breastfeeding mother gets reinforcement from inside her body, too; several hormones reinforce bonding every time you nurse.

Some environmental pollutants have been found in human milk, but experts say human milk is still the best option because of all the advantages of breastfeeding for baby and mother. Also, cows that produce the milk for most of the formula that is sold are exposed to many of the same environmental pollutants that mothers are. In addition, some dairy cows are treated with drugs that have been found in milk samples.

Most health care professionals are all for breastfeeding today, and they encourage you to do it. But don't look to them automatically for practical help. The advice of some hospital nurses and doctors is not always helpful. (This may be because many of them do not have personal experience in breastfeeding.)

You will receive the best help from other women who have successfully breastfed. There's an art to breastfeeding that can only be gained by experience. The women who are most successful with breastfeeding have friends or relatives who breastfed.

Bottle-feeding has advantages, too. It may be more convenient for you and your life-style. Bottle-fed babies usually don't eat as often. Anyone can feed the baby, which is a help mostly for mothers who work away from home. And your baby probably won't wake up as much at night.

If you don't nurse your baby, you'll have to suppress the milk that naturally forms in your breasts after childbirth. The usual way to suppress milk is to not stimulate your breasts (that is, don't express milk) and to wear a tight bra. Use either cold (ice bag wrapped in a towel), heat (hot water bottle), and/or aspirin to relieve the pain. Many women are offered a drug (Parlodel, TACE, delmadione, among others) to specifically dry up the milk in the breasts. These drugs are often not effective and they may have negative side effects, such as a short drop in blood pressure, seizures, nausea, dizziness, and blood-clotting. Although a Food and Drug Administration advisory group called for the ban of these drugs more than a decade ago, about 700,000 bottle-feeding women annually are given these drugs after childbirth.

The nurse told me my breasts were too small, and my doctor told me that I was too little to nurse such a big baby. When I asked him how women managed to nurse twins, he said most of them couldn't. You can imagine my relief when my sister-in-law showed up. She nursed all of her kids and got me started.

I love bottle-feeding and find the idea of breastfeeding repulsive. My sister-in-law nursed her kids, and it seems like that's all her babies ever did. I work part-time and never have doubts about whether or not my baby will take a bottle from someone else. Sometimes it's my husband who feeds the baby, sometimes it's a sitter.

Chronic Fatigue Syndrome (CFS)

What It Is

Chronic fatigue syndrome (CFS), once called Epstein-Barr virus or chronic mononucleosis, is characterized by flulike, bone-weary fatigue that lasts six or more months (sometimes years) and that doesn't go away with rest and is not the result of any other disease.

Signs and Symptoms

Other symptoms, according to the Centers for Disease Control and Prevention, include any eight of the following symptoms that persist for six months or more and that developed over a period of hours or days:

- Mild fever or chills
- Sore throat
- Painful lymph nodes
- General muscle weakness
- Muscle discomfort

- Prolonged fatigue after exercise that once was normally tolerated
- Painful joints
- Headaches
- Sleep disturbances
- Neuropsychological complaints, such as visual disturbances ("seeing spots")
- Depression
- Excessive irritability
- Confusion
- Difficulty thinking
- Forgetfulness
- Inability to concentrate

MAKING THE DIAGNOSIS

There is no standard test to diagnose CFS, so evaluation begins with a thorough history and physical exam, which includes urine and extensive blood tests. As CFS has become better known, other tests, such as neuro-psychiatric testing, exercise testing with oxygen-consumption measurements, abdominal ultrasound, and cranial magnetic resonance imaging (MRI), have been used to rule out other diseases as well as to confirm CFS.

The woman most likely to have CFS is allergic to some type of inhalants, drugs, or food. In some surveys, more than half of women with CFS have allergies and about one third had a previous bout of mononucleosis, a disease that is caused by the Epstein-Barr virus and that usually lasts about four to six weeks. CFS has been diagnosed more in women than men (although the gap may be closing) and more often in people who are white and between the ages of 25 and 50, although it has been reported in infants and the elderly.

CFS can resemble other illnesses, including anemia, hypoglycemia (a blood-sugar disorder), mononucleosis, systemic lupus erythematosus (see "Lupus" on page 391), fibromyalgia (chronic muscle pain and stiffness), and rheumatoid arthritis (chronic pain and swelling in the joints of the hands and feet). What they all have in common is fatigue. This confusion occurs, in part, because CFS symptoms fit other disease profiles. In addition, many physicians are not familiar with CFS.

CAUSES

Although the disease itself may not be new, our understanding of CFS is still in its early stages. No one knows for sure what causes CFS, so no one knows whether it's contagious. Some research shows it may be, because it has appeared in clusters of people in reports from eight countries, including the United States, over the past 50 years.

Some scientists believe that CFS is an immune-system disorder or is linked to exposure to the live rubella virus used in German measles vaccines in the late 1970s. It may be triggered by some version of the Epstein-Barr virus, but this virus is also associated with other diseases, including Hodgkin's disease, and 90 percent of the population carries the Epstein-Barr virus in a latent form.

CFS may be triggered or kept alive by a combination of viruses, or it may be a new virus, as yet undiscovered. Or CFS may be caused by depression, some researchers claim, because people with CFS have a higher rate of lifetime depression. (On the other hand, it must be depressing to have CFS.)

Other trigger possibilities are a combination of stresses, for instance, the loss of a loved one or a job, a malfunctioning immune system, or the controversial Candida yeast (sometimes caused by chronic use of antibiotics). (See "The Immune System" on page 9 and "The Chronic Candida Controversy" on page 534.) Other possibilities are genetic predisposition, and environmental toxic overload from paint, paint thinners, wood strippers, polluted air, and the combined effect of chemicals of all kinds.

TREATMENT OPTIONS

The drug ampligen is experimentally used to treat CFS, but it doesn't have FDA approval yet. In the past, researchers have unsuccessfully experimented with a variety of cures, including acyclovir, the drug used for herpes, because the Epstein-Barr virus linked with CFS is a herpes virus. As there is no specific treatment for this disease, individual symptoms are treated. Examples are antidepressants for depression, painkillers for headaches, stress-reduction techniques to delay or eliminate relapses (see suggestions on how to relieve stress on page 55), and gamma globulin, a blood product, to boost the body's immune system.

Find a doctor who helps you find relief from symptoms and who takes the disease seriously. If you think you might have this disease, it would be wise to contact a CFS organization or your local medical school to find a doctor experienced with this disease. (See "Chronic Fatigue Syndrome" on page 571 in the Resource Directory.)

HOME REMEDIES YOU CAN TRY

- *Get adequate rest and good nutrition* (see "Food" on page 26).
- *Exercise a small amount every day*, though not to overexertion.
- *Ration your energy.*
- *Find emotional support with friends or family, and/or contact a CFS self-help group.*
- *Look into nontraditional treatments*, such as acupuncture and Chinese herbs for pain relief, visualization, and vitamin C. (See "Acupuncture" on page 82, "Meditation" on page 59, and "Chronic Fatigue Syndrome" on page 615 in Recommended Reading.)

WHY CFS IS NOT A "YUPPIE" DISEASE

The association of CFS with well-educated, white professionals has resulted in its nickname, the "yuppie flu." However, yuppies are probably the most likely to be successful in getting an accurate diagnosis because they are persistent, willing to get many opinions, believe they have a right to know, and have either the income or insurance to pay for the extensive medical testing.

Although the Centers for Disease Control and Prevention classified CFS as a new disease in 1985, some doctors still do not think CFS is a disease and believe rather that the symptoms are all in the patient's head. (See "Keep the Role of Attitude in Perspective" on page 68.) This attitude is unfortunately not that unusual with diseases that are difficult to diagnose and confirm. If you know there is something wrong with you, keep looking for treatment until you find someone or something that makes sense to you and is helpful.

I was stricken with an ailment I decided was the flu. Within two months, rather than improving, I had become severely ill. An appalling weakness prevented me from walking. I soon was unable to take a shower, my arm ached from the effort required to brush my teeth.

I came home from having a hysterectomy and I slept on the couch from St. Patrick's Day (March 17) to June. My ex-husband sued for custody of our daughter and he got it. I couldn't take care of her. I had to sell my furniture. I lost my apartment.

Cosmetic Surgery

What It Is

Cosmetic surgery is surgery almost always performed for the sake of appearance. It involves the reshaping of normal parts of the body. Plastic surgery can also be used to correct flaws resulting from burns, accidents, or birth defects.

Types Available

The most common cosmetic surgeries for women are:

- *Face-lift*. Excess skin is removed, and sometimes underlying muscles are tightened, while remaining skin is stretched and tightened.
- *Forehead lift*. Lines and wrinkles are modified by removing excess skin and tightening and stretching the remaining skin.
- *Eyebrow lift*. A section of skin is removed just above the sagging area of the eyebrow, and the outer portion of the eyebrow is lifted.

• *Eyelid lift.* Fat and excess skin around the eyes are eliminated to remove wrinkles, bags, and pouches.

• *Permanent eyeliner.* The rim of the eyelid is surgically tattooed.

• *Nose surgery.* Nasal bone and cartilage are reconstructed and any excess removed and reshaped.

• *Chin surgery.* A small silicone implant is inserted to augment a receding chin. This procedure is often performed with nose surgery to improve a woman's profile.

• *Double-chin surgery.* Fat deposits beneath the chin (often called a "double chin") are removed and the underlying muscles and skin of the upper neck are tightened.

• *Breast reduction.* Reducing the size of large breasts relieves weight-bearing pain. This procedure is not usually performed purely for cosmetic purposes.

• *Breast augmentation.* Implants are inserted to enlarge small breasts or to restore a more natural appearance after mastectomy.

• *Breast lift.* This procedure is used to reposition saggy breasts.

• *"Tummy tuck."* Abdominal skin is reduced and tightened to provide a firmer abdomen and narrower waist.

• *Liposuction.* Fat is vacuumed from beneath the skin through a hollow tube. This procedure, which can only safely remove four or five pounds of fat at one time, can be used on "love handles" and fat on the hips, buttocks, thighs, abdomen, arms, calves, knees, and under the chin.

Some procedures qualify as cosmetic surgery, even though they are nonsurgical:

• *Collagen injections.* Collagen, a structural protein, is injected under the skin to raise and puff the skin, smoothing out isolated wrinkles and small scars. It is not approved for enlarging otherwise normal facial features, such as lips. If you are considering collagen injections, the FDA (which reports that 30 percent of these procedures result in known side effects) warns that you must be tested for an allergy (symptoms are rash, hives, joint and muscle pain, headache, and sometimes difficulty in breathing) to the substance first. And if you are allergic to a number of substances anyway, you may want to reconsider getting these injections.

• *Dermabrasion.* Sanding removes the outer layer of skin and gives the face a smoother texture. This technique removes superficial scars and age lines.

• *Chemical peel.* This is the same as dermabrasion, except it's performed by a controlled burn with a caustic solution.

POSSIBLE COMPLICATIONS

Each of these procedures has potential risks, although it's believed that most women are pleased with the results. It's also true that cosmetic surgery problems may not show up for years, and even when they do, women may not realize that the surgery or the product used (such as a breast implant) is the source of their problems. Individual stories about bad outcomes, however, are truly terrible, with some women having many operations to correct the original cosmetic surgery. The full risk of any procedure will depend on the reliability and extent of the procedure, your surgeon's skill, and your individual body's response.

No one knows how many women have died as a result of these operations, because no government agency has kept track. Cosmetic surgeons readily admit that their surgery is not 100 percent safe; no form of surgery ever is. That's why many surgeons do not accept every person who seeks their care. Some people have too many health risks — like obesity, diabetes, heart disease, or smoking — to make surgery advisable.

Any of the surgeries may be done incorrectly or, even when performed correctly, may leave undesirable scars. Tummy-tucks leave long, thick abdominal scars, for example, facial peels can cause infections and scarring, collagen injections can trigger autoimmune diseases, and all facial cosmetic surgery can cause temporary or permanent nerve damage, hemorrhages under the skin, infections, or reactions to anesthesia.

• *Liposuction.* This is the most common cosmetic procedure, and it may cause permanent skin discoloration, severe pain, infection, rippling of the skin, excessive blood or fluid loss, coma, and occasionally death.

• *Breast surgery.* Breast reduction causes several long scars per breast, may result in reduced nipple sensation or none at all, and makes breastfeeding impossible. A breast reduction or breast lift may also leave you with uneven breasts.

• *Breast implants.* Along with whatever pleasure they may give you, breast implants are a guaranteed life-long problem. Getting them inserted is only your first operation. Silicone gel implants never last a lifetime. And even if you don't get sick with them, implants ordinarily require several expensive out-of-pocket surgeries and/or replacements about every five to seven years.

Implants can cause painful baseball-hard breasts from the hardening of the scar tissue around the implants. This is yet another reason for repeat surgery — to break up the scar tissue. The silicone inside these breast implants can leak out slowly or rupture into other internal organs, including the lymph nodes which circulate throughout your body. Implants can also cause inflammation and internal scarring of the breast as well as visible external scarring.

Silicone gel implants sometimes move and shift, leading to allergic reactions and nonmatching breasts. Implants interfere with the flow of breast milk, often making breastfeeding impossible, and sometimes implants alter nipple sensation. And at least one implant brand is controversially linked with cancer in lab animals.

Breast implants may also cause inaccurate mammogram readings, which may mean breast cancer may be more advanced before it's recognized. Breast implants also increase your risk for several diseases including scleroderma, a potentially serious (though rare) connective tissue disease that affects the skin and can damage other organs, rheumatoid arthritis, and systemic lupus erythematosus. A new addition to the breast implant side-effect list is a list of symptoms — chronic fatigue, inability to swallow, rashes on upper chest, and hair loss — not associated with any known disease. Scientists now speculate that all of these autoimmune diseases are the result of antibodies produced in reaction to the silicone in these women's bodies.

Thirty years and one to two million inserted breast implants later, the FDA in 1992 ruled that silicone gel implants can only be used in women requiring breast reconstruction after a mastectomy, in women with serious breast malformations, and in women who for medical reasons require replacement of previously implanted silicone gel implants. In addition, a limited number of women can have silicone gel implants for breast enlargement — the reason for 80 percent of implants in the past. This group will be required to enroll in an FDA-controlled trial research study.

Saline breast implants are still on the market, but they have their problems, too, including potential rupture, hardening, pain, need for replacement operations, and difficulty with mammogram readings. Another option, though expensive (estimated $20,000 per breast), is autologous breast reconstruction in which a woman's own body tissue (abdomen, back, thigh, and buttocks) is used to reconstruct a breast. However, this experimental approach can have unpredictable results, too, as demonstrated by troublesome side effects that have shown up after fat has been injected into other parts of the body, such as facial wrinkles.

If you currently have breast implants, it's important to know, according to the FDA, that implants don't last a lifetime, they leak silicone into your body even if they have not ruptured, and it is not known how often implants rupture. Take special care in obtaining mammograms to avoid both implant rupture and misleading x-rays. (See "Mammogram" on page 100.)

Find out what kind of implant you have, get at least annual checkups from your physician to check for signs of any complications, and keep accurate records. (To find out the current status of breast implants, to enroll in the FDA study, or to ask any other question about implants, call the FDA Breast Implant Information Line on page 573 in the Resource Directory. See also information about medical devices on page 73 and International Implant Registry on page 587 in the Resource Directory.)

I [a woman later diagnosed with lupus, arthritis, and scleroderma] had always been a body-conscious person. Implants just seemed an easy thing to make my body better. One morning, my hair started coming out in big clumps. I got a rash on my face and neck and chest area, and I woke up so tired I could barely get myself out of bed.

There's always a percentage of the population that won't tolerate anything foreign put into the body. I think they're blowing things out of proportion. The reconstruction made it easier for me to live with the mastectomy. I don't feel I'm in many little pieces now. It looks good and feels good.

I went to Johns Hopkins, had an MRI scan and they said no, the implants look fine. Eight weeks later I had them taken out anyway. The doctor found both had ruptured long ago and silicone was all over the inside of my chest.

How to Decide

Cosmetic surgery can be considered successful if it meets your expectations. In general, cosmetic surgery is especially appreciated by people who have prominent scars or disfigurement from accidents or birth defects. They have the most to gain and probably the fewest expectations. Those women who had a "normal" appearance before surgery and later said that the surgery met their expectations often feel their appearance has been enhanced and their self-confidence increased.

Disadvantages are:

• *The operation is not always successful, or the results may not meet your expectations.* An unknown number of women are not satisfied with the work of cosmetic surgeons. Some problems are evident right away, but some don't surface until many months or, more likely, years have passed, as in the case of high-cheekbone silicone implants that expand and move or breast implants that harden and become infected, for example.

Doctors usually speak only of their successes, and they are not required to publish complaints or report them to the government or list the malpractice suits that have been filed against them. Nor do county and state medical societies have to tell you about these statistics either.

In 1990, the U.S. National Practitioner Data Bank began to collect information on its own. It provides data about physicians' and dentists' serious errors in diagnosis and treatment to hospitals, licensing agencies, and other medical groups. Consumers cannot access this data bank. Even if you could, it would likely be incomplete as the information gathering only began in September 1990. Prior problems are not listed. You can, however, go to the courthouse of the county in which the surgeon you are considering resides or does business, and speak with the court clerk about checking in their records for previous court cases that indicate malpractice suits. Another source of information is the Lexus-Nexus computer data network which is often used by lawyers.

• *It hurts.* Many women who have had cosmetic surgery comment on the severity of the pain. They say they didn't realize it would hurt so much, even though they were told it would. Even if your mind is already made up, make sure you hear all the information you're given.

• *Your surgeon is likely to underestimate the pain, recovery time, and the possibility of complications in comments to you.* Part of the reason for this is that his (97 percent of cosmetic surgeons are male) view is different. It's not his body, so he doesn't have the personal experience of either pain or recovery — especially with breast operations. And there's a fine line in his mind between a complication and a common outcome. For instance, you may call a droopy lower eyelid a problem, but it is so common after certain kinds of eye surgeries that for your surgeon, droopiness is routine, not a complication.

• *You'll have to alter your life for several weeks or several months,* or at least until the bruising begins to fade. After liposuction, women are wound tightly in tape and wear support garments, like girdles, for many weeks. After a face-lift, you can't use cosmetics or moisturizers for at least two weeks, or hair-coloring products, mousses, a blow dryer, or astringents for two months. You also can't wash your face or your hair for 10 days, and you'd best stay out of the sun for several months, and quit smoking, if you are a smoker, for a while to help healing. Not surprisingly, many women experience a period of depression after a face-lift.

• *The desired look may not last long.* Except for ear and nose surgery and the application of permanent eyeliner, cosmetic surgery is not forever. Collagen, as an example, only lasts for a few months, and face-lifts usually last five to eight years. On the other hand, your skin won't look normal for one year after liposuction, and you can get the fat back anytime you gain weight.

If you are trying to make up your mind about a procedure, know that the pain and inconvenience of cosmetic surgery are not worth it if you are doing it because someone else wants you to do it for their sake, not yours. Many women who let themselves get talked into surgery later regret it.

Cosmetic surgery was once only the choice of movie stars or millionaires. Today, an estimated one million people every year, including those in ordinary professions and often of modest means, as well as teenagers, get cosmetic surgery. They spend thousands of dollars which are not reimbursed by insurance and do not qualify as a tax deductible medical expense. For some, going to the cosmetic surgeon is sometimes the next step after the hairdresser.

Often the woman who has cosmetic surgery is a college-educated professional who says she wants to either keep up with younger colleagues or look as young as she feels, and she has a right to do that. Getting cosmetic surgery for the boardroom, not the beach, probably accounts for much of the 60 percent increase in cosmetic surgery in the past ten years. (If you have decided that cosmetic surgery is for you, see "Surgery" on page 95 and "Cosmetic Surgery" on page 615 in Recommended Reading.)

I got my eyes fixed for me. My husband thought I was crazy, and my sons thought it was a waste of money. ("We like you the way you are, Mom.") I had already decided that no one had to agree or approve.

Don't let anyone tell you this doesn't hurt. My face is aching. My eyes are tearing, with the lids tugging at the sutures. My vision is blurred. I am wrapped in a turbanlike bandage, and my neck hurts each time I try to turn over. My forehead throbs.

I wish I had found out more about the aftermath of cosmetic surgery. I had my chin reshaped and when I woke up from surgery, my neck was a swollen mass from just beneath my eyes to my shoulders. I had my jaw wired together for six weeks and, obviously, couldn't eat. But what I hadn't thought about was that I couldn't talk either. When I did say something, people would treat me like I was retarded. That was an insight. The only thing my surgeon had ever told me about the aftermath of surgery was that if I had a good attitude I wouldn't have any trouble. Can you believe that?

My body was entirely black and blue where the machine had sucked out fat. For days I couldn't walk because of the pain. Finally, almost a year later, I did look terrific, but by then I had started to gain more weight.

My husband talked me into the surgery so that I would look like "the woman he married." Like a fool, I did it. He wasn't the one who had to stay hidden for two months because of the bruises. I'll never do that again.

Some of my friends have had cosmetic surgery and encourage me to have it, too. They tell me that every woman has a desire to change her appearance through cosmetic surgery. I laugh and say that sounds like something their doctors told them. Why should I get something fixed that's not broken? I exercise, eat well, and take vitamins. That's my style.

HOW TO GET THE MOST SUCCESSFUL COSMETIC SURGERY

There are no guarantees with cosmetic surgery, but there are steps you can take to help ensure you have a satisfactory experience:

• *Avoid any surgeon who is not a board-certified cosmetic surgeon.* This eliminates obstetrician/gynecologists and general surgeons even though legally they can perform cosmetic surgery. Exceptions would be dermatologists and ophthalmologists who perform certain specific procedures within their area of expertise. Be aware, however, that terrible results can and do still occur even when you choose a qualified, board-certified plastic and reconstructive surgeon.

Cosmetic surgery is very lucrative. Fees are high and ordinarily are paid in full in advance. Any medical school graduate with a state M.D. license can take weekend courses in liposuction, for instance, and run an ad in the paper the next week. Protect yourself from inexperienced physicians. Check the *Directory of Medical Specialists* at your local library for names of board-certified cosmetic surgeons in your town, or contact the "Cosmetic Surgery" organizations listed on page 572 in the Resource Directory.

• *Look for someone who has performed the operation that you want hundreds, not dozens, of times.* If the procedure is so new that no one has that kind of experience, realize that the operation is experimental and no one knows what all the consequences may be. For example, many permanent eyeliners were tattooed on women's eyelids before it was discovered that one of the consequences was the permanent loss of eyelashes for some women.

• *Alert the surgeon to your medical history*, including any chronic problems that you have or drugs that you take regularly. Discuss your surgery with your regular doctor, too.

• *Ask to see before-and-after photographs of previous patients who chose the operation that you want.* Remember, however, that you'll likely see the best pictures only, not the ones that didn't work out so well.

• *Get a second opinion* from another board-certified cosmetic surgeon about whether the procedure will yield the results you want.

• *Ask to see your before-and-after look in a computer imaging system* in which your surgeon projects your image on one screen and then repeats it on another, making changes on the second screen with a stylus to show you how you would look after surgery.

• *Ask for the names of other women who have had the surgery you want.* These women can give you realistic detail about recovery after the surgery.

• *Get a full explanation of the procedure.* Before you agree to do it, find out what it feels like, how long it takes, whether it requires local or general anesthesia, what the expected results and possible risks are. Be aware that if the surgeon is reluctant to give you details or seems rushed now, the lack of forthcoming information will likely only get worse after the surgery.

I had liposuction done on my stomach, hips, inner thighs, and knees. I was told that I would have "some discomfort for a few days," but I ended up in severe pain for three weeks. My arthritis doctor says that I should have never undergone the procedure.

CYSTITIS: *see* Urinary Tract Infections (UTI)

Diethylstilbestrol (DES)

What It Is

DES is a synthetic form of the female hormone estrogen. It was administered in pills (including prenatal vitamin preparations), injections, and suppositories for 30 years beginning in the 1940s. It was manufactured by more than 200 companies, an estimated five million U.S. women took this drug, and its peak use was probably in the 1950s.

DES was commonly prescribed to pregnant women who had a history of miscarriage, premature birth, or slight bleeding during pregnancy, because it was thought that the drug would prevent or stop these occurrences. It was also given to many other pregnant women, including those who had morning sickness or diabetes and those who planned to bottle-feed to reduce breast engorgement.

Possible Side Effects

Not only did DES fail in its preventive function, which research showed as early as the 1950s, but it also caused physical problems later for some of the women who took the drug during pregnancy and for some of the offspring of DES pregnancies. (See "Diethylstilbestrol" on page 616 of Recommended Reading.)

Women who took DES during pregnancy have a greater chance of developing breast cancer. The good news is the increased risk is probably small. Most women who took DES probably don't know that they did so, because it was given in the days when most women didn't ask the name of a drug they were given nor did their physicians offer the information. If you don't know whether you were given DES, it will not be easy for you to find out by checking medical records made 20 to 40 years ago. In spite of that, there are thousands of lawsuits against several DES manufacturers.

Risks to the daughters (and sons) of women who took DES during their particular pregnancy range from body changes to susceptibility to certain sexually transmitted diseases.

Side effects include: childbearing problems (including higher rates of infertility, ectopic pregnancies and premature births); structural abnormalities, such as the cervical "hood" (an extra ridge of tissue that may make it impossible for the woman to use a diaphragm) or a T-shaped uterus (which

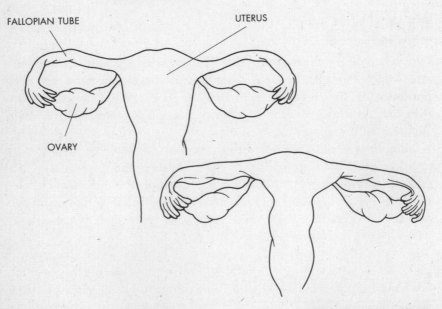

NORMAL UTERUS

FALLOPIAN TUBE

UTERUS

OVARY

DES T-SHAPED UTERUS

may cause premature labor, miscarriage, ectopic pregnancy, or infertility because of menstrual irregularities or failure to ovulate); and adenosis, the unusual presence of glandular tissue in the vagina, which is the most common vaginal change and which is often no longer visible in women over 30.

Despite these problems, most DES-affected women are able to give birth to healthy babies, though it's important to get early and complete prenatal care.

The presence of abnormal tissue on the cervix (called *dysplasia*) occurs twice as often in DES-daughters, and is a potential precursor of cervical cancer. Also common in DES-daughters is *carcinoma in situ*, a noninvasive, treatable cancer on the surface of the cervix. Clear cell adenocarcinoma and squamous cell cancer of the vagina or cervix are rare cancers found in less than 1 percent of these women, and they are usually treatable if discovered early. (See "Cervical Cancer" on page 234.)

In addition, DES-daughters are more likely to be troubled by herpes and genital warts, herpes especially, because their vaginal and cervical structural abnormalities make them more susceptible. The same is true of pelvic inflammatory disease when it's sexually transmitted. (See "Sexually Transmitted Diseases" on page 493 and "Pelvic Inflammatory Disease" on page 441.)

Finally, some of these women have emotional problems, including depression, anxiety, and low self-worth, probably as a result of concerns about reproductive functions. Many DES-daughters are helped emotionally and in other ways by the information and support of self-help groups. (See "Diethylstilbestrol" on page 574 in the Resource Directory.)

Reports of risks to the sons of women who took DES during their particular pregnancy are rare, but side effects may include infertility due to sperm abnormalities, small and/or undescended testes, abnormally small penises, and testicular cancer.

WHAT TO DO IF YOU SUSPECT THAT YOU MAY BE A DES-DAUGHTER

If you know or suspect that your mother took DES when she was pregnant with you, you may want to have a DES exam. (It's suspected that over half the people exposed to DES are not aware of the problem.) Find a physician who is familiar with the changes that DES causes and has much experience in examining women who have those changes. Contact DES organizations for physician referral, or call a local medical school for suggestions.

The physician will do the following, in addition to a regular pelvic exam:

- *Feel your vaginal walls.*
- *Take a Pap smear* from both the cervix *and* the vagina. (See "Pap Smear" on page 105.)
- *Examine your vagina and cervix with a colposcope,* an instrument that magnifies the image of the cervix 10 to 40 times. While lying on your back with your feet up in stirrups, a speculum will be inserted into your vagina to make your cervix visible. The colposcope will then be positioned at the opening of your vagina and your physician will look through the eyepieces at the magnified view of your cervix. It is possible then for small samples of cervical tissue to be removed for biopsy, and for photographs to be taken.
- *Stain parts of your vagina and cervix* with a cotton swab that contains iodine, so that adenosis tissue becomes visible.
- *Take a tissue sample, perhaps, for a biopsy* (this procedure feels like a pinch), if she's still unclear about the condition of your vagina and cervix.

If you have some DES-related changes, you will be asked to return for regular checkups, so that further changes can be monitored.

You may also want to avoid the following:

- *Cervical surgery,* unless you get an opinion from a DES expert.
- *The Pill,* because it's an additional source of synthetic estrogen, and some researchers think it may increase your risk for breast cancer.
- *Tamoxifen,* a drug chemically related to DES, which is used to treat breast cancer. Sometimes it is also used experimentally to prevent breast cancer.

Dilation and Curettage (D & C)

What It Is

A D & C involves two procedures. During *dilation*, the cervical opening is gradually widened, using progressively larger metal rods. *Curettage* is the gentle scraping of the uterine lining with a spoon-shaped, sharp instrument called a curette that is inserted through the dilated cervix.

A D & C, which usually lasts about 15 to 30 minutes, most often is performed in a hospital operating room because of the use of general anesthesia. You will be anesthetized, your legs will be put into stirrups, and your vaginal area and inner thighs will be cleansed with an antiseptic solution. Your doctor will then give you a pelvic exam and insert a speculum into your vagina so that the cervix can be viewed. Then she will dilate your cervix with metal rods and remove the uterine lining. If appropriate, uterine tissue will be further examined at a laboratory.

Women often have some bleeding for a week or two after a D & C, and it's wise to avoid tampons and intercourse during that time because the cervix will not be entirely closed and the uterus is more vulnerable to infection. Your next menstrual cycle may be early or late, as well as profuse

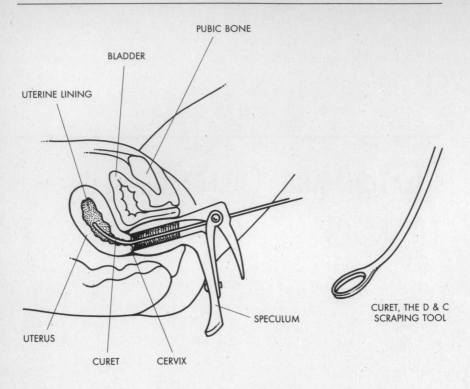

PUBIC BONE

BLADDER

UTERINE LINING

UTERUS

CURET

CERVIX

SPECULUM

CURET, THE D & C
SCRAPING TOOL

HOW D & C IS PERFORMED

for a cycle or two. Contact your physician if you develop a fever, foul-smelling vaginal discharge, persistent abdominal pain or cramps, faintness or dizziness, or if you bleed profusely.

WHY A D & C MAY BE NECESSARY

A D & C is performed for the following reasons:

• *Diagnosis and/or treatment of abnormal uterine bleeding.* Many doctors will perform a D & C to rule out endometrial (or uterine) cancer, especially when excessive bleeding occurs in early menopause, though this can be normal for many women. Abnormal uterine bleeding is also not to be confused with the monthly bleeding of postmenopausal women who take estrogen replacement therapy that includes progesterone. Endometrial cancer accounts for 6 percent of women's cancers (1 percent of cancer deaths). An endometrial biopsy is less invasive and as effective a procedure as a D & C in ruling out endometrial cancer (see "Uterine Cancer" on page 233).

• *Diagnosis and treatment of polyps.* Polyps (noncancerous growths) within the uterus can cause abnormally heavy or irregular menstrual flow. D & Cs to remove polyps are now often being replaced by simpler office procedures.

• *Removal of incomplete miscarriage.* Sometimes tissue is left in the uterus and doesn't come out on its own. This is a health hazard for women who require treatment. However, not every miscarriage necessitates a D & C. An ultrasound scan may help prevent an unnecessary D & C, especially in women in their 20s and 30s whose miscarriage occurred three months or earlier into pregnancy. (See "Miscarriage" on page 487 and "Ultrasound" on page 476.)

• *Removal of an intrauterine device (IUD).* Ordinarily an IUD can be removed with office instruments. (See "Intrauterine Device" on page 208.)

• *Abortion.* D & C abortions are rare. More than 90 percent of U.S. abortions are performed by the simpler suction curettage.

POSSIBLE COMPLICATIONS

Women who have a sexually transmitted disease, such as gonorrhea or chlamydia, or who had pelvic inflammatory disease in the past are the most likely to develop a pelvic infection after a D & C. (See "Pelvic Inflammatory Disease" on page 441 and "Sexually Transmitted Diseases" on page 493.)

Other risks are bleeding, sometimes leading to a hysterectomy (see "Hysterectomy and Oophorectomy" on page 354); perforation, or puncture, of the uterine wall; and damage to the bladder and/or intestines. In addition, adhesions (the growing together of usually separate tissue) and scarring of the uterine lining may result from repeated or overly vigorous D & Cs. Cervical incompetence (the inability of the cervix to remain appropriately closed during pregnancy, causing premature labor) is also a risk. This, too, is more likely to happen with repeated and/or overly vigorous D & Cs.

As with any procedure using general anesthesia, there is the risk, though small, of side effects from the anesthesia itself, ranging from nausea to cardiac arrest and death.

ALTERNATIVE TREATMENTS

A D & C is not 100 percent reliable as a diagnostic procedure. Statistics show that in 10 to 15 percent of cases, an inaccurate diagnosis is made even when a woman goes ahead and has a D & C. While performing a D & C, the physician can't see the uterine lining, and only about half of the surface of the uterine lining is removed, so some things can be missed.

• *A wait-and-watch attitude.* This is probably most appropriate for women who are in their 20s and 30s with menstrual irregularity and no other signs of disease.

• *Hysteroscopy.* A hysteroscope is a tiny viewing instrument that is inserted into the uterus through the vagina. It allows the physician to look inside the uterus for lesions and abnormal cells and to identify the precise location (unlike the "blind" D & C) before obtaining a tissue sample with a small instrument. Although it is usually performed in a hospital, this procedure may be performed with local anesthesia in a doctor's office and is considered a more accurate diagnostic procedure than a D & C.

• *Suction curettage.* In this procedure, a small pump is used to "vacuum" the uterine lining instead of scraping it with a curette. This is an office procedure that usually requires a local anesthetic at most. A possible disadvantage is that it does not necessarily provide the same amount of tissue samples as a D & C.

• *Endometrial biopsy.* During this procedure, a sample of tissue is collected with a small plastic tube (cannula). While you are on your back with your feet in stirrups, the physician will insert a speculum into the vagina and hold the cervix open with an instrument called a tenaculum. Then the tissue sample is taken. This procedure does not require stretching of the cervical opening and usually does not involve the use of anesthesia. It is used most often to diagnose irregular bleeding and is as effective as a D & C in ruling out endometrial cancer.

• *Ultrasound.* An ultrasound scan is an alternative to a D & C for locating a "lost" IUD.

HOW TO DECIDE

Many women have a D & C recommended to them at some time during their lives. When it happens to you, get specific reasons why you need a D & C now, and why the safer and perhaps cheaper alternatives are not an option. Request a second opinion about your need for surgery. (See "Surgery" on page 95.) Ask if the reason your doctor gives for your D & C will cease to be a problem after menopause.

About the time my periods became irregular, I occasionally had weeks of heavy bleeding. My gynecologist told me to have a D & C, or better yet, a hysterectomy. When I went to another doctor for a second opinion, she told me that she couldn't find anything wrong and that the bleeding would stop when I was finished with menopause. And it did.

Eating Disorders

Anorexia

What It Is

Anorexia, which affects 1 percent of U.S. women, is an eating disorder in which a person starves for an extended period of time.

Signs and Symptoms

Symptoms are this person's personal belief that she is heavier than she really is; the loss of 25 to 50 percent of her original weight, which is not due to any known illness; and amenorrhea (no menstruation). A woman with anorexia typically does not believe she looks too thin, even though observers may find her appearance shocking, and she probably exercises excessively. In addition, many, but not all, women with anorexia have an obsession with food, especially as more weight is lost, and they shun the flavor of fat. They know the exact amount of calories in everything they eat, and they often hoard food. People who have anorexia believe that eating very little is normal.

Consequences of anorexia vary and are the result of starvation. Most, but not all, disappear when the person's body resumes a normal weight. They are: slowed pulse (persistent resting pulse of 60 or less); low body temperature with icy hands and feet; low blood pressure; low white cell count; hyperactivity and euphoria alternating with lethargy and depression; dry, thin hair that may fall out; dry skin covered with downy fuzz; dry mouth; constipation and bloating; digestive difficulties; muscle cramps; tremors; infected gum tissue; lots of cavities; general weakness; brittle fingernails that split, peel or crack; difficulty in concentration; infertility; vaginal dryness and vulnerability to vaginal infections or urinary tract infections; irregular heartbeat; and — rarely — a heart attack. (See "Vaginal Infections" on page 532 and "Urinary Tract Infections" on page 515.)

Another consequence is osteoporosis. Even after recovery, there can be long-term, osteoporosis-like damage to the bones, and some women with anorexia have unusual spinal-compression fractures. (See "Osteoporosis" on page 431.) It's not clear why this happens, but estrogen deficiency and malnutrition are suspect. Less than 10 percent of these women eventually die of anorexia. Those who do usually die because of life-threateningly low levels of potassium, which is necessary for normal heart function.

CAUSES

Women with anorexia show a malfunction of the hypothalamus, which is a region of the brain that affects sex hormones and eating behavior. Experts say it's not clear if the abnormal functioning is a cause of anorexia or an effect. Also, occasionally diabetes triggers anorexia. Some experts suggest that there may be a genetic link that must be present, along with environmental factors, in order for someone to become anorectic. Although anorexia is not common among sisters, it shows up more in identical twin sisters, suggesting a genetic link.

It's believed by many experts that anorexia is caused by a desire for power and control that is satisfied by not eating. In fact, we usually admire historical figures who starved themselves for "a greater good." Certain Catholic women saints and Mahatma Gandhi are just a few examples.

However, the woman with anorexia has physical changes in her brain that may be either the cause or the result of starvation, as well as deficiencies in zinc and essential fatty acids that keep her from wanting to eat. Whether and to what degree anorexia is a psychiatric disease remains controversial and varies from woman to woman.

TREATMENT OPTIONS

Some young women who are treated for anorexia will return to their normal weight after treatment when a variety of methods are used, including eating more and getting bed rest and therapy. Recovery is quicker if the starvation lasts only six to nine months and if she is not yet totally preoccupied with food.

Suggesting anorexia's link to specific deficiencies, a zinc sulfate supplement in a regular dose has sometimes restored normal eating completely, even after years of anorexia. The most successful treatment for anorexia, many experts claim, may be to use a variety of methods starting with getting the person to eat, since a more normal weight is essential for any change to occur. A starved brain cannot respond to logic or therapy.

This is often accomplished with a combination of bed rest and high-calorie whole foods. Then this is followed by therapy and close follow-up. Some women are treated with a variety of drugs, including tranquilizers and other antidepressants, because some health professionals believe eating disorders are a form of depression. It's not known if this is effective long-term. Psychotherapy can include individual, group, and/or family therapy. Training is often offered in behavior modification, nutrition, and assertiveness.

Because it's the most successful strategy for quick weight gain, force-feeding via a tube down the throat or a needle in a vein is sometimes used, though this may be intensely demeaning, and it may be followed by medical complications. Women with anorexia who are successfully persuaded to eat will sometimes resort to binge eating patterns after they gain weight.

The hormone cortisol, which is released by the adrenal glands, becomes unbalanced in the body of a person with anorexia. At a Florida clinic that treats people with food disorders success is claimed for drugs that lower this adrenalinelike hormone. Cortisol is what gives women with anorexia such high energy, but it also shrinks the decision-making frontal lobe of the brain. At this clinic, some clients begin eating normally within a week after starting treatment with drugs that lower the body's cortisol. (See also "How to Overcome Anorexia or Bulimia" on page 326 and "Eating Disorders" on page 616 of Recommended Reading, particularly Werbach.)

BULIMIA

WHAT IT IS

Bulimia (or bulimia nervosa), which affects overall about 1 percent of U.S. women—2 percent of college students—is an eating disorder that includes binging and purging of prodigious amounts of food. For many people, binging means eating a dozen cookies at one time, or eating a bigger meal than usual (Thanksgiving dinner). The women with true bulimia, however, will eat 2,000 to 5,000 calories in a brief period, and some consume 50,000 calories in a day, or the caloric equivalent of five gallons of ice cream.

SIGNS AND SYMPTOMS

Symptoms are an irresistible urge to eat large quantities of food, especially sweets and other refined carbohydrates; vomiting after eating (often with Ipecac syrup, a liquid toxic to the heart that induces vomiting and is meant to be used for accidental poisoning); and excessive use of laxatives, diuretics ("water pills"), and "diet" pills. Along with these symptoms is a fear of becoming fat. Binges usually occur late at night after dieting all day, at times of stress, or during unstructured time. They may occur several times a month or as many as a dozen times a day. Some women who have bulimia also exercise excessively.

Consequences of binging and vomiting are: menstrual irregularities; ovarian cysts (see "Ovarian Cysts" on page 437); swollen glands in the neck beneath the jaw; sore throat or sinus infections; dry mouth; tooth decay and loss of tooth enamel; puffy, splotched face; bags under eyes; fainting spells; blurred vision; tremors; rapid or irregular heartbeat; stomach and abdominal discomfort; muscle cramps and weakness; numbness; bruises; scars and/or teeth marks on the back of the hand; and depression.

Common side effects of laxative abuse are: dependency on the product; loss of muscle tone in bowel; dehydration; tremors; weakness; fainting spells; rectal bleeding; abdominal pain and/or distention; constipation; and diarrhea. Common side effects of diuretic abuse are: permanent, irreversible kidney damage; dry mouth; coated tongue and cracked lips; dependence on the drug, with water retention on withdrawal from pills; dehydration; muscle weakness; fainting spells; irregular heartbeat, heart attack, and occasionally death.

Women with bulimia who use laxatives may eat 50 to 100 tablets a day, a dose that could kill a person whose body is not accustomed to that amount. Many regular dieters use laxatives, too, in the mistaken belief that laxatives cause weight loss. They don't. Even when women have four to six quarts of laxative-induced diarrhea, the calories remaining in their bodies are reduced by only 12 percent. Although laxatives barely reduce calories in the body, they (just as diuretics will) definitely reduce body fluids and minerals to dangerously low levels. Those women with bulimia who use diuretics are at increased risk for heartbeat irregularities. Side effects of excessive use of diet pills are anxiety, high blood pressure, and even, rarely, a cerebral hemorrhage.

CAUSES

It's believed that bulimia, like anorexia, is caused by a desire for power and control over food. However, brain scans of women with bulimia are different than those of women who do not have this disorder, and women with bulimia have unusually high levels of the brain chemical vasopressin, which researchers say suggests a physical component. Women with bulimia also have the reinforcement of physical craving for refined carbohydrates, sugar especially, combined with the repetitive pleasure of eating fast and vomiting violently. As with anorexia, the role of psychiatric disease associated with bulimia is controversial and varies from woman to woman, but clearly these women are also showing the psychological effects of a nutrient-deficient diet.

TREATMENT OPTIONS

Traditional treatment is behavior modification, psychotherapy, and perhaps drugs. However, some research shows that some women can recover from bulimia with a switch to a nutrient-dense diet. That includes whole foods only with vitamin C, B complex, and multivitamin supplements. This diet omits alcohol, caffeine, refined sugar, white flour, flavor enhancers, most salt, and cigarettes. This supplies adequate nutrition and stabilizes blood sugar – insulin levels (reducing the body's need to binge). (See Werbach on page 616 for more nutritional information and also "How to Overcome Anorexia or Bulimia" on page 326.)

PHYSICAL EXPLANATIONS FOR ANOREXIA AND BULIMIA

Many researchers think eating disorders are only psychological, but there are definite physical aspects of both disorders that are often overlooked or minimized. What may have been an innocent diet for the woman with anorexia or the vomiting after a too-big meal for the woman with bulimia becomes a relentless habit, due at least in part to alterations in body chemistry that now demand the new behavior. Binging is a biological consequence of dieting.

Extreme dieting can produce a high and reduce anxiety in some women. Women with bulimia often have low levels of serotonin, the brain chemical that tells us we're full. The woman with bulimia has to vomit; she needs that familiar physical sensation. After awhile, she no longer tastes the food; it's the purging that's addictive.

The more we vomited ourselves into emptiness, the more we needed to eat. I didn't understand for a long time that the act of vomiting causes a sudden drop in blood sugar which, in turn, produces a craving for more food. And so it would begin all over again leaving us, ultimately, weakened and depressed.

A TYPICAL PROFILE

Bulimia and anorexia occasionally occur in the same person, though not at the same time. Women with either kind of eating disorder may have begun with a diet to take off five to 20 pounds, they may have lost a friend who perhaps moved away, or they may feel they lost a parent through divorce. They may have quit eating as the result of the end of a romance, or they may have left home. Women with either anorexia or bulimia think about food all the time.

Some women with eating disorders come from a family where there's lots of talk about dieting. They are nearly always female, white, and from upper middle-class or upper-class families. They have a poorly functioning appestat, the internal monitor that tells us when we're hungry and when we're full, and may exercise excessively even after they are injured. They are often perfectionist overachievers with low self-esteem and are from high-achieving families. They believe that there is an ideal American body shape and that size and shape are the most important features in a woman.

Typically, these women were model children, compliant, making few independent decisions, feeling helpless about life events, and they may have had difficulty asking for help. Usually women with these eating disorders rarely express anger, and they often come from a family in which there is an alcoholic or a compulsive eater. (This is truer of bulimia than it is of anorexia.)

Women with these eating disorders are dissimilar in that those with anorexia tend to be younger. There are, of course, exceptions to the age guidelines. Women in their 60s have occasionally sought treatment for both disorders. Women with anorexia spend little money on food, while those with bulimia do just the opposite.

Women with anorexia have severe weight loss and may be ballet dancers, models, jockeys, or in other professions that require unnaturally low weight. (Of course, not all members of these professions have eating disorders.) Women with bulimia may not lose any weight at all, and are more outgoing, have more friends, and are more sexually active than women with anorexia, who are more introverted and keep to themselves. Women with bulimia often appear to be successful, self-confident super-women of normal weight. Most are well-adjusted, some researchers claim, and lead outwardly normal lives.

Unlike bulimia, anorexia is impossible to hide. The families of these young women may not realize at first that there's a problem, because their daughter wears baggy clothes, or she says she's had the flu and that's why she lost weight. But sooner or later, parents usually see their child's dilemma. To add to the pain of watching a daughter, or occasionally a son, seemingly waste away, some parents are then accused by many health professionals, as well as other family members or friends, of being the cause of the anorexia. Researchers claim that there's not enough evidence to prove that. Though some families are hypercritical or display disturbances in relationships, such as alcoholism or abuse, others do not fit this pattern.

When my daughter was a high school sophomore, I think she was at least mildly anorectic. We had just moved from another state, and she hated leaving her friends and her old school. The only classes she liked at the new school were the P.E. classes. Her brothers noticed she looked so thin, and I noticed that her menstrual periods had stopped. She didn't eat much and when she did, it was carrots and salads. After several months of this, she said she wanted to go to a therapist because she was so unhappy. She did go, and shortly after that, began to eat regularly, gained back her weight, and became more like her old self.

I began to worry about my weight when I was only eight. My older sister was obese and my mother was always dieting. I knew it was terrible to be overweight. . . . But when I was 15, I found the one diet that really worked. I stopped eating. At first, it was great. When I got down to 109, people were impressed: "What discipline," they said, and "Boy, you look terrific." But losing weight didn't solve my problems. That summer, I went to camp and lost 30 pounds. When I came home, I was skin and bones. I weighed 80 pounds, and couldn't think about anything but food.

From as early as I can remember . . . all the women who surrounded me talked anxiously about the pros and cons of their physiques. Hefty thighs, small breasts, a biggish bottom—there was always some perceived imperfection to focus anxieties on.

Of course, I had my breakfast. I ate my Cheerio.

She woke me up, crying hysterically. She said she couldn't take it anymore. She told me she had been throwing up and that she needed help. I asked her what she was talking about. . . . "I've been putting a toothbrush down my throat for three years." To think that I was with my daughter every day for three years and I didn't know she was throwing up.

We discussed the "superwoman syndrome"—that attempt to be the perfect friend, lover, hostess, student . . . and perfect looking. And binging, I saw, was my form of defiance. But if you're living life as the perfect woman, you won't cuss, you won't get drunk or laid or drive too fast. No, in the privacy of your own room you'll eat yourself out of house and home. But how dare you be defiant? And so you punish yourself by throwing it up.

My 30-year-old sister wants to have a baby, but she never manages to get pregnant. She went to a fertility specialist who told her that she was anorectic and that's why she doesn't menstruate. She says she likes the way she looks, is full of energy, and what's his [the doctor's] problem?

HOW TO OVERCOME ANOREXIA OR BULIMIA

If you've been told by many people that you're too thin, and you exercise strenuously to keep your weight down while eating little, you may want to consider making some changes. Whether you do that by yourself, or with a friend or two, or with a professional counselor, following are suggestions:

• *Eat whole foods*, especially complex carbohydrates, like grains and beans. If you have had anorexia, eat small amounts of high-quality foods throughout the day and avoid refined carbohydrates, like white flour and refined sugar. Bulimia can't exist without junk food, because the more refined carbohydrates we eat, the more we want. One doesn't have to have bulimia to recognize that reaction. By avoiding these foods, you'll break the craving you have for them. (Remember the nutrient-dense diet discussed earlier?)

• *Decide for yourself and by yourself that you really do want to make a change.* If someone else decides for you, it's always easy to sabotage treatment. Why use up your time and theirs doing that? They may win a few battles, but you'll win the war.

• *Avoid people who have anorexia or bulimia and spend time with people who have the behavior you want.*

• *Find other ways besides eating or not eating, or exercising many hours a day, to meet your needs.*

• *Accept your body.* You don't need to look like anyone other than yourself.

• *Try to stop the behavior by yourself.* Health care professionals say that's difficult, if not impossible, for many women. But some women do it. It's easier if you've had anorexia or bulimia only a short while.

• *Set yourself up for success.* If you have bulimia, eat regularly. Extreme hunger is a natural trigger for binging, whether you have bulimia or not. It's the body's message to you that it wants food fast. If you want to stop "exercise bulimia" (excessive exercising instead of, or along with, eating too much), some experts suggest that you turn to friends instead of turning to food or exercise, and that you keep a diary recording your feelings about eating and working out.

• *Contact an eating disorder organization* (see "Eating Disorders" on page 577 in the Resource Directory).

• *Get some counseling.* Check with your health insurance company to find out if they will pay for this. Find a counselor with whom you feel comfortable. Your chances of recovery are much greater if you feel at ease. (See "How to Find a Therapist" on page 51.) All people, of course, do not respond to the same treatment. As with a number of other ailments, no one solution works for everyone.

• *Consider an eating disorder clinic.* They are springing up everywhere, and some are better than others. Call the ones in your area and ask them what their treatment program consists of, how much experience they have, and what their cure rate is. Ask them for an initial interview before you commit yourself to a program, which may be long-term and may cost thousands of dollars.

• *Get a physical exam that focuses on the particular consequences of your condition.* You may be suffering multiple vitamin and mineral deficiencies. Health care professionals who have a lot of experience in dealing with your particular problem are more likely to diagnose your needs.

If you're like most women with anorexia or bulimia, you will recover. Perhaps many of you will always have a tendency to occasionally think about repeating these behaviors — much like former smokers occasionally think about what it would be like to have another cigarette — but that doesn't necessarily mean you'll do it. Or that a momentary lapse means you failed. A new way of eating and a new way of looking at your body can become just as much a habit as was the anorexia or bulimia.

S even days a week my daughter got up to run six miles in the morning, usually while it was still dark. When she started, we admired her persistence. We felt we had an athlete in the family for the first time. But we became concerned when she started skipping food mid-day and going to aerobics classes on her lunch hour. She finally decided on her own to talk to a therapist, and now she exercises moderately and eats more.

I threw away my "skinny clothes." I bought new, pretty, colorful clothes in my true size and felt free from the tyranny of belts that pinched, buttons that popped open, and zippers that required pliers to close.

I 've been an anorectic for about three years now and I've never thrown up and I never take laxatives; I just didn't eat. But I know for three years I didn't like being it. . . . I just took it on myself and I said I'm going to do it, you know, I'm going to put on weight. I'm not going to do it for other people who look at me and say, "Put some meat on your bones." I'm going to do it for myself.

I became a member of Overeaters Anonymous . . . and I am finally coming to grips with a lifelong problem of compulsive binge eating and a 25-year problem of intermittent bulimia. More important, OA has provided me with tools that bring me more and more peace of mind.

One of the last things I learned in therapy was that a lapse back into bulimia does not mean a relapse. No one gives up binge/purging all at once, once and for all, with no slips or missteps. Each time I lapsed, I asked myself what I could learn from the episode so I would be better prepared to deal with the trigger event the next time it appeared.

I went downtown to a professional counseling center and made an appointment with an eating disorders specialist. I wanted the counselor to help me be normal. . . . The counselor told me I was trying to cope with overwhelming problems by turning to food. Her words made sense to me. Then she said I had options and choices; there were other ways to work on problems besides eating and vomiting. This thought was new to me, and I pondered it for days.

I consider myself lucky to have escaped from my seven years of bulimia with only a handful of medical complications: heartbeat irregularities, dental problems, digestive disturbances, and menstrual and hormonal difficulties. Others I know have suffered ruptured esophaguses, goiters, ovarian destruction, intestinal ulcers, and completely eroded teeth.

ENDOMETRIOSIS

WHAT IT IS

Endometriosis — *endo* (inside) and *metra* (uterus) — is a disease in which fragments of the uterine lining attach themselves to organs inside the pelvic cavity. These fragments imitate the menstrual cycle by bleeding as menstruation begins as if they were still inside the uterus. Since this blood has no way to leave the body, painful cysts form.

Endometriosis usually affects the ovaries (60 percent of the time) and the fallopian tubes, often causing pain and scarring.

SIGNS AND SYMPTOMS

In some cases, endometriosis causes no symptoms. However, many women who have endometriosis report several of the following symptoms: menstrual cramps, often growing worse over the years; diarrhea and bowel upsets; nausea or vomiting; dizziness; shorter menstrual cycles (27 days or less) with heavy or longer (week or more) menstrual flow; constipation; fatigue; ovarian cysts; low resistance to infections; low grade fever; and

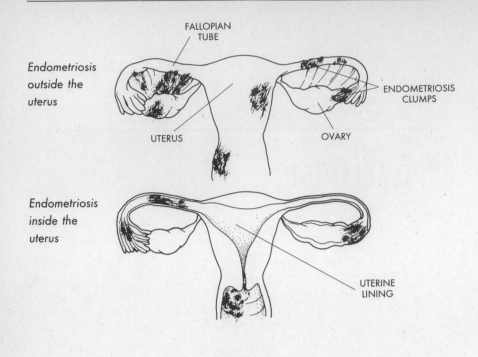

Endometriosis outside the uterus

FALLOPIAN TUBE

ENDOMETRIOSIS CLUMPS

UTERUS

OVARY

Endometriosis inside the uterus

UTERINE LINING

ENDOMETRIOSIS

pain. Endometriosis can be very painful. Most women have symptoms each month, including painful sex, pain during midmonth ovulation, and painful urination. The pain may occur only during menstruation or it may occur at other times, too. The degree of pain is not related to the extent of the disease.

Endometriosis often causes infertility. This is due, in part, to adhesions and scarring around the ovaries and the fallopian tubes that causes interference with normal ovulation. Endometriosis is the cause for 30 percent of women's infertility, and the longer you have this disease or the more extensive it is, the more difficult it is to conceive. (See "Infertility" on page 364.)

CAUSES

Although there are several theories, the cause of endometriosis is unknown. Women are seven times more likely to have endometriosis if they are related to other women who have it.

This disease was recognized as early as 1600 B.C. in an Egyptian papyrus that described some common endometriosis symptoms, among them painful menstruation and infertility. But only in the past two decades or so has endometriosis been recognized more widely, with an estimated five million U.S. women having this disease.

There are several reasons for what appears to be an increase in the occurrence of endometriosis. One is more accurate diagnoses, due to physicians' growing knowledge and to the use of better diagnostic tools. Another is that women have earlier menstruation, fewer pregnancies, and later menopause now than they did only a few generations ago. Ovulation is a major trigger in endometriosis.

The most popular theory for how endometriosis occurs is that bits of uterine tissue and menstrual blood somehow back up in the fallopian tubes, instead of coming out entirely through the vagina during menstruation, and then attach themselves to the ovaries, parts of the tubes, or to other organs in the abdomen. This wayward material clusters in clumps as small as a dot or sometimes as large as an orange. These growths become a dark color and are sometimes referred to as "chocolate cysts."

Another theory is that endometriosis is spread through the blood or lymph systems, which might explain why endometriosis growths are occasionally found in other parts of the body far from the pelvis, for example, in the lungs. Though the most common triggers for endometriosis are ovulation and menstruation, occasionally a cesarean, the birth control device IUD, or tubal ligation will stimulate the onset of this disease, too.

Even these theories of how endometriosis occurs do not explain why it happens. The answer may be that it is an immune system malfunction and/or a hormonal problem. It is believed that pregnancy along with breastfeeding usually causes endometriosis to subside because of the hormonal changes in the body that prevent ovulation. This is temporary relief, but the relief menopause provides is permanent because it's the end of menstruation and ovulation.

MAKING THE DIAGNOSIS

Since endometriosis is often confused with other diseases — bladder infections, pelvic inflammatory disease (PID), ectopic pregnancy, ovarian cysts, cancer, appendicitis, and diverticulitis, among others — the only accurate diagnosis is made with either laparoscopy, a surgical procedure usually performed in a hospital under general anesthesia (see "Laparoscopy" on page 173), or magnetic resonance imaging, which is performed with a machine that uses a very strong magnetic field. MRI of the abdomen and pelvis is reported to be 96 percent accurate, so it now increasingly replaces laparoscopy as the initial diagnostic approach.

TREATMENT OPTIONS

• *Estrogen and progesterone.* These are hormones used in the Pill, but when used for endometriosis they are sometimes taken in higher dosages. The Pill, even at usual doses, is frequently effective for mild endometriosis because of its antiovulatory effect. (See "The Pill" on page 181.)

• *Danazol* (sold as Danocrine in the United States) is an anabolic steroid, a synthetic derivative of the male hormone testosterone. (See "Anabolic Steroids" on page 39.) Treatment with this drug costs more than $100 a month. It appears to be most effective if the endometriosis is mild, and it may clear up mild endometriosis over several months. About half the women who use Danazol report relief, but this relief usually lasts only as long as the drug is taken. Birth control is still necessary while using this drug, because not all women will stop ovulating, and birth defects are probable for the child of a woman who becomes pregnant while taking danazol.

Common side effects are: weight gain, water retention and bloating, menopausal-type symptoms (hot flashes and vaginal dryness), depression and irritability, and masculinization, including hairiness, decrease in bust size, deepening of voice, loss of head hair, increased muscular development, and enlargement of clitoris. Other side effects that are sometimes reported are: muscle cramps, headaches, skin problems, including acne and oiliness in skin or hair. Some side effects are irreversible.

• *Newer drugs. Gonadotrophin-releasing hormone (GnRH),* which produces a medical oophorectomy, or removal of the ovaries, reduces pain and endometriosis growth. Side effects are similar to those of Danazol. A nasal spray, *Synarel (nafarelin),* suppresses the secretion of estrogen. Side effects of this drug include hot flashes, vaginal dryness, decreased sex drive, headaches, and insomnia. It's likely that after treatment is completed (6 months), a relapse in symptoms will occur. *Lupron (leuprolide)* is an injection given monthly. The *goserelin implant (Zoladex),* a ⅓-inch device that is implanted under the skin and not yet approved by the FDA, releases the drug over 28 days.

• *Transcutaneous electrical nerve stimulation* (TENS). This is a pain-management technique that involves passing a weak electric current into nerve fibers just beneath the skin via one or more electrodes to relieve the pain of this disease.

• *Laparoscopic surgery.* This not only is the best way to know for sure if you have endometriosis, it is also the most common surgical procedure used to remove pelvic scar tissue caused by this disease. However, for one third of women, surgery will need to be repeated, because the endometriosis will return. Occasionally laser surgery is used in conjunction with laparoscopic surgery and is reputed to result in a quicker recovery period for women.

• *Hysterectomy*, removal of the uterus, sometimes accompanied by *oophorectomy* (removal of the ovaries), is considered the ultimate solution, especially for women with endometriosis involving organs outside the pelvis. However, estrogen replacement therapy (ERT), which is necessary after removal of the ovaries, will reactivate the endometriosis 5 percent of the time. (Sometimes this is avoided by delaying the use of ERT for several months after the operation.) ERT is given to women who've had both their uterus and ovaries removed surgically to reduce or eliminate menopausal symptoms, like hot flashes or vaginal dryness, and to prevent osteoporosis later on. (See "Hysterectomy and Oophorectomy" on page 354 and "Estrogen Replacement Therapy" on page 337.)

I am 55 now and for the last 15 years, I've had a normal "feeling fine" everyday existence. It's been like a rebirth to health. The surgery not only cured the medical problem but was the final proof that I had not imagined the discomforts all those years and that was a mental lift.

I was definitely diagnosed as having endometriosis 15 years ago at the age of 19. . . . I have had seven surgeries over the last 13 years . . . but I'm still suffering from the disease. I've had a total hysterectomy with both ovaries removed that was supposed to have cured me completely. However, the estrogen therapy prescribed has caused the endometriosis to come back. I am currently on medication trying to get rid of the disease once again. . . . It seems every doctor has his own definite opinion on treatment and cure.

HOME REMEDIES YOU CAN TRY

There is no cure for endometriosis. Many women use several approaches to cope with it, often combining home remedies with medical treatment, and permanent relief is not always achieved.

• *Exercise regularly* to reduce your risk for having endometriosis in a severe form, strengthen your immune system, and alleviate depression (a side effect of some of the drugs and surgery recommended for endometriosis and also a familiar companion of many women who are dealing with a chronic ailment). (See "Exercise" on page 41.)

• *Reduce dietary fat*, especially saturated animal fat and hydrogenated vegetable oils. They appear to stimulate the production of certain types of prostaglandins. These are normal hormonal secretions that occur during the menstrual process. When they are released in excess, however, they cause menstrual cramps, a common complaint of women with endometriosis. (See "How to Find Fat in Your Food" on page 29.)

• *Eat foods especially rich in vitamin E and the mineral selenium, the B vitamin complex, especially B_6, calcium and magnesium, and vitamin C.* (See "The Anti–Breast Cancer, Healthy Heart Diet" on page 28 for foods associated with these vitamins and minerals.) Some women also find it helpful to take evening primrose oil, which is used successfully by some women who have premenstrual syndrome (PMS). (See books marked with an * on page 604 under "Food" in Recommended Reading for specific dosages.)

• *Try acupuncture and Chinese herbs*, acupressure, and meditation, which are helpful for many women, especially for pain relief. (See "Acupuncture" on page 82, "Accupressure" on page 56 and "Meditation" on page 59.)

I have talked to many women who have endometriosis and the one conclusion I have drawn is that the disease is different for different women. And likewise, the treatment that works for one woman may not work for someone else. My own treatment was a long process of trial and error, and trying out things I wasn't sure I believed in. I don't think it's the answer for everybody. But maybe hearing about this can get a few other people started on their own way. We all seem to be explorers in unmapped territory.

I find I feel much better physically and emotionally if I exercise strenuously and regularly. I really have to force myself and must have the discipline from a class. I'm taking aerobic dancing; it helps keep my weight down and keeps my muscles toned and strong, and I flow off a lot of frustration and anger, which really helps keep me "normal." . . . I walk very much, too, which is good for my mental state, as well as my body.

I wanted to get pregnant and my gynecologist suggested that I have surgery to remove the endometriosis, and then use fertility drugs if the surgery wasn't enough. I decided to try acupuncture because a friend of mine used it, and it worked. I started to feel good and was pregnant within the year, but it took Chinese herbs, major diet change, exercise, and vitamin therapy along with the needles.

WHY ENDOMETRIOSIS IS NOT A "CAREER WOMAN'S DISEASE"

A widespread myth is that career women are more likely to have endometriosis. One reason offered to support this myth is that career women have fewer pregnancies (during which endometriosis usually subsides). However, the working woman in her 30s is probably not more likely to have endometriosis; she's more likely to have it diagnosed. As with other difficult-to-diagnose diseases, the woman who is most likely to get both accurate diagnosis and effective treatment is a woman who believes she has the right to know what's wrong with her body; who acts with confidence and persistence, no matter how many times she's not helped; and who can pay medical fees, either from insurance or personal income.

White affluent women in their 30s who have postponed childbirth are not the only ones who have endometriosis. It's also been diagnosed in women of other races, from their teen years to their 40s.

This disease was confirmed by the sixth doctor I went to and I wish I'd seen him before Jack, my fiancé, took off. . . . Jack said he loved me and that he'd do anything to help, but he didn't love what he'd been hearing from doctors: that my pain was from V.D.!

I think the worst thing about endometriosis is the anxiety and uncertainty I experience the week before each period. I'm always wondering, "How bad will it be this time," "Should I cancel all of my appointments for next week?" and "Will I be able to make my midterm exam?" . . . Being an active college student can be very difficult.

WHAT TO DO IF YOU SUSPECT THAT YOU HAVE ENDOMETRIOSIS

Get an opinion from a health care provider who has a lot of experience in *successfully* treating women with endometriosis. Then think about getting a second opinion, as endometriosis is so often confused with other diseases. (See "Get a Second Opinion" on page 95.)

Put your age and the extent of your endometriosis into perspective. Are you in your 40s and near menopause? If so, you may want to wait and see what happens as symptoms of endometriosis fade when you quit menstruating. But perhaps your endometriosis is too painful now to wait. Or are you in your 20s or 30s and want to have children in the future? Then you may want to consider options now that stop the spread of this disease, whether you're in pain or not.

Contact "Endometriosis" organizations or your local medical school for physician referrals. (See "Endometriosis" on page 579 in the Resource Directory and also on page 616 in Recommended Reading.)

M y endometriosis was discovered during surgery to remove a cyst that did not exist, but large masses of endometriosis did.

W hen I was younger, I thought the pain was just normal cramps, and I thought that's what everybody had. It wasn't until I was suffering quite a bit that I really began to be concerned. But my main problem right now is that my husband doesn't believe any of this period stuff. He thinks I'm imagining all this and that it's in my head. He thinks women use their pain for extra attention. I don't know if he's capable of understanding what's involved with endometriosis.

ESTROGEN REPLACEMENT THERAPY

WHAT IT IS

Estrogen replacement therapy (ERT), also known as hormone replacement therapy or HRT, is a drug designed to supplement or provide the body's supply of estrogen, a reproductive hormone naturally produced by the ovaries. Frequently in the United States, estrogen is combined with progesterone, another reproductive hormone, in ERT. Production of estrogen gradually slows down at menopause because our bodies are no longer in the baby business and don't need as much estrogen. After surgical removal of the ovaries (oophorectomy), estrogen levels drop dramatically, rather than gradually.

Usually ERT involves taking estrogen pills for three weeks, and progesterone (or progestin) for seven to 10 days. Other approaches include estrogen only (if the woman has had her uterus removed), both hormones daily, or a hormone-free week within each month-long cycle. Estrogen is also available in a vaginal cream as well as in a silver-dollar-sized skin patch, similar to a Band-aid. The theoretical advantage to the skin patch is that estrogen will bypass the liver, reducing the likelihood of side effects.

When ERT is used because a woman has had her ovaries surgically removed, the effect is better when the male hormone testosterone is added (although this gives some women male characteristics including aggression, voice deepening, and hairiness) because it mimics the natural process of menopause. The bodies of women with naturally occurring menopause automatically produce more androgen after menopause, which may be the reason for increased sexual desire for many postmenopausal women. (See "Hysterectomy and Oophorectomy" on page 354.)

ERT is traditionally considered most effective if it's started within three years of menopause, whether it's a naturally occurring or a surgically induced menopause. Women who have had their ovaries surgically removed are encouraged to take ERT at least until the age of natural menopause, age 50 or so.

WHO SHOULD (AND SHOULDN'T) CONSIDER ERT

Women who benefit the most from ERT:

• *Have had both ovaries surgically removed.* Women in this category who do not take ERT have twice the normal risk of heart disease and are at greater risk for osteoporosis.
• *Are at high risk for osteoporosis.* (See "Osteoporosis" on page 431.)
• *Find the symptoms of menopause* (such as hot flashes and vaginal dryness) *especially disruptive.*

Women with the following histories should *not* take ERT, or should take it with extreme caution:

• *Cancer of breast, uterus, or reproductive tract or close family history* of one of these cancers
• *Diseases involving the liver or gallbladder*
• *Blood-clotting disorders and active thrombophlebitis*
• *High blood pressure, heart disease, and heart attacks* (See "Heart Disease" on page 348.)

Women who are also advised to use ERT with caution have:

• *Experienced side effects from the Pill* (See a list of side effects of the Pill on page 184.)
• *Used diethylstilbestrol (DES) or are DES-daughters* (See "Diethylstilbestrol" on page 309.)
• *Undiagnosed genital bleeding*

• *Endometriosis* (some forms of ERT make this condition worse). (See "Endometriosis" on page 329.)

• *Migraine headaches, diabetes, or asthma.* (See "Migraine Headache" on page 419.)

Smokers are also advised to use ERT with caution.

POSSIBLE SIDE EFFECTS

Use of ERT will probably always wax and wane as new discoveries are made. ERT began its popularity in the United States in the 1960s as a "youth pill," *the* solution for that misnamed "deficiency disease" called menopause. In those days promoters said ERT would smooth wrinkles, keep bodies slim and sexy, and decrease suicide and alcoholism, to name just a few items in a list of more than two dozen menopausal "symptoms" and "cures" offered by some drug companies and some physicians.

ERT use dropped in the 1970s when information about its association with increased risk for cancer of the uterus emerged. Then in the mid-1980s, drug companies launched an ad campaign for the use of ERT based on its ability to prevent osteoporosis. Following that, a new campaign in the late 1980s promoted ERT's possible protective advantage against heart disease. By the early 1990s, ERT was one of the top selling prescription drugs in the United States.

ERT is associated with a five to ten times greater risk of uterine (endometrial) cancer, especially if estrogen alone is used. Consequently women on ERT are more likely to have a hysterectomy (to avoid uterine cancer). The longer a woman has taken ERT and the stronger the daily dose, the greater the risk. After 10 to 15 years of ERT use, the uterine cancer rate is 20 times higher than that of women who don't take the drug. (See "Uterine Cancer" on page 233.)

There is also an increased risk for breast cancer in women who have used ERT for at least five years. Women who have had hysterectomies with their ovaries removed, who are in their early 50s and who also have a mother, sister, or daughter with breast cancer are at an additional higher risk for breast cancer.

The combination ERT is the most commonly used in the United States, because U.S. doctors believe it's safer. However, Swedish research in 1989 showed that the estrogen-progestin ERT (in a slightly different chemical form than is used in the United States) increased the rate of breast cancer fourfold after four years of use, whereas the estrogen-alone formula doubled the breast cancer rate. On the other hand, U.S. research generally shows no increase in the breast cancer rate. In addition to this maybe cancer risk, combination ERT is associated with increased cholesterol levels with perhaps increased heart disease risk as well as symptoms of premenstrual syndrome, breast lumps, and menstrual-like monthly bleeding. (This may taper off, but don't count on it. You may be wearing pads or using tampons for many years.)

ERT is also associated with a twofold risk for gallbladder disease. Hair loss, nausea, uterine fibroid growth, edema and weight gain, headaches, an allergic rash, and/or yeast infections, monilia, or vaginitis are all possible consequences. (See "Uterine Fibroids" on page 522 and "Vaginal Infections" on page 532.)

It's believed that estrogen-containing creams and skin patches have fewer side effects, but as the estrogen from these products is absorbed into the bloodstream, there can still be unknown side effects.

I took estrogen pills when my doctor discovered I had osteoporosis. The pills made my hair fall out, which is a side effect a lot of people don't know about. I quit taking them because I wasn't interested in going bald. My sister just couldn't understand why I let that bother me. She said I could buy wigs, which is what my doctor had told me, too.

HOW TO DECIDE

The U.S. cultural view of menopause has two sides. One is the disease version, with some physicians (and others) believing that menopause is an endocrine deficiency that requires medication. The other approach is that menopause is a normal process with advantages and disadvantages, although unquestionably some women have more unpleasant symptoms than do others. If you have not had a surgical menopause, including the removal of your ovaries (this requires ERT for the best functioning of your body), you can decide which group you're in, and act accordingly.

Advantages of ERT are that it reduces or eliminates hot flashes and restores vaginal lubrication in those women who experience dryness. It may also decrease or eliminate related symptoms of burning, itching, and pain with intercourse.

ERT often halts the bone loss caused by osteoporosis. Fractures of the vertebrae are reduced 90 percent, in some studies, and hip and wrist fractures are reduced 60 percent when ERT is begun within a few years after menopause. (Some studies also show that a calcium-rich diet and regular exercise maintain adequate bone strength. See "Menopause" on page 395 for nondrug options.) When ERT is begun later, it may halt the progression of bone loss, although it won't take your bone density back to where it was at the beginning of menopause. One of the ways to help you make up your mind about ERT is to get your bone density measured. (See "Bone Measurement Test" on page 109.)

Whether or not taking ERT protects a woman from heart disease remains controversial. Some research shows that it does (particularly with women who have had their ovaries removed or women who already have heart disease); some shows that it doesn't. Until randomized clinical trials are performed, no one knows. Natural menopause, however, does not increase your chances of heart disease, as some researchers once believed, nor does the use of ERT increase your longevity or improve your memory.

Discuss the possible side effects of ERT with your physician *before* starting treatment. Unless you plan to take ERT until your death (or about 30 years or more), there is a rebound effect for almost all women. That means every possible ERT advantage (the avoidance of bone loss, plus the elimination of hot flashes and vaginal dryness) will not persist if you stop taking the drug. Bone loss occurs again after ERT is discontinued, and it may occur more rapidly than if ERT had not been taken at all. In fact, in the most comprehensive study to date, there was little difference in bone density in 75-year-old women who had taken ERT for as much as 10 years after menopause and those who hadn't used the drug at all. Since hip fractures typically occur around age 80, for those women who choose ERT, non-stop use of this drug is required for maximum life-long bone strength. Hot flashes usually come back more intensely than ever. (Many women go on and off ERT, but that's obviously not a good idea.) Some U.S. research indicates that ERT improves women's moods. On the other hand, British studies found that the mood-improving or "mental tonic" side effect of ERT is a classic sign of drug dependency.

A few women avoid the hot-flash rebound effect by going off ERT over a long period of time by taking smaller and smaller doses, but don't count on your body being that cooperative because that outcome is unpredictable. It's unknown if the rebound effect of bone loss, or the potential heart disease protection, or the effects of mood change can be avoided in the same way by taking smaller ERT doses over a long period of time. What is known is that all women who take ERT and then quit have a likelihood of some rebound (some return of symptoms).

ERT is a trade-off of health benefits and problems. Which concern is stronger to you depends on your personal medical history (ERT seems to have more benefit for women who have had oophorectomies and, to a lesser degree, hysterectomies) as well as your attitude about health care in general (are drug options the first thing you would try or are they the last?). If you choose to take ERT, you will need careful, semiannual medical supervision for the rest of your life. Because of the rebound effect, it's not wise to start ERT with the idea of using it only for a short period, although many women apparently do just that. In one study, 40 percent of ERT-users stopped taking the drug after only eight months.

If you use ERT, use it wisely. Ask your pharmacist for a copy of the patient insert for the particular drug you are taking. You may also want to ask your doctor or pharmacist what else is in your ERT prescription. Occasionally other drugs, like tranquilizers, are included as well. Avoid generic drugs for ERT, as some versions are not effective.

Get your semiannual physicals and endometrial biopsy (if you still have your uterus). This is a procedure in which a small tube is passed through the opening of the cervix into the uterus to gather a small amount of the uterine lining. Have a biopsy *before* you start taking ERT so you know what they are like. Many women find that this is painful, which makes them reluctant to have regular exams after they start taking the drug. However, all women who take ERT need to be followed closely since this drug effects your body from your hairline to your toes.

If you choose ERT, work with your doctor to find the lowest possible dose for you, and eat a well-balanced diet to offset some of the potential side effects of the drug. (See "Estrogen Replacement Therapy" on page 616 in Recommended Reading.)

After starting ERT, see your physician immediately if you have any of the following toxic symptoms: pain in calves or chest, sudden shortness of breath, severe headaches, breast lumps, or jaundice (yellowing skin).

I love taking my estrogen pills. They keep me wet, but they don't do a thing for my wrinkles. You people can whine all you want about how I'm going to get cancer—I don't care. Since my latest divorce, I've had a very active sex life, and there's no way I'm going to get in the clinch with some guy and then whip out my tube of lubricating jelly, and say, "Wait a minute, I've got to get some of this on." No way!

My mom tried to quit estrogen after taking it for about ten years. But that didn't last; her hot flashes were horrendous, much worse than they were before she ever started the pills. About that time her doctor gave her a hysterectomy, because of the changes in her uterus. He said that she couldn't get uterine cancer then, and she could take ERT the rest of her life.

He [her physician] started her on Premarin in a cycle of three weeks on and one week off medication. After about six weeks, Alma noticed that all her symptoms had eased up. She continued to take Premarin for about four years. Her physician was very cautious and conservative and always decreased dosage whenever symptoms lessened. By the age of 45, all symptoms, as well as monthly periods, had ceased. Alma is now 62, and says that she has never had a recurrence of any of her symptoms.

The biopsy hurt a lot. When I went home I felt traumatized and cried for a while. I felt as if my body was invaded and it made me emotional. I never felt that way after a pelvic exam.

FATIGUE

WHAT IT IS

Fatigue is feeling tired, drained, exhausted all the time.

SIGNS AND SYMPTOMS

Symptoms vary from mild to severe, and in addition to tiredness, they are: low motivation, reluctance to be physically active, feelings of inadequacy, and little or no sexual desire.

CAUSES

Nearly all women experience fatigue at some time in their lives, whether during an illness or while managing several jobs (family, career, housework). Men experience fatigue, too, but they don't report it as often as women do, nor are their symptoms the same.

The cause — or more likely, the combination of causes — will vary from woman to woman. Some women experience fatigue from allergies, before their menstrual period starts, or from the body changes of pregnancy and childbirth. Women who have babies who are awake around the clock or women with small children are often lethargic, as are women who are caretakers for sick or disabled people.

Some women will be fatigued because they work too much (especially at unrewarding jobs), others because they are bored and work too little. Some feel fatigue after too much caffeine causes a letdown, as a result of crash dieting, or from leading too sedentary a life.

Others develop vitamin deficiencies from eating poorly; some have heavy menstrual periods that result in anemia. Some are worn out as a reaction to smoking or from drugs, including the Pill, antihistamines, or sleep aids. Some have a chronic condition, like lupus, diabetes mellitus, hypothyroidism, or heart disease, that leaves them tired. It's not unusual to feel fatigue with the onset of a cold or the flu. Emotional problems, especially depression and anxiety, cause fatigue (or maybe it's the other way around — fatigue causes depression). And an unknown number of women who are bone-weary tired for at least six months may have chronic fatigue syndrome (see "Chronic Fatigue Syndrome" on page 295.)

The woman most likely to feel fatigue is younger, and likely to be a mother of small children. That's true whether she works outside the home or not. New mothers who go back into the work force within six months of childbirth, as most mothers do today, are likely to be fatigued.

I was tired the whole decade we were having kids. And I know why. I probably never had a full night's sleep. I took for granted that being bone-weary tired was normal. Today I know better. My daughters are having their own children now, and I tell them how to find ways to get enough sleep, including asking their husbands to do well-defined, specific chores.

HOME REMEDIES YOU CAN TRY

• *Get enough sleep daily.* Of course, if that were easy to do, you would probably be doing it already. Think of ways to increase the amount of sleep you get by as little as 30 minutes more each 24 hours. As you increase your sleep, the amount you accomplish in a day may take less time and be done more cheerfully, because you are functioning better. Don't assume that you will always need the same amount of sleep. Pregnant women and women who are sick, for instance, need more. Take brief naps midday, if your schedule permits (and if they don't cause insomnia).

• *Exercise on a regular basis.* Some women leave fatigue permanently behind when they start a three-times-a-week exercise program. It increases upper body strength, reduces reports of aching shoulders in office workers, and may increase your sense of well-being. For many women, this is the only change they have to make not to feel tired all the time anymore. (See "Exercise" on page 41.)

• *Eat well and avoid fatigue triggers,* like too much caffeine, refined sugar, or fatigue-producing recreational drugs. Eat a diet rich in the B vitamins, vitamin C, and vitamin E. (See Werbach on page 616 for more nutritional information.)

• *Ease your workload,* if that seems to be part of the problem.

• *Do something interesting* that you've been putting off, if boredom is your problem.

• *Do something for yourself.* Look at the most expendable part of your day or week, and whittle away time for yourself. Arrange to have your own time, no matter what your work load is, to meet your needs, not just those of others. Consider yourself that important. Learn to say no. Other people do; watch how they do it and copy them. You can put your needs first, depending on your life situation, if only for 15 to 30 minutes each day.

• *Learn stress-relieving techniques.* In some studies, more than half of the women surveyed report that they lead stressful lives. Use visual imagery to create the future that you want. Try meditation, massage, or a hot bath, among many options. (See suggestions to relieve stress on page 55.)

If home remedies don't work for you, you may want to get a medical evaluation to determine if your fatigue is related to a hidden disease. Pay attention to other symptoms that you might have, too, and describe them to your doctor. This will help you avoid being told inappropriately that your fatigue is all in your head, a diagnosis that many women have reported. (See "Fatigue" on page 616 in Recommended Reading.)

GENITAL WARTS: *see* Sexually Transmitted Diseases

GONORRHEA: *see* Sexually Transmitted Diseases

HERPES: *see* Sexually Transmitted Diseases

Heart Disease

What It Is

Although there are a variety of heart problems, the leading form of heart disease for women, as with men, is *atherosclerosis,* in which the passageways through the coronary arteries becomes narrowed and roughened by fatty deposits called plaques. Healthy arteries are flexible, elastic, and strong with a smooth inside lining, allowing for the easy flow of blood.

Atherosclerosis is the major cause of stroke and heart attack in the United States and is often associated with older men. However, more women die of heart disease than of any other ailment, including cancer, and it's the leading killer of women over 65. It's found in all economic levels and races, though women who are less than five feet tall are more likely to have heart disease. (It's believed they may have narrower coronary arteries to begin with, leaving them more vulnerable to blockage.)

A heart condition that occurs twice as often to women as it does to men is *mitral valve prolapse* (MVP): An abnormality of one of the heart valves occasionally produces a murmur that can be heard with a stethoscope. Heart palpitations are the most common symptom. Others are: chest pain, light-headedness, fatigue, dizziness, and occasional numbness of the hands.

Usually MVP does not require treatment, but occasionally it will cause serious progressive heart disease, including heart valve leakage which requires treatment. (See Anderson on page 616 in Recommended Reading.)

SIGNS AND SYMPTOMS OF ATHEROSCLEROSIS

Heart disease is called a silent killer because it has no symptoms until the coronary arteries are so damaged that blood flow is restricted. Atherosclerosis can affect circulation to different parts of the body and can cause:

• *Angina* (or angina pectoris). Angina is a warning sign of atherosclerosis. An angina attack feels like a fleeting, tight, crushing pain in the chest, is the result of arteries narrowed by a passing spasm, and does no permanent damage. When angina attacks come frequently and are not the result of physical exertion, they can be a sign of an impending heart attack.

• *Heart attack* (or myocardial infarction). A heart attack occurs when coronary arteries become blocked and the blood supply to one region of the heart is cut off. Without an adequate blood supply, a portion of heart muscle can be injured or die. The most important symptom of a heart attack is an anginalike pain that doesn't go away and doesn't respond to nitroglycerine, the usual treatment for angina. Other symptoms are shortness of breath, fainting, nausea, vomiting, intense sweating, a sense of doom, and pain that extends beyond the chest to the left shoulder and arm, back, and sometimes teeth and jaw.

• *Stroke* (or cerebrovascular disease). Unlike a heart attack that is caused by blocked coronary arteries, a stroke is caused by blocked blood flow in the brain. Your brain requires 20 percent of your blood and oxygen, so a blood clot in an already narrowed artery due to atherosclerosis can cause damage in the affected area, sometimes in a matter of a few minutes. Symptoms of a stroke are double vision, slurred speech, inability to move an arm or leg (usually on same side), loss of sense of balance, uncoordination, or difficulty with swallowing.

• *Transient ischemic attack.* This is a temporary reduction of blood flow to the brain with milder versions of stroke symptoms and can be a forerunner of a stroke, just as angina is a warning for heart attacks.

MAKING THE DIAGNOSIS

Atherosclerosis is generally diagnosed through its severe consequences. Diagnosis of a heart attack, along with symptoms, is usually made with a combination of blood tests and an electrocardiogram (EKG), which is a painless test that produces a graphic record of the heart's electrical impulses detected by means of 12 to 15 electrodes attached to different parts of your body. A stroke is diagnosed through symptoms as well, along with use of computerized axial tomography (CAT) scanning, which uses x-rays, or magnetic resonance imaging (MRI), which uses a very strong magnetic field.

CAUSES

Several risk factors contribute to the development of atherosclerosis. Among them are:

• *High blood pressure* (or hypertension). Blood pressure is the force with which your blood pumps through your blood vessels. That rate is measured in two numbers, the higher *systolic* reading and the lower *diastolic* reading. When those numbers are elevated, it's called high blood pressure. Normal blood pressure is usually considered to be 120/80, but what's considered normal is age-related, with 140/90 considered normal for average middle-aged men. It's not clear what is the normal range for average middle-aged women. Borderline hypertension for men ranges from 150/90 to 160/100. Severe hypertension, which 20 percent of all people with hypertension have, is defined as 200/115. Elderly African-Americans are more likely than any other group to have hypertension. Blood pressure is enormously variable, so several readings should be taken for accuracy.
• *Smoking*
• *Obesity*
• *A sedentary life-style* (U.S. government defines this as fewer than three 30-minute walks per week.)
• *Diabetes*
• *High serum cholesterol*
• *Family history of heart disease*
• *Stress*

TREATMENT OPTIONS

Both heart attacks and strokes require immediate attention. How much damage is sustained depends on what part of the body is affected and how soon treatment is begun. A number of drugs (beta-blockers, anticoagulants, clot-busters, clot-stoppers, and blood thinners) are used to reduce the risk of recurrent problems.

Medications can alleviate some of the problems associated with heart disease, but no drug can reverse the damage that has been done to diseased arteries. (See "Preventive Measures You Can Try" below for a method that can reverse the damage.)

Lasers and catheters can be used to burn, weld, or pare plaque from artery walls. A defibrillator is a permanently implanted electrical device that jolts the heart back to a normal rhythm when necessary, and a pacemaker stabilizes a too-slow heartbeat. There are also heart surgery options, like coronary bypass surgery (new veins are grafted onto the heart so the old ones can be bypassed), carotid endarterectomy (the removal of large obstructions), and balloon angioplasty (used to open up narrowed blood vessels), all of which are controversial and overperformed in the opinion of many physicians.

Many treatments have been tested nearly exclusively on men, so their success and consequences may be different for you. Sometimes even with equivalent treatment, women are more likely to die after a major heart attack. If you are interested in surgery, find a surgeon who has a lot of experience in treating women for heart disease. (See "Heart" on page 616 in Recommended Reading and on page 582 in the Resource Directory.)

PREVENTIVE MEASURES YOU CAN TRY

Deaths from heart disease in the United States have decreased in past years, but heart disease is still the No. 1 killer of women. You're five times more likely to develop heart disease than you are to be diagnosed with breast cancer, for example. Furthermore, heart disease is ten times more likely to be the cause of your death than is breast cancer. Given this scenario, and since it is difficult to undo the damage of heart disease, prevention is of critical importance. Heart disease is, in many cases, fully preventable.

• *Quit smoking and avoid passive smoke.* The risk for stroke and heart attack increases with each cigarette smoked daily (and, no, low-tar cigarettes don't help). Happily, it also decreases with each day you don't smoke, regardless of how old you are when you quit. Smoking is considered the major trigger for most heart attacks, apparently is a greater risk for women than men for unknown reasons, and is more devastating when combined with obesity. (See "Tobacco" on page 605 in Recommended Reading.)

• *Maintain a reasonable weight.* (See the "right" weight chart on page 429.) Obesity, particularly abdominal, is a risk factor for heart disease, as is so-called yo-yo dieting. (See "Obesity" on page 424.)

• *Exercise regularly*. Exercise not only improves your circulation, but it is key in maintaining a normal weight. (See "Exercise" on page 41.)

• *Make dietary changes for you and your family*. (Heart health begins in childhood, and problems may appear as early as the teen years.) A low-fat diet helps you maintain your appropriate weight, which aids in keeping your blood pressure normal and your cholesterol level low as well. A diet rich in Vitamin E also reduces the risk for heart disease. (See "The Anti–Breast Cancer, Healthy Heart Diet" on page 28 for details.)

• *Reduce stress* (see suggestions for relieving stress on page 55) and job strain — if possible. Job strain occurs when you have very little control over day-to-day decisions along with high psychological demands.

• *Maintain a helpful network of friends and family*. Heart disease risk is lower in women who have healthy support networks and who work at jobs they like. (See "Friends and Family" on page 44.)

• *Do all of the above and reverse existing artery damage*. In a 1989 study, one group of women and men who were diagnosed with heart disease actually reversed their condition by not smoking, eating a vegetarian diet, exercising moderately (walking for a half-hour daily or one hour three times a week), and spending an hour a day on stress relievers (such as yoga and meditation), and group support. (See Ornish on page 616 in Recommended Reading.)

• *Monitor your serum cholesterol levels if you know you have a problem*. Cholesterol is a fatty substance produced either by the body or ingested in foods of animal origin, such as meat, butter, eggs. It is present throughout the body and is necessary for health. A low-cholesterol diet is helpful in preventing heart disease because it reduces fat, not because it reduces cholesterol. The cholesterol content of the food that you eat has little effect on the cholesterol level in your blood. The most effective way to reduce the cholesterol in your blood is to lose weight through regular exercise and a low-fat diet. Despite these facts, we are saturated with low-cholesterol reports and products, leaving many of us with cholesterol phobia.

If you decide to be tested (which may be particularly helpful for women with a genetic history of heart disease), see "Cholesterol Test" on page 109 for information on how to make sure your test results are as accurate as possible.

You also may have heard of more controversial ways of preventing heart disease, including:

• *Estrogen replacement therapy (ERT)*. Since it's rare for premenopausal women to die of heart disease, it's believed that women's hormones, estrogen in particular, provide the protection. As an additional indicator of estrogen's role, women who have had their ovaries (the producers of the body's estrogen) removed are at increased risk for heart disease. (See "Hysterectomy and Oophorectomy" on page 354.)

Some research indicates in fact that ERT does reduce the incidence of stroke and heart disease. However, other research shows that the use of ERT doesn't make a difference for women who have had a natural menopause with ovaries still intact. And so far the research has been on the ERT drug that uses estrogen only, which is not what most women take. The hormone replacement therapy of choice in the United States for women with a uterus is a combination of estrogen and progesterone. No studies have yet evaluated this combination's effect on heart disease. (See "Estrogen Replacement Therapy" on page 337.)

• *Aspirin.* There are no conclusive studies that show whether women benefit from taking aspirin as a heart-disease preventive, though 1991 research suggests they may. In that study the women who took one to six aspirins per week had 25 percent fewer first heart attacks. Those who benefited the most were past 50 and had special risk factors for heart disease. If you're considering taking aspirin, be sure to discuss this drug's side effect with your health care provider. (See "Aspirin" on page 33.)

• *Alcohol.* The issue of alcohol's effect on heart disease is very controversial. At least eight studies suggest that moderate drinking (three to nine drinks per week) is good for heart health. Other studies show, however, that moderate alcohol use doesn't improve your heart disease risk at all and may make it worse. (See "Alcohol" on page 37.)

I t used to be that my friends and I were always worried about the Pill. Then we got older, and it was breast cancer. Now it's high cholesterol we talk about when we get together. The last time we played cards, half of them were comparing their blood cholesterol levels. I can't even enjoy a steak anymore without worrying about all that fat gooing up my arteries.

Hysterectomy and Oophorectomy

What They Are

A hysterectomy is the surgical removal of the uterus. A total hysterectomy removes the cervix as well. An oophorectomy removes the ovaries. A total hysterectomy with bilateral salpingo-oophorectomy removes the uterus, cervix, fallopian tubes (or salpinges), and both ovaries. A radical hysterectomy, in addition, removes the upper part of the vagina and some lymph nodes.

A hysterectomy can be performed either through an incision in the lower abdomen or through the top of the vagina. A vaginal hysterectomy produces no abdominal scar, probably causes less pain, and usually requires a shorter recovery time. However, it's usually only used for uterine prolapse (see "Uterine Prolapse" on page 527).

The abdominal procedure, which is used 75 percent of the time, is required for women who have adhesions from previous abdominal surgery, pelvic inflammatory disease, or large uterine tumors. This surgical route allows for a better view of the pelvic organs.

If the ovaries are removed along with the uterus, that shuts down the production of estrogen. This hormonal shock results in hot flashes and vaginal dryness within days. These are symptoms that take place over several years, not a couple of days, in a naturally occurring menopause, and symptoms usually occur gradually and are less severe.

WHY A HYSTERECTOMY MAY BE NECESSARY

Most hysterectomies are performed for the following three reasons:

• *Uterine fibroids*, small lumps of tissue that are usually harmless, but may require surgical intervention if they are causing significant symptoms such as pelvic pain, excessive uterine bleeding, recurrent miscarriages, and infertility. Uterine fibroids are the leading reason for hysterectomies for all races, but it is particularly true for African-Americans. (See "Uterine Fibroids" on page 522.)
• *Prolapsed uterus*, which is one that has fallen or slipped down from its usual position.
• *Endometriosis*, a condition in which uterine lining tissue migrates and grows in clumps on nearby organs, such as the ovaries or fallopian tubes or around the bladder or rectum. (See "Endometriosis" on page 329.)

Other reasons for hysterectomies are:

• *Heavy uterine bleeding*, especially if it's severe enough to require a transfusion (see "Menopause" on page 395).
• *Precancerous uterine-lining changes*, which vary in their severity.
• *Cancer of the uterus, cervix, or fallopian tubes* (see "Cancer" on page 231).

WHY AN OOPHORECTOMY MAY BE NECESSARY

• *Cancer of the ovaries* (see "Ovarian Cancer" on page 234).
• *Pelvic inflammatory disease* (PID), which can affect fallopian tubes and ovaries, causing severe pain (see "Pelvic Inflammatory Disease" on page 441).
• *Endometriosis*, which has traveled to the ovaries.
• *Ovarian cysts*, which are nearly always harmless, and require removal only when cysts are malignant or are exceedingly large (see "Ovarian Cysts" on page 437).

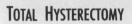

TOTAL HYSTERECTOMY

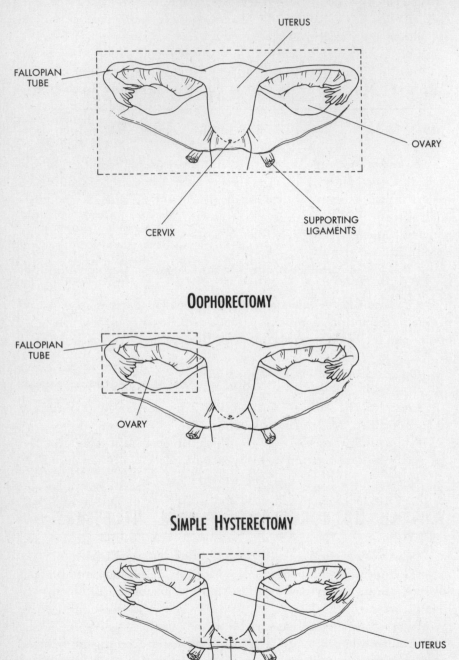

UTERUS

FALLOPIAN
TUBE

OVARY

CERVIX

SUPPORTING
LIGAMENTS

OOPHORECTOMY

FALLOPIAN
TUBE

OVARY

SIMPLE HYSTERECTOMY

UTERUS

CERVIX

POSSIBLE COMPLICATIONS

A hysterectomy can be life-saving in correcting severe problems such as obstetric hemorrhage, cancer of the uterus, vagina, or ovaries (an oophorectomy would be performed for this), or other cancers that have spread to the uterus. It also can provide relief from excessive menstrual bleeding, pain from endometriosis, or discomfort from a severely prolapsed uterus.

Other advantages include an increased sexual desire for 10 to 15 percent of women who have a hysterectomy, and no menstrual period or need for birth control for all. Another benefit from an oophorectomy is the prevention of ovarian cancer, a devastating and usually lethal disease. Ovarian cancer, however, is rare. (Fewer than 1 percent of women who keep their ovaries after a hysterectomy develop cancer.)

Disadvantages are that most women have one or more complications after a hysterectomy with or without an oophorectomy and there is a long period of recuperation (although women are often told four to eight weeks is typical), sometimes as long as a year, although this varies from woman to woman.

Reports of this operation's effect on sexual response are mixed, and what a woman experiences may vary depending on why she had the procedure and how extensive it was. (Keeping the cervix, for instance, makes it less likely a hysterectomy will interfere with sexual response.) About half the women who have hysterectomies report a decrease in sexual appetite. (See "Oophorectomies, Hysterectomies, and Sex, or Why Some Women Feel Like Eunuchs Afterwards" on page 362.)

After the hysterectomy, other organs may shift because the uterus kept everything in place. Prolapse, or a falling out of position, of the bladder, rectum, and vagina are common occurrences even though a prolapsed uterus is often the reason for the hysterectomy. This may result in hospital readmission within two years for surgical repairs. In addition, when you have both of your ovaries removed, you have an increased risk for carpal tunnel syndrome, a painful condition of the wrists; heart disease including a heart attack; interstitial cystitis, a chronic disease of the bladder; osteoporosis; and growth of facial hair. (See "Carpal Tunnel Syndrome" on page 244 and "Interstitial Cystitis" on page 387.)

Major surgery always carries some risks. Transfusions are required during 5 to 15 percent of hysterectomies due to hemorrhage. Pelvic, kidney, and bladder infections (see "Urinary Tract Infections" on page 515), blood clots in pelvic or leg veins, urinary incontinence, which is usually temporary, and damage to internal organs, like bowel, bladder, or ureter, are also possible. And death, the ultimate disadvantage, is a risk for one in 1,000 women who have hysterectomies, primarily due to side effects from anesthesia.

Women who have only hysterectomies continue to have functioning ovaries, therefore, they are not menopausal, though some women experience hot flashes and vaginal dryness. Women who do not have these symptoms may experience an earlier, more troublesome menopause, due to a drop in hormone production from the ovaries (a possible side effect of removal of the companion organ, the uterus), which results in menopause at 44 to 45 years, instead of the usual 49 to 50 years.

After an oophorectomy, ovarian remnant syndrome, which is rare, occurs when functioning ovarian tissue is left and/or extra scar tissue forms around the remaining tissue, causing cysts and perhaps pain during sex. Posthysterectomy syndrome, which is thought to be due to an endocrine imbalance, is a combination of hot flashes, urinary symptoms, extreme fatigue, headaches, dizziness, insomnia, and depression. Although many women do not report depression, those who do are more likely to have had an emergency operation, an abdominal hysterectomy, or to have experienced decreased sexual desire after the operation.

The estrogen replacement therapy (ERT) that is offered rarely alleviates all symptoms, especially sexual malfunctioning, nor can it replace all the systemic functions of the ovaries. Better options for many women, especially after an oophorectomy, are carefully monitored estrogen, progestin, and androgen hormone replacement and sexual retraining. (The addition of the male hormone testosterone, however, may result in male characteristics of aggression, voice deepening, and facial hair growth.) (See Cutler on page 617 in Recommended Reading.)

ALTERNATIVE TREATMENTS

Know what your alternatives are. You may be able to avoid a hysterectomy by finding a doctor skilled in an alternative treatment. Today there are more treatment options than ever, including:

• *Hysteroscopy* (also known as endometrial ablation). A hysteroscope contains a tiny lens, light, and opening for surgical instruments and is inserted through the vagina into the uterus. This instrument and the tools used with it, including lasers, can eliminate excessive bleeding, uterine fibroids, and growths caused by endometriosis.

• *Myomectomy*. In this operation the uterus is not removed. Instead, the fibroids are cut out and the remaining uterus is reconstructed to as near normal as possible. If the results are good, total uterine function will be retained including the ability to conceive. In France, physicians are far more likely to recommend myomectomy over hysterectomy for the removal of uterine fibroids because it is considered culturally important to keep the uterus. Myomectomies, however, are more expensive, more difficult to perform than a hysterectomy, and about one fourth of the time new fibroids will grow in the uterus within ten years. (See Payer on page 617 in Recommended Reading for information about the European use of this procedure.)

• *Dilation and curettage (D & C).* This is a simpler operation that involves scraping out the uterine lining. A D & C can be used for precancerous uterine-lining changes and heavy bleeding. (See "Dilation and Curettage" on page 313.)

• *Laparoscopy.* With this simpler procedure, misplaced tissue due to endometriosis or infected tissue from pelvic inflammatory disease (PID) is scraped away. Some surgeons now offer a combination of laparoscopy and vaginal surgery to avoid abdominal hysterectomy. This combined approach, however, apparently increases postoperative pain, cost, and operating time. (See "Laparoscopy" on page 173.)

• *Drug therapy.* Sometimes medications can be used, at least for a limited amount of time, to treat endometriosis, PID, precancerous uterine-lining changes, and uterine fibroids.

• *Surgical realignment of the uterus.* This operation resuspends the uterus back in its proper place and can be used for a prolapsed uterus.

HOW TO DECIDE

Get a second opinion. Most hysterectomies are elective, and reasons for performing them will vary from surgeon to surgeon. Reflecting individual physician beliefs, hysterectomy rates vary from region to region, too. As an example, the rate for hysterectomies in New York State is less than half what it is for the southern states. (See "Get a Second Opinion" on page 95.)

One third of all U.S. women have a hysterectomy by the time they're 60, a rate that's the highest in the world. Hysterectomies are second only to cesareans as the most performed surgery in the United States, and two thirds of hysterectomies are performed on women under the age of 45.

Sometimes a hysterectomy is exactly what you need, but sometimes it's not. No one knows how many hysterectomies are unnecessary, since most are performed for quality of life, rather than to save one's life. The Centers for Disease Control and Prevention claims 15 percent of hysterectomies are questionable, and a Blue Cross/Blue Shield study said their number is 33 percent. In the end it's up to you to decide for yourself. Only 10 percent of hysterectomies are considered literally life-saving, so the other 90 percent are elective and possibly unnecessary. If your hysterectomy is not a matter of life and death, you have a difficult decision to make. Believe that you have a right and the knowledge to make the choice about having a hysterectomy.

Although we live in a time that celebrates consumer rights and information, women's questions often disappear when doctors mention the word "cancer." And that's a word that comes up in hysterectomy discussions with doctors even when there's no sign of cancer in your body, and your pelvic organs show no disease of any kind.

HOW TO AVOID AN UNNECESSARY HYSTERECTOMY

Ask questions. Don't assume you'll be automatically given all appropriate information. Doctors often only give optimistic "best case" scenarios when they encourage you to have a hysterectomy. Example: "You'll feel great in six weeks and your sex life will be better than ever." It's up to you to get the other side of the story unless you live in California (or perhaps a few other states by now) where there are informed consent laws that require that you be told risks, length of hospital stay, recovery time, costs, and alternatives to hysterectomy.

If you feel that you may forget all of your questions once you're in your doctor's office if you hear the "c" word, then take along a friend who can ask questions for you. Some questions are: Why do I need a hysterectomy now? What would happen to my body if I didn't have it? Will my problem (fibroids or bleeding, for example) go away after a natural menopause? What are the alternatives to a hysterectomy? What are the risks? What can you do for me if any of these complications happen to me?

Don't be in a hurry to have the hysterectomy unless your condition is life-threatening. Beware of doctors and friends who tell you "just get it over with." The fact that your friends/your mom/your neighbor all had a hysterectomy doesn't mean that it's the best decision for you.

Since a hysterectomy at my age (30) seems like such a drastic step, I have consulted another doctor. This second gynecologist asked what symptoms I wanted to alleviate by surgery, and he mentioned several, including loss of urine and poor sexual relations. When I told him I had none of those symptoms, he said he saw no need for surgery either now or ever, as long as I remain symptom-free.

He says that the chances of the distention (uterine prolapse) worsening to the severe point the first doctor foresees are practically nil. How could two doctors disagree so totally?

I underwent an unnecessary hysterectomy one and one-half years ago and have had nonstop troubles since day one. The time span between the discovery of my "problem" and the actual surgery was only six weeks—hardly long enough to see if nature would help my condition.

When my condition (endometriosis) was finally diagnosed, the disease had already eaten a hole through my uterus causing severe, painful internal bleeding. After a hysterectomy and removal of one ovary, I functioned well for a period of 18 months. Then the remaining ovary became diseased and the endometriosis rampaged throughout the abdominal and pelvic area. Surgery was performed again to remove the second ovary.

How to Get the Safest Hysterectomy

- *Prepare for surgery* (see "Surgery" on page 95).
- *Avoid the removal of healthy ovaries*, because it is associated with more side effects and profound changes. Understand your personal risk for ovarian cancer (are there family members with the disease, for instance?); then weigh the risks versus benefits for you. If you decide to keep your ovaries, write on the hospital's consent form that your ovaries must be left in. Some doctors take them out as a matter of routine, sometimes without telling you in advance, especially if you are past a certain age, which could be 45, 50, or 55, depending on your doctor. (A 1989 U.S. government report showed that there has been an increase in the number of oophorectomies.)

Ignore your doctor's negative comments about your healthy ovaries. (Some women have been told that they were "sentimental," primitive," or "unsophisticated" to want to keep their ovaries.) Or better yet find a doctor who agrees with your preference to keep your ovaries.

It's normal for you to want to keep your ovaries, and you don't have to defend that wish any more than men have to defend keeping their testicles (the male version of ovaries) to avoid cancer of the testicles.

- *Arrange to keep your cervix if it is not diseased.* As the cervix produces half your lubrication, keeping your cervix reduces the severity of vaginal dryness. Most U.S. women have their cervixes removed with a hysterectomy to avoid the occurrence of cervical cancer. Read the description of cervical cancer risk factors and decide for yourself what's best in your case.

• *Line up supporters*, and/or contact a hysterectomy support group. (See "Hysterectomy" on page 584 in the Resource Directory and "Hysterectomy and Oophorectomy" on page 617 in Recommended Reading.) Research shows that you'll experience less depression and a quicker recovery.

• *Know details about what the operation will do and what it won't do.* The less you know, perhaps the more anxious you'll be — and the more likely it is that you'll be depressed later.

OOPHORECTOMIES, HYSTERECTOMIES, AND SEX, OR WHY SOME WOMEN FEEL LIKE EUNUCHS AFTERWARDS

Many doctors say that there's no physiological reason why a hysterectomy would affect a woman's sexual response. But that's not what many women say.

The intensity of your sexual pleasure can be enhanced by your uterus, which contracts rhythmically during orgasm and excretes pleasure-enhancing substances, by the network of veins and their supply of blood to your pelvic area, and by your cervix which produces some of the lubrication for your vagina. A hysterectomy removes the uterus, reduces the network of veins because many of them are tied off, and often includes the removal of your cervix.

Women who have had their ovaries removed, however, are castrated. Like eunuchs in harems, they have little or no sexual desire, arousal, or fantasies. To help you return to normal sexual functioning, take estrogen and androgen hormone replacement. Many doctors believe that estrogen replacement therapy (ERT) will restore your sexual feelings and desires. However, that's often not true. Women who receive testosterone along with ERT report more sexual feeling than women who receive only ERT. Try a sexual retraining program. This can include visual imagery, muscle tension exercises, relaxation techniques, and sexual fantasy. (See Wigfall-Williams on page 617 in Recommended Reading.)

I had a hysterectomy and kept my ovaries. But ever since my surgery, sex has not been the same and I rarely reach a climax. I went back to my doctor, but he told me the problem is all in my mind, and other women have better sex after the operation.

They sent me home on a low dose of estrogen, and when I came back for my six-week checkup (after having a hysterectomy and oophorectomy), the doctor said, "Oh, by the way, you can resume sexual relations now." That was the problem. There was nothing, just nothing. I'm not aroused. Nothing is going on.

The only loss I'm aware of is that the sensitive but anatomically impossible cord that always seemed to link my breasts and my clitoris became a bit less sensitive — but I'm retraining it.

INFERTILITY

WHAT IT IS

The medical definition of infertility is the inability to conceive within a 12-month period. Many women who are labeled infertile by this definition do get pregnant given more time. One in 12 U.S. women is infertile, and infertility is about equally divided between women and men.

CAUSES

Infertility can be caused by diseases, some forms of birth control, life-style choices, and medical operations and procedures. It also occurs for unknown reasons. Until a woman becomes pregnant the first time, she doesn't know if she's fertile. But never having been pregnant is not, by itself, an indication of infertility. It's merely an unknown factor to be fully understood later.

Following are common reasons given for women's infertility. Some women have one factor in the list; some have several; and some have none and are still unable to conceive. It is often not easy to pinpoint the exact reason or reasons for infertility, which is the source of part of the frustration many women experience.

• *Endometriosis.* With this disease, uterine lining tissue attaches to other pelvic organs, often causing pain and scarring. Infertility becomes more likely as endometriosis progresses. (See "Endometriosis" on page 329.)

• *Pelvic inflammatory disease (PID).* This disease can leave scarring and blockage of the fallopian tubes. At least 25 percent of women who have PID become infertile. (See "Pelvic Inflammatory Disease" on page 441.)

• *Sexually transmitted diseases (STDs).* The most likely STDs to cause infertility are gonorrhea and chlamydia. Chlamydia alone causes 100,000 women each year to become infertile. It's possible that you have had an STD and did not know it at the time it occurred because you didn't have visible symptoms. STD-caused infertility is 10 times more common in black women. (See "Sexually Transmitted Diseases" on page 493.)

• *Ectopic (tubal) pregnancy.* This is a pregnancy that attempts to grow in a fallopian tube instead of the uterus. At least one in five women who has had one tubal pregnancy will be infertile because of pelvic scarring. And of those who subsequently become pregnant, only one in three will carry the pregnancy to term. (See "Ectopic Pregnancy" on page 488.)

• *Age.* Women's fertility probably peaks at around age 30. That means that statistically all women in general become pregnant more quickly in their teens and 20s than they do later. That doesn't mean women don't become pregnant after that; obviously, millions do. But women in their 40s, for instance, do not ovulate every month even though they menstruate. And the older one gets, the more opportunities there are to develop diseases or physical conditions that could interfere with fertility. Consequently, it's no surprise that one in five women between the ages of 40 and 44 is infertile. No one knows beyond population statistics how fertile an individual woman is if she has not attempted to get pregnant in the past.

• *Menstrual irregularities.* Some women, from their earliest menstrual cycles, never ovulate on a regular basis even though they may menstruate monthly. Other causes of irregular ovulation are: anorexia, bulimia, and intense, frequent exercise — especially for women who weigh less than 110 pounds. (See "Eating Disorders" on page 318.)

• *Birth control.* There are three kinds of birth control that may affect your fertility. One is the Pill, because it can cause "Pill amenorrhea," or the absence of menstrual periods after stopping the Pill. One fourth of former Pill users take more than 13 months to become pregnant, and amenorrhea may last from a few months to a few years. The Pill rarely causes permanent infertility, however.

Another is the intrauterine device (IUD) because it is associated with pelvic inflammatory disease (PID). Some research shows that IUD users are three to four times as likely as nonusers to experience infertility, and the risk is greater for women under the age of 25, because they are more susceptible to PID.

The third birth-control method that may affect your fertility is the diaphragm. In one study, infertile women who had used a diaphragm for one year before attempting to conceive had a greater chance of having abnormalities of cervical mucus. (See "The Pill" on page 181, "Intrauterine Device" on page 208, and "Diaphragm" on page 200.)

• *Smoking.* Women who smoke, especially more than 15 cigarettes a day, take longer to become pregnant and are less likely to have a full-term birth, particularly if they have not had a child before.

• *Marijuana use.* Regular use of marijuana (about four times a week or more) may interfere with ovulation. (See "Marijuana" on pages 38 and 452.)

• *Habitual use of nasal decongestants.* Sometimes these products, which are used to dry up nasal secretions, also have a drying effect on other mucus membranes in the body, including cervical mucus. This may inhibit conception.

• *Regular exposure to nitrous oxide.* Also known as "laughing gas," nitrous oxide is usually administered with oxygen to reduce anxiety in dental patients. (It's also used in hospitals, ambulances, and veterinary clinics.) Dental assistants who are exposed to nitrous oxide five or more hours per week are not only more likely to be infertile, but appear to have a higher rate of miscarriage.

Our son Joshua, almost four and a half, was unplanned, unexpected, and conceived while I used a diaphragm. When he was a year old, we tried to conceive again. At first we discovered a luteal phase defect after I stopped nursing him. Recently I had surgery to remove the endometriosis that stole my fertility in one short year.

When I was 30 I went to an infertility specialist. He told me I wasn't getting pregnant because I seldom menstruate. I told him my periods had never been regular. He said that might change if I would eat more (I weigh 96 pounds), and if I quit exercising several hours a day. But I'm afraid I would get fat if I followed his instructions!

After conscientious use of birth control during my 20s, I was shocked not to be able to have a baby on demand. After I stopped taking the Pill, it took

18 months for me to get pregnant. However, after that birth (twins), I later got pregnant very easily.

One in three infertile women is unable to conceive because of a procedure, a product (like the IUD), or drugs (like the Pill) that were prescribed for her by her doctor. They were all offered in good faith with no intent to cause a problem then or later. Infertility can be caused by:

• *Cervical conization*, an operation that removes part of the cervix and is used to diagnose cancer. Other operations on the cervix may reduce fertility, too.

• *Dilation and curettage (D & C)*, a surgical procedure in which the interior of the uterus is scraped using a curette. (See "Dilation and Curettage" on page 313.)

• *Myomectomy*, an operation that removes uterine fibroids. (See "Myomectomy" on page 525.)

• *Cesarean*, a surgical childbirth, which can cause damage to internal organs, scarring, and perhaps endometriosis. (See "Cesarean Birth" on page 267.)

• *Pelvic or abdominal surgery*, because of possible internal scarring. Those operations ironically include procedures used to correct infertility.

• *Diethylstilbestrol (DES)*, a drug that was given to pregnant women from the 1940s through the 1970s theoretically to prevent miscarriages. If your mother took DES while pregnant with you, this may be an infertility factor for you. DES-daughters often have structural abnormalities of the vagina, cervix, or uterus. Some also have more difficulty in conceiving, as well as in carrying a pregnancy. DES-daughters have a higher rate of ectopic pregnancies, miscarriages, and premature births. However, an estimated 70 percent will eventually be able to have a child. (See "Diethylstilbestrol" on page 309.)

I was miserable after I had an emergency cesarean when I was 30. Nothing went right with that birth except the baby. She's wonderful! Now four years later I discover that I'm infertile because of all the internal pelvic scarring due to that operation. I'm heartsick!

Male infertility can be caused by:

• *Sperm irregularities.* Low sperm count, or less than 20 million sperm per cubic centimeter of ejaculate (about one-fifth teaspoonful), may be counteracted by the simultaneous artificial insemination of several specimens to achieve pregnancy. Poor sperm motility is when at least half of the sperm when viewed under a microscope are not swimming properly. Another irregularity is sperm that is adequate in volume, but creates an allergic reaction to the mate's vaginal flora. This can often be remedied with artificial insemination placed well up into the uterus, bypassing the woman's vagina. Some sperm irregularities might be caused by the mother's exposure to DES when she was pregnant with this son.

• *Varicocele.* This is a varicose vein in the testicles that slows sperm production. It can be treated surgically and causes about 25 percent of male infertility.

• *Sexually transmitted diseases (STDs).* STDs can cause blockage of the male reproductive tract.

• *Smoking.* Sperm levels are much lower in smokers than they are in nonsmokers, and vitamin C supplementation has been shown to increase sperm counts. (See "The Smoker's Diet" on page 35.)

• *Marijuana use.* Regular use of marijuana (about four times a week or more) can cause inadequate sperm count and motility, a condition that is usually reversible.

• *Drug or alcohol use.* Even certain prescription drugs like Tagamet (for ulcer treatment) and occasionally antibiotics like penicillin and tetracycline can have an adverse effect on sperm.

• *Exposure to environmental pollutants.* Lead, cadmium, and certain pesticides can compromise sperm health.

• *Childhood mumps.* Mumps can damage one or both testicles, causing sterility.

MAKING THE DIAGNOSIS

The first test for infertility is usually a postcoital exam. It occurs during the fertile days in your menstrual cycle. You and your partner have intercourse and within a few hours you go to the doctor's office, where a vaginal smear is taken to determine how well your partner's sperm fares. (Does it look healthy? Does it move well with your vaginal flora?) These tests are nearly always performed to determine the fertility of both women and men. Many couples find the postcoital exam stressful, especially if one partner is identified as the source of the difficulty. Although this test has been performed this way for 125 years, studies show that sperm tests are not reliable. In fact, a newer test, the sperm penetration assay, is not a good indicator either of a man's fertility.

Also helpful in making the diagnosis is an ovulation chart you make by charting your body temperature on a graph to determine if or when you ovulate. In addition, your mate can get his semen checked in a variety of tests that analyze the amount of sperm, motility (how well sperm moves), and the sperm's ability to penetrate cervical mucus, among others.

The following tests can also be used to determine the cause of infertility:

• *Endometrial biopsy.* In this office procedure, a tiny sample of endometrial lining is obtained and analyzed to determine if ovulation is taking place and if hormone levels are normal.

• *Serum progesterone test.* With this blood test, progesterone levels are determined.

• *Laparoscopy.* This surgical procedure is often used to determine whether ovulation is occurring, to repair pelvic scarring, to perform biopsies, and to locate and treat endometriosis. It's also sometimes used in conjunction with other fertility treatments, including artificial insemination, in vitro fertilization, and embryo transfer. (See "Laparoscopy" on page 173.)

• *Hysterosalpingogram.* This is an x-ray of the uterus and fallopian tubes, after insertion of an opaque dye, used to determine if there is any blockage.

With the exception of African-American women whose rate of infertility has increased for unknown reasons, the infertility rate for all U.S. adults hasn't changed significantly in the past two decades. What has changed is the belief that something can be done about it. And that's true. Fertility technology, a phenomenon of the 1980s, has made the difference for many infertile couples, especially for those who are white, married, college-educated and over age 25, because they can pay for it.

Although this technology — including fertility drugs, in vitro fertilization, and its handmaiden, surrogate motherhood — is much in the news, only one in 1,000 infertile women has used any of it, in part because of its high cost. However, for those who can afford it financially and emotionally, fertility technology is an alternative to stoic acceptance of a childless life or adoption. (See "Infertility" on page 617 in Recommended Reading.)

HOME REMEDIES YOU CAN TRY

If you have had difficulty becoming pregnant, you may find the following home remedies helpful:

- *Eat a well-balanced diet*, especially rich in zinc and vitamins E and C.
- *Boost your immune system*. (See "How to Stay Healthy" on page 25.)
- *Avoid drugs of all kinds*, including cigarettes, alcohol, and excessive amounts of caffeine.
- *Avoid negative stress*, since infertile couples are found to be more stressed than other couples. (See "Stress" on page 54.) Since failing to conceive month after month can be very stressful, set a time limit during which you will allow nature to "take its course." During that time, try to be philosophical about any setbacks. After that time, consider a consultation with health care professionals, including M.D.s and/or acupuncturists. (See "Acupuncture" on page 82.)

TREATMENT OPTIONS

Following is a description of different medical treatments for infertility, including the more established options, as well as the newer fertility technology. Couples who have difficulty conceiving may use one or more of these methods, and some methods for some couples will be more successful than others.

- *Planned sex during the woman's fertile time*. Every woman who conceives does so during her fertile time. Most women become pregnant without knowing the exact day when they ovulate. If they aren't using birth control (and sometimes even when they are), they'll conceive in a matter of months. But for women who are experiencing a delay in conceiving, the first step to becoming pregnant is determining their fertile time and having intercourse then.

The same methods (charting body temperature, observing cervical mucus changes and other keys to ovulation) used in natural family planning for avoiding pregnancy will also let you know when to have intercourse to get pregnant. (See "Natural Family Planning" on page 212.)

For many years, this information was all the help that was available to infertile couples. But for many couples, having intercourse at the woman's fertile time is only the beginning of the solution. One or more of the new fertility technologies will be the next step.

• *Antibiotics.* These drugs are not new for general healthcare, but they are new as an early treatment for infertility. They can be helpful in treating sexually transmitted diseases that can affect the fertility of both women and men, if not treated.

• *Artificial insemination (AI).* Artificial insemination is usually done in an AI clinic or doctor's office. Sperm is inserted into a woman's vagina or into her cervix, usually by means of a syringe, although it's occasionally now performed with laparoscopy.

In the United States, approximately 30,000 births (less than 1 percent of all births) occur annually as a result of AI, and the husband is the sperm donor about half the time. Sperm banks try to match the physical characteristics of the sperm donor (for example, race, hair color, and eye color) to those of the father-to-be. Although the technique of artificial insemination has been known and used for 40 years, AI didn't become popular until the 1960s.

Artificial insemination is used most by couples in which the male is infertile, but single women — particularly childless career women — use AI, too. (See "Infertility and the Law" on page 385 for information about parental rights.) Individual sperm banks may choose to provide artificial insemination to married couples only, but that's not true industry-wide.

Donors are paid up to $125 for each sample. AI costs the consumer from $400 to $1,600 or more, depending on where you get it (some sperm banks charge more than others), and on how long it takes you to conceive. It often takes four to six months (two artificial inseminations per month). About 90 percent of artificially inseminated women conceive within one year, and women who are younger than 35 take fewer sessions.

AI is mostly an unregulated industry, which includes 11,000 physicians and 400 sperm banks. The American Fertility Society (AFS) guidelines are:

  ○ *All sperm specimens should be frozen for six months and the donor retested for disease* at the end of that time before the specimen is used in AI. Several diseases have been transmitted to women via AI, including: AIDS, hepatitis B, genital herpes, gonorrhea, and chlamydia. Pregnancy is easier to achieve with fresh sperm, but thawed and tested sperm is safer.

  ○ *Sperm donors should be no more than 40 years old* to avoid passing on age-related hazards.

  ○ *No donor should father more than 10 children* to minimize the risk of intermarriage.

Providers of AI are not required in most states to follow AFS and government recommendations about testing and the use of frozen sperm, so it's up to you to find the safest source. (See "Artificial Insemination" on page 554 in the Resource Directory and "Infertility" on page 617 in Recommended Reading for more information.)

If you're considering AI, find the facility that uses the safest techniques, that tests donors for a variety of diseases, and that obtains a genetic history so that you can avoid passing genetic diseases on to your child. A 1988 review of AI in the United States showed that although the procedure is mostly done by obstetricians/gynecologists, sperm bank personnel are the most careful and offer the safest AI. Most sperm banks offer anonymity to their donors unless they agree in writing that the child may contact them on reaching the age of 18.

• *Corrective surgery.* Certain surgical procedures are used in the treatment of infertility, but ironically they may also contribute to infertility because they may cause scarring in the pelvic area. *Tubal insufflation* is a procedure used to determine if the fallopian tubes are open, and *uterine suspension* is an operation that moves the uterus a little within the abdominal cavity to theoretically better enable the woman to become pregnant. Another operation is *ovarian wedge resection*, which may restore the function of diseased ovaries. In addition, there are several procedures to open blocked fallopian tubes.

• *Fertility drugs.* Fertility drugs stimulate a woman's pituitary gland to release hormones that trigger the ovulation process. They are useful for women who don't ovulate or who ovulate irregularly. However, these drugs may cause superovulation, resulting in a multiple-birth pregnancy. Often more than one drug is used. During the course of treatment, women are monitored by their physician for ovulation, temperature, and cervical mucus changes. The monthly cost of these drugs ranges from $25 to $1,500. Fertility drugs are sometimes used with males, too, with the intent of increasing sperm count.

Four of the most commonly used fertility drugs are listed below. The first two, Clomid and Pergonal, are appropriate only for ovulatory problems and are sometimes used in combination.

Clomid (clomiphene). This drug is the most commonly used and is taken by mouth for five to eight days. Possible side effects are similar to the side effects of the Pill. They are: nausea, vomiting, insomnia, vision problems, headache, irritability, breast tenderness, intense mood swings, and sensitivity. Clomid may not be appropriate for women with large fibroids or ovarian cysts. There is a 40 percent chance of pregnancy, with a 10 percent chance of conceiving twins. (Chances of a woman having twins without taking fertility drugs is about 1 percent.)

Pergonal (human menopausal gonadotropin). This is the next most commonly used fertility drug and is prescribed for women who don't respond to Clomid. Pergonal is sold in 50 countries and used by an estimated 9,000 U.S. women every year. It is taken by injection for nine to 12 days. If you take this drug, you must be carefully monitored with daily ultrasound (see "Ultrasound" on page 476) and pelvic exams, along with blood work. Side effects occur rarely, but can be severe, and are: ovarian enlargement, ovarian cysts, abdominal swelling, and weight gain. There is a 20 to 80 percent chance of pregnancy, with a 20 to 40 percent chance of conceiving twins.

Parlodel (bromocriptine). This drug is used by women who have elevated prolactin levels and is taken by mouth every day of the month. The intent is to take the drug until ovulation returns, then to stop the drug, and then get pregnant before your prolactin level increases again. Side effects are: nausea, nasal stuffiness, dizziness, low blood pressure, and headache. There is a 65 to 85 percent chance of pregnancy. The miscarriage rate with Parlodel, similar to the use of Pergonal, is higher than it is for the general population. Parlodel has been available for fertility treatments and has been used for that purpose for 10 years, although it is not approved by the Food and Drug Administration for that use.

GnRH (gonadotropin-releasing hormone). This treatment is released by a pump, which mimics the action of the pituitary gland, and is used with women who do not respond to Clomid. The battery-run pump is three inches by four inches and is strapped around your waist. It's attached to a catheter which is inserted under the skin in your arm. The pump is used daily until ovulation occurs, which often takes one to two weeks. Pregnancy rates vary. Possible side effects are bruising or infection at the needle site, as well as a risk for ovarian cysts.

• *In vitro fertilization (test tube babies).* This process (literally fertilization in glass) begins with the use of fertility drugs to stimulate ovulation. Next, mature eggs are removed from a woman's ovary and fertilized with sperm in a petri dish (a shallow, transparent, covered dish commonly used in laboratories), creating a microscopic embryo (or embryos). Finally, this embryo is then surgically inserted into the woman's uterus.

Newer methods use either the single egg that is produced in a monthly cycle or immature eggs from a woman's ovaries. Both of these procedures eliminate the need for fertility drugs.

In vitro fertilization is often used when a woman's fallopian tubes are blocked and a fertilized egg cannot travel to the uterus in the usual way. It also may be used when the man's sperm count is low, or when the woman has endometriosis.

The first "test tube," or in vitro, baby was born in 1978. About 15 years later, in vitro has created about 20,000 babies in the United States alone. Each procedure—and it usually takes several—costs about $7,000 to $9,000 with prices increasing regularly. If in vitro is going to be successful (only 10 percent of women who use it become pregnant and give birth), it's likely to happen after only a few attempts. Those who do conceive are likely nonsmokers and are most often in their 20s or 30s, and of those, 20 percent will have a multiple birth, usually twins.

In some research centers, clinics freeze extra embryos that are formed during one procedure so that if one embryo doesn't work, another thawed one might later. Several births have been reported from thawed embryos, including twins. (See "In Vitro Fertilization" on page 618 in Recommended Reading.)

Following are newer versions of, or alternatives to, in vitro fertilization:

GIFT (gamete intrafallopian tube transfer), also known as *ZIFT (zygote intrafallopian tube transfer)*. Instead of fertilization occurring in a petri dish, the egg and sperm are mixed together and injected into one of the woman's fallopian tubes either vaginally or with laparoscopy. The cost is $3,500 per month, and the success rate is similar to that of in vitro fertilization. This technique is most often used with couples who have unexplained infertility.

Partial zona dissection. Before the eggs and sperm are combined in a petri dish, the extracted eggs are placed in a solution that makes it easier for the protective outer layer, which includes enzymes, to be pierced by sperm. This procedure can be used when sperm are malformed, immobile, or scarce, but no one knows what long-term effects there are.

• *Donor eggs.* This is the female equivalent of sperm donation. The egg donor is given pregnancy drugs and then her eggs are surgically removed and placed in a petri dish with the sperm of the recipient's mate. Each attempt costs about $10,000 and when successful, the resulting early embryos are transferred into the recipient's uterus. Like donors for artificial insemination, egg donors are paid a fee ($2,000 is average) and are matched to the infertile spouse for ethnic origin, hair and eye color, height, weight, and blood type. Most clinics prefer to use eggs from an anonymous donor, but a few request that the recipient bring her own donor. (Some women have found this to be difficult and embarrassing.) This process is used with women who carry an inherited disease, who don't have ovaries, or who have ovaries that don't produce eggs or produce defective eggs. Donor eggs have been used in successful pregnancies in several women as old as 55 who were past menopause.

• *Embryo adoption, or "Rent-A-Womb."* This is a process that begins with in vitro fertilization, but instead of the embryo being surgically placed into the wife's womb, it's inserted into a second woman's womb. When a woman enters into an embryo adoption arrangement, she doesn't provide any genetic material. She does, however, provide the living conditions in the womb for the baby. During those nine months what she eats and drinks and her state of health affect the fetus. (See "Surrogate Mothers" on page 381.)

I remember the "trying" days. The accoutrements remain fresh in my mind. The basal thermometers, the jagged graphs designed to pinpoint the exact moment of ovulation, the endlessly understanding books claiming, "You, too, can have a baby!" . . . Monitoring of functions was paramount. Once I had to drive a bottle of my newly deposited semen to the hospital. . . . But mostly, there was the trying itself. The synchronized sessions on the couch, the scheduled dalliances in the bed. . . . There always was the sense that this one was going to be the one. That raised the stakes, redoubled the hope. . . . Then my wife's period would come. It became a wrenching cycle.

W hen I saw the syringe, I almost jumped off the table in last minute panic. But, once again, my desire for a child kept me in place and I watched the "stranger's" semen enter my body. The procedure itself is not painful, but the emotional turmoil is quite strong.

W e tried to go with [a donor who had] my husband's appearance— blondish-red hair and five feet, 10 inches. It amazes me; everyone says Gabriel looks just like his dad.

I [sperm donor for 11 children] signed an agreement saying these children could reach me when they're 18. It's like a time capsule.

W e just look at it [conceiving quintuplets after using a fertility drug] as divine will. It's awe-inspiring. And I guess it shows God's got a sense of humor. . . . Our expenses and all will be high, but we'll manage. After seeing them [the quintuplets] in the sonogram, I just don't know what I'd do if one of them didn't make it.

M y doctors say I'm doing fine when I ask, but won't give details. It [in vitro fertilization] feels at first like a cold, clinical way to have a baby. The doctors seem busy, impersonal and uninformative. It's ironic to go to all this trouble to have something we went to all that trouble to avoid for years. . . . I am depressed, wondering when it'll all be resolved.

HOW TO MAKE THE BEST USE OF INFERTILITY TECHNOLOGY

The infertility industry doesn't have to prove that its methods are safe or effective. For example, only 10 percent of the women who try in vitro fertilization ever give birth to a live baby, but the procedure is very much in demand despite its low success rate. Infertility technology is also seductive; once you start trying new procedures, it's hard to stop. (See "Don't Be Seduced by Medical Technology" on page 71.) Moreover, clinics want you to keep coming back. One U.S. infertility clinic reportedly has a sign that reads, "You never fail until you quit trying."

Following are some suggestions to help you make the best use of this technology:

• *Protect yourself by deciding in advance how you'll handle tricky issues and how far you'll go.* Maybe you'll be one of the lucky ones. Maybe you'll get your healthy baby with a minimum amount of investment in fertility technology. If so, you won't have to deal with most of the following issues. But maybe you'll be like most women who use in vitro and similar procedures, the process will take more emotion, time, wear and tear on your body, and money than you thought it would.

What would you do if you ended up with leftover embryos like the Tennessee couple who divorced after creating seven embryos and couldn't agree on custody? What would you do if you become pregnant with more fetuses than you can safely carry? If you abort three fetuses, for instance, and keep two, how will you feel? Since the in vitro procedure doesn't work nine times out of 10, how would you feel when it doesn't work for you? When will you stop — how many times are you willing to try?

How secure are you with the experimental quality of all of these procedures? On the one hand, there is no evidence that babies born from this technology have any more birth defects or problems than babies conceived and carried in the usual way. That includes multiples, too. On average they have more problems than singleton babies, but that's true no matter how the babies were conceived. On the other hand, not enough time has passed to know what the long-term problems might be for the babies. Ultrasound hasn't been proven safe, x-rays are definitely not considered safe for fetuses in the first trimester, and there's some question about the effect on fetuses of exposure to powerful fertility drugs. There's some question about their effects on you, too. A controversial report in 1993 showed a threefold increased rate of ovarian cancer with the use of fertility drugs, in particular, Pergonal and Clomid.

None of us can possibly know everything in advance when it comes to pregnancy, but you can think about these basic issues you may be facing in pursuing a pregnancy.

Since many techno-baby success stories are multiple births, be prepared for premature births and long hospital stays for you while you're pregnant and for the babies after they're born. Almost half of twins are born prematurely, and triplets on average spend four to six weeks in intensive care. Plan in advance to get help for you and your babies. (See "Twins, Triplets, and Quads" on page 570 and "Premature Birth" on page 569 in the Resource Directory. See also "Caregivers" on pages 114 and 557.)

• *Find a clinic with doctors who have as much experience and success with your particular infertility problem as possible.* Look for physicians who have completed at least two years of specialized training in infertility, in addition to a residency. Ask what your chances for success are given your age. (In one study, women aged 39 or younger, for instance, were three and one-half times more likely to become pregnant using GIFT than women 40 or older.)

Ask what percentage of women have live births for any procedure you are considering, not how many get pregnant. The pregnancy rate alone is misleading, since that will always be much higher than the number of babies actually born, due to miscarriages and other pregnancy losses. Ask how many in vitro procedures they will use before reevaluating your chances for a successful pregnancy. (Some clinics reevaluate after two failed in vitro attempts; others keep going as long as you're willing to do it.) Fertility clinics do not offer warranties — you don't get your money back if you don't get pregnant or if you miscarry.

Half of U.S. fertility clinics have not reported any births. No more than a handful of the 170 or so U.S. clinics are responsible for two thirds of the test-tube births. The best clinics have take-home-baby rates of 20 percent. (See "Resolve, Inc." on page 584 in the Resource Directory for infertility specialists referrals.)

• *Find out how much the procedures that you need will cost.* Most insurance companies won't pay the whole cost of these procedures, but some may pay for a part of the expense. The nine states by 1992 that required insurance companies to pay at least a portion of the costs for fertility technology were Arkansas, California, Connecticut, Illinois, Maryland, Massachusetts, Hawaii, Rhode Island, and Texas. Many more states are considering similar laws.

• Stop when you want to stop, and get support from family and friends for your decision.

I had surgery three times, took fertility pills, and was treated for endometriosis with a pill that put 20 pounds on me and gave me hot flashes. After a year, I had a positive pregnancy test. I must have told 300 people in three days I was finally pregnant. It turned out that I wasn't, and I don't think I have ever been so disappointed. I used to cry every time I saw a pregnant woman. The stress of waiting, trying, being disappointed, and hoping was almost too much for me to bear.

I am grateful that I can choose to fight infertility because of doctors and patients who have preceded me. Maybe I won't get a miracle baby, but I know that I will be glad that I had the privilege of trying.

Last January, our dream came true. We finally were pregnant. Joy was cut short when my amniotic fluid began to leak. As hard as we think it is to get pregnant, it is even harder to be pregnant and lose your baby. Should we try again, could I cope with a repeat, should I accept the fact that we may never have our baby? Does hope flare eternal?

I'm numbed by the pain, amazed that I'm so fragile. I never thought I could be emotionally crippled by anything. I want to be a mother, plain and simple. I can't face the possibility of failure. It's a matter of self-preservation. It's a matter of freedom—freedom from want.

We decided with our doctors to put back four embryos to increase the chance of having one. I had panic attacks when I heard it was triplets, but I [mother of triplets after 11 years of fertility treatments] would rather have my hands full than empty.

ADOPTION

Adoption is the process through which a child born to one woman becomes the legal responsibility and child of another woman and, usually, her husband. (Occasionally the adoptive parent is single and/or homosexual.)

Although this is the oldest known solution to infertility, adoption by strangers didn't become common in the United States until the 1920s. Individual states regulate all adoptions, except those of Native American and foreign-born children, which are regulated by the federal government.

One quarter of U.S. babies are born to single women, but only 2 percent of those are given up for adoption. That's a turnaround from several decades ago when nine out of 10 babies of unmarried mothers were given up for adoption, and the supply of babies available for adoption was greater than the need.

Fewer unmarried women give up their babies today for adoption because single motherhood has lost much of its "sinful" stigma, and welfare payments make it possible for some to financially survive. Other single women, especially those in their 30s, are financially secure and choose to get pregnant and raise a child on their own.

The babies most in demand for adoption are healthy, white infants, but the most readily available babies belong to other races or are handicapped. Women who give up their babies for adoption often do it with the hope that their infant will have a better life with an adopting couple. Research has shown that adopted children usually live in two-parent homes with higher family income and education than the U.S. norm.

Another source of adoptive infants is other countries. About 75 percent of the 10,000 foreign-born children who are adopted each year are from Asia, and more than half of those are from Korea. (See "Adoption" on page 550 in the Resource Directory for organizations that specialize in foreign-born children.)

Traditionally, adoption was based on absolute secrecy. Other than a few medical facts about the biologic mother, perhaps her age and a little background, neither the biologic mother nor the adoptive couple knew anything about each other. Perhaps that method better suited a time when there were more babies available than couples to adopt them.

Today biologic mothers who give up their babies often make more demands of the adopting couple. Most mothers who relinquish their babies now choose independent adoptions (which are illegal in a handful of states), instead of working through traditional adoption agencies. This is not shared parenthood; the adoptive parents are still the legal parents of the child. But the biologic mother may choose the adoptive parents, and sometimes she may have an agreement with the adoptive parents to occasionally see the child as she or he is growing up, although the adoptive parents are not legally bound to do this.

Adoptions, "open" or traditional, usually cost the adopting parents between $8,500 and $12,000, although if the arrangement is made through a state agency, adoptions occasionally don't cost the adoptive couple anything. Mothers who give up their babies for adoption have one month to change their minds, and some do — to the dismay of the adopting parents. If you're considering adoption, shop around. Ask agencies what their fees are, the length of waiting time, and how many adoptions they handle each year. Find out all you can about the health of the prospective baby's biological parents, too. (See "Adoption" on page 617 in Recommended Reading.)

I have the good fortune to live on a block where there are three adopted children. One of them came from India. When she arrived, she was three months old but barely weighed six pounds. As the months went by, this frail baby flourished physically and psychologically. Now she is an adorable, healthy toddler. . . . The other adopted babies on the block came from Korea.

*E*ach and every time the phone rings you put your heart on your sleeve. I flew to California to meet with one birth mother. She really wasn't sure what she wanted to do, and I found it very traumatic to go that far to be rejected.

*I*f it hadn't been an open adoption, I wouldn't have given her up. . . . I can picture [the adoptive couple] holding her. I know what their house looks like. I knew I could call her. It was a tremendous sense of relief.

*A*t 26 I got pregnant, had my son, and gave him up for adoption. . . . Although I have not seen him since, I have learned from that experience one very valuable lesson. Decisions affect the rest of our lives; there is no way to have any decision we make end its effect when the immediate results of the decisions are finished.

I was my parents' only biological child. My two brothers were adopted after I was born. One of my brothers could kiss my parents every day for adopting him. He says he could have spent his life growing up in foster homes, but our parents saved him from that. But that's not how my youngest brother feels. He's upset and longingly wants to know who his birth parents are. I spoke to him on the phone the other night and when I said something about Dad, my brother said, "He's your dad, not mine."

SURROGATE MOTHERS

A surrogate mother is a woman who carries a pregnancy for another woman. The surrogate mother enters into a contract with a man to become pregnant by artificial insemination with his sperm for the sole purpose of providing him with a baby which will be legally his. The baby born from such an arrangement is genetically one half this mother's and one half the donor father's.

A newer and more expensive version of surrogacy involves a rent-a-womb arrangement, also known as gestational surrogacy, in which the surrogate mother has no genetic link to the baby. (See "Embryo Adoption" on page 374.)

The concept of surrogacy is not new, though the first publicized U.S. surrogate arrangement occurred only about a decade ago. Dating back to Biblical times and earlier, there have been many instances of concubines or slaves who have carried owners' babies. For many centuries wet nursing (breastfeeding another woman's baby) was another arrangement in which a woman "rented" a part of her body and was considered entirely ordinary.

Some say that perhaps as many as 5,000 U.S. babies have been born in surrogate arrangements. Others say there have been many more thousands of these arrangements. No one knows the exact figure because surrogacy arrangements do not have to be reported. (See "Infertility and the Law" on page 385.) In U.S. surveys, approval of surrogate motherhood, especially among the young and well educated, has increased steadily since 1983. (See "Surrogate Motherhood" on page 618 in Recommended Reading for pro and con information about surrogacy.)

The typical person who buys the services of a surrogate mother is in his late 30s and well educated, as is his mate. The total cost to the purchasing couple may be as much as $35,000 (more for gestational surrogacy). The typical surrogate mother is married, in her 20s, Christian, has at least one child, and has a high school education. Although surrogate motherhood candidates score high in empathy, only 15 percent would do it without pay. These women also like to be pregnant and may have been adopted themselves, given up a baby for adoption, or had an abortion.

Much of the criticism of surrogate motherhood is directed at its "unnaturalness," the appearance of baby-selling and the obvious social-strata difference between surrogate mothers and the purchaser-fathers. Yet the appeal of surrogate motherhood is multifaceted. Most couples find that it's quicker and theoretically easier than the usual adoption, though more expensive. It allows for the man, and occasionally the woman (either through a relative, such as a sister, or in a "rent-a-womb" arrangement), to have a genetic link with the child.

The typical pair who arrange for a surrogate birth is a childless married couple in which the wife is permanently infertile. Other people who have made surrogate arrangements are single men, homosexual couples, and heterosexual fertile couples. In 1987, both a homosexual couple in Kansas and a single man in California arranged surrogate births. And in Virginia, a married couple in their late 40s missed having kids around after their two children were grown, so they arranged the surrogate births of two more.

Sometimes surrogate mothers negotiate for visiting rights with the child; others may never meet the purchasing couple before or after the birth. In most cases the surrogate and purchasing couple meet initially and perhaps during the pregnancy, maybe even during the labor, but never again after the birth. Currently, at least 24 agencies operate as surrogate "match-makers" in the United States.

If you and your partner are considering hiring a surrogate mother, one strong advantage is that the baby has a genetic link to one of you. A strong disadvantage, however, is that the natural mother may decide to not give up the baby. Surrogate mothers sometimes underestimate the impact of their feelings about the baby, and some have great difficulty in giving their child to someone else. This may be particularly true with those surrogate mothers who never had a baby before, but it's also true with women who have had other children, especially if the other children are excited about the new sibling.

If your surrogate mother can't go through with the arrangement, you may then have a genetic link with a child you will not be able to see, much less raise. When fathers have taken these cases to court, outcomes have been mixed. The father retained custody of "Baby M" in the 1987 New Jersey case, but the surrogate mother has visitation rights, and there are other cases in which the father had to settle for shared custody with the surrogate mother. When the purchaser father and his mate divorce, settlement is complicated and may involve the surrogate mother, too.

The surrogate mother usually earns $10,000, over and above whatever expenses are incurred for the pregnancy and birth. She may feel a great deal of satisfaction for giving the gift of life to another couple. If her egg is used, she may value extending her genetic link into the world.

A desire to be pregnant is one of the strong motivations of women who choose to become surrogate mothers. The flip side of this is that women who like pregnancy enough to become pregnant for someone else are probably at a higher risk for feeling especially attached to the baby. The reality is that pregnancy and birth are always a major event in a woman's life, no matter whether the baby was planned, unplanned, or contracted for. A woman's feelings about a particular pregnancy, and a particular baby, are unpredictable. It may be easier for surrogate mothers to willingly have a baby for someone they are related to, because they will always have a tie with that person.

It should be noted that some surrogate mothers readily relinquish custody, essentially never looking back. They derive satisfaction from their contribution and accept the consequences.

If you enter into an agreement with a surrogate mother, you may draw up a contract that includes stipulations about the pregnancy, such as medication use and the requirement for an amniocentesis, and the agreement to an abortion if that test shows the fetus to be abnormal.

It's often written into surrogate contracts that the father, who is paying the surrogate mother to have his child, is responsible for the child if the pregnancy lasts more than four or five months, even if the baby has birth defects. The responsibility for such a child is either dependent on the father's good will to honor the contract or on the decisions of the court to which the surrogate mother and the purchaser-father may appeal.

O ur attitude is that there can never be too many people in your life who care about you. . . . I told Matthew [her 5-year-old, adopted son born through a surrogate arrangement] that she [the surrogate mother] carried him and gave birth to him, but she let us raise him — like a gift. Now we talk to her on the phone [and] we write.

I was the center of attention during my surrogate pregnancy. I was important then. Once I had the baby though, it was "Bye-bye, Sally." I called the baby's adoptive parents once when I traveled to the state where they live. Ice cubes on the phone — they sure didn't want to hear from me.

M y son has a mellow disposition. Part of that might be the result of my husband's genes, but it could also have come from this baby's real mother. She was a no-nonsense lady. I have nothing but respect for her.

N ine months of my life is not that much to give to a couple. They're borrowing one tiny little egg and some space. I'm not giving that much of myself, but I'm giving a lot to them.

We birth mothers call it the big sleep, and eventually they will all wake up from this denial and realize what they've done. It just took Mary Beth Whitehead [the surrogate mother in the 1987 "Baby M" case] less time than most of us.

I had told myself all along that it would be easy but it wasn't. . . . It was hard for me to take the money. I rationalized that we'd use it to get something for the kids because if the money was just for me I'd feel as if I'd sold her.

My older sister, Carolee, had a hysterectomy when she was 21. . . . Although we wanted to have another baby, and I was already 33, we decided that Carolee and Ernie's desire for a child should come first. . . . After hours of a very difficult labor, I gave birth to my sister's baby.

I felt their joy, but it was different from mine. I never thought of him as my child. I was carrying him for another couple. Even to this day I have no second thoughts. I'm happy for the couple.

WHAT DO THE CHILDREN THINK?

It is too soon to know much about children born with the help of fertility drugs, in vitro fertilization, donor eggs or embryos, and surrogate arrangements, because these options are so recent. Many children born by the in vitro technique are twins, triplets, or members of even larger multiples and, consequently, are often premature, small, and of low birth weight. But one study of preschool toddlers showed no difference between in vitro–born children and others. Some children born with help from an anonymous donor and artificial insemination resent being the offspring of an unknown father who sold his seed to a sperm bank.

There's no perfect formula to please every child about her or his roots. Many parents who raise their own 100-percent-biologic children can attest to that.

INFERTILITY AND THE LAW

Along with opportunities for great joy, infertility technology has created extremely difficult legal tangles. Among them are:

• *Leftover embryos.* In the in vitro fertilization process, excess embryos are almost always created. In fact, it's estimated that tens of thousands of these embryos are stored in tanks of liquid nitrogen in the United States. (In England and France, on the other hand, the number is far less because the number of embryos created at one time is restricted to three.)

Once a healthy embryo is inserted successfully into a woman, what happens to the leftovers? In parts of the United States and in some other countries, they can be used for research for a limited number of days. In the United States there's been at least one case in which custody of seven embryos was an issue in a divorce case. In Australia, there was a question about who had custody of the embryos of a couple killed in a plane crash. Most states do not have regulations about embryos as yet, but Louisiana does. It gives embryos the same rights as persons, and six other states prohibit research on embryos. Currently, there is no U.S. national policy regarding frozen embryos.

• *Paternal rights.* In 30 states, if a woman is successfully artificially inseminated and if she is married, her husband's name is put on the birth certificate as the father, if he signs a statement acknowledging the child. But what if the woman is not married? Does the donor have paternal rights? In California, if the woman has a physician perform the insemination, she's protected against the sperm donor claiming any rights. However, if she finds a donor on her own, she's not protected, and in one case, the sperm donor demanded — and won — visitation rights.

• *Birth parents rights.* With adoption, the biologic mother has one month after the birth to change her mind about giving up her baby. Once she signs the adoption papers, however, the child irrevocably belongs to the adoptive parent(s). Since the 1970s, most states require that the unwed father of the baby not only be notified of adoption procedures, but have a right to a hearing to discuss those procedures.

• *Surrogate mothers.* The surrogate mother signs a contract with the purchaser father to provide him with a child who will be his. The father's mate then legally adopts the child after birth. No state has a law legalizing surrogacy contracts, 18 states ban or severely limit surrogate arrangements, and many other states are considering laws.

Great Britain allows occasional surrogate-mother arrangements, but has outlawed payment for them. France and Germany prohibit them altogether. Norway, Sweden, and the Netherlands are currently considering bans on surrogate arrangements. Australia's 1984 fertility-technology law states that fertility procedures can occur only in government-approved facilities, that in vitro fertilization may be used only as a last resort, and that it can only follow 12 months of other fertility treatments.

No money can be paid for donated sperm, eggs, embryos, or surrogate mother arrangements. And the "adoption" of unwanted embryos is encouraged. Although the legality of who is responsible for embryos is mostly an unclear issue, there are many thousands of frozen embryos worldwide.

Interstitial Cystitis (IC)

What It Is

Interstitial cystitis (IC) is a painful, chronic inflammation of the bladder wall. The lining and elasticity of the bladder wall are reduced because it has become scarred and stiff. A severely IC-afflicted bladder may hold only two or three ounces, which is less than a third of the capacity of a normal bladder.

Signs and Symptoms

Symptoms of IC mimic an acute urinary tract infection and include a frequent need to urinate, often with 50 to 100 trips a day to the bathroom. (There's some pain relief with urination when the problem is IC, although there is not when the problem is a urinary tract infection.) IC is also characterized by an urgent need to urinate, accompanied by intense pain and pressure in the lower abdomen. Another symptom is pain in the urethra and vagina, including painful sex, since vaginal penetration increases the pressure on the bladder.

IC is often confused with urinary tract infections (see "Urinary Tract Infections" on page 515). Today IC is suspected when you have what is thought to be a urinary tract infection, but no bacteria are present in a urine culture, and antibiotics don't give relief.

Urination frequency keeps many women with IC unable to hold a job. They are also often fatigued, probably because they get so little sleep at night.

MAKING THE DIAGNOSIS

Several diagnostic procedures are used, mostly to rule out other conditions, but the IC diagnosis is only certain with cystoscopy, a procedure in which a thin instrument is inserted into the urethra to view the inside of the bladder and examine it for scarring.

IC is a progressive disease that ranges from mild to very severe, and nine out of 10 people who have it are women. In the United States the number is estimated to be nearly half a million. Typically, it takes about four years after symptoms are first felt and from two to five physicians to get an accurate diagnosis. The difficulty of diagnosis occurs because many other conditions and diseases have to be eliminated first, such as anatomic defects, endometriosis (see "Endometriosis" on page 329), as well as any other bladder or kidney disorder.

IC is often believed erroneously to be a psychological ailment. It is diagnosed more often in middle-aged women than in younger women, but perhaps only because that's the age when symptoms have progressed far enough that these women are persistent in getting an accurate diagnosis.

As with other difficult-to-diagnose diseases, the woman who is most likely to obtain both diagnosis and treatment for IC is a woman who believes she has the right to know what's wrong with her body, acts with confidence and persistence, no matter how many times she's not helped, and can pay medical fees, either from insurance or personal income. If you think that you might have IC, you'll have to work both to find a physician who knows about it and to find the right combination of treatments for you. (See "Interstitial Cystitis" on page 618 in Recommended Reading and on page 584 in the Resource Directory.)

The pain used to make it hard to walk, much less exercise. I have to be aware of what I eat and drink. I've gotten relief, but all I've done is put the disease on hold. It took five doctors and many thousands of dollars to get the correct diagnosis.

My most outrageous false diagnosis was my problem was psychological, and I didn't want sex with my husband. If I hadn't been married happily for years to a wonderful man, I might have believed this doctor, if only because I wanted someone to be successful in figuring out my problem.

Causes

The causes of IC are not clear, but it's believed by some researchers that it is the result of a bladder injury. Some women with IC have a history of urinary tract infections earlier in their lives, and some researchers believe certain antibiotics used to treat urinary tract infections may contribute to or cause IC. Environmental factors, like chemical pollutants, and the Epstein-Barr virus (linked to chronic fatigue syndrome — see "Chronic Fatigue Syndrome" on page 295) are also suspected. In addition, researchers wonder about a hormonal link, because IC often begins, or gets worse, after an oophorectomy, the removal of the ovaries, or gets better (or worse) during pregnancy and with use of the Pill.

Treatment Options

There is no cure for IC. However, many women receive some relief, often from a combination of treatments. Some options combat frequency of urination, others focus on pain with 75 percent receiving some relief.

In one procedure, the bladder is distended by filling it with water, under general anesthesia, to stretch it. This improves the bladder's capacity.

Different drugs are used to help the bladder wall regenerate, including the most popular Rimso 50 (dimethyl sulfoxide). Others are Clorpactin and silver nitrate. Some women use narcotics, antidepressants, and antihistamines to ease the pain, though their use is controversial.

Transcutaneous electrical nerve stimulation (TENS) is also used to relieve pain, as is the reduction of bladder nerve endings. For a few women, the pain is so severe that they choose from a variety of surgical options.

HOME REMEDIES YOU CAN TRY

Since IC symptoms ordinarily come and go, do what you can to keep the flare-ups to as few as possible, though the reality is the return of symptoms is often unpredictable. Specific foods are troublesome to some, but not all, women with IC. Because an IC pain reaction to food usually occurs in about 20 minutes, you'll know by trial and error if the foods and beverages on the following lists are troublesome for you. Try the following and see what works for you:

• *Avoid foods high in acid.* They are: alcohol, citrus fruits, tomatoes, apples, cantaloupes, carbonated drinks, cranberries, grapes, guava, peaches, pineapple, plums, strawberries, and vinegar.
• *Avoid foods high in tyrosine, tyramine, tryptophan, and aspartame (NutraSweet).* These include: diet drinks and other products sweetened with NutraSweet, avocados, bananas, brewer's yeast, canned figs, champagne, cheeses (hard and soft), chicken livers, chocolate, corned beef, cranberries, fava or lima beans, mayonnaise, nuts, onions, pickled herring, pineapple, prunes, raisins, rye bread, saccharine, sour cream, soy sauce, and yogurt. (See discussion of aspartame on page 30 and Gillespie on page 618 in Recommended Reading.)
• *Take one teaspoon of baking soda in water once a day.* This may decrease the burning sensation you feel in your bladder.
• *Drink lots of clear liquids.*

LUPUS

WHAT IT IS

Lupus is a chronic inflammatory disease that affects the connective tissue, the network of fibers throughout the body that binds together and supports other tissues and organs. Lupus is an autoimmune disorder, in which the body's own immune system attacks the connective tissue.

There are three kinds of lupus. *Discoid lupus erythematosus (DLE)* is the most common and also most mild form that mostly affects the skin, usually from the upper chest on up, causing raised, scaly skin areas. The second form is *systemic lupus erythematosus (SLE)*, which affects the internal organs and systems of the body. This type varies in severity, but is potentially fatal. The third kind is *drug-induced lupus*, which has the same symptoms as systemic lupus. Usually when the particular drug is stopped, the disease goes away.

SIGNS AND SYMPTOMS

Lupus usually has a combination of symptoms, and they often come and go. Common signs, particularly when they occur together, are:

- Arthritislike joint pain and/or swelling and redness that sometimes lasts for a day or two, then moves on to another part of the body.
- Red skin rashes, which can be mild and fleeting or more severe, sometimes developing into ulcers, scabs, and scars. A common rash is called the "butterfly rash" because it appears in the shape of a butterfly across the cheeks and bridge of the nose.
- Sensitivity to the sun
- Unexplained chronic or recurrent low fever
- Hair loss (including temporary bald spots)
- Anemia (see "Anemia" on page 158)
- Pale or purple fingers or toes from cold or stress
- Depression
- Fatigue
- Nausea, vomiting, and abdominal pain
- Enlarged lymph nodes in women who are in the active phase of SLE
- Problems with kidneys and bladder

CAUSES

Researchers think the cause of lupus may be a combination of heredity and environmental triggers, although all that's known for sure is that the disorder is not contagious. There is a genetic link, as it often runs in families, and there may be a hormonal link, too, because it's more likely to occur during the childbearing years. (Most women with lupus are able to have successful pregnancies, especially if they are monitored closely. Although there's a slight increase in the rate of stillbirths, worsening of lupus symptoms during pregnancy is not common. However, the disease frequently flares after the baby is born.)

The triggers that may release an as yet unidentified virus that induces lupus flare-ups in some women are: sunlight, infection, injury, surgery, overexertion and exhaustion, nervous tension, emotional upsets, and certain drugs, including the Pill (see "The Pill" on page 181), infection-fighting sulfa compounds, antihypertensive hydralazine, and procainamide, a drug used to control irregular heartbeats.

MAKING THE DIAGNOSIS

Nine out of 10 people who have lupus are women, and it's more common among minorities, especially African-American women. As with other difficult-to-diagnose diseases, a woman with lupus may be told that it's all in her head after other diseases have been ruled out, and it may be years before she gets an accurate evaluation.

(See "Lupus" on page 618 in Recommended Reading and on page 586 in the Resource Directory. If you are African-American, see White on page 610 in Recommended Reading. Also contact the rheumatology or immunology department of your local medical school and ask for a physician referral.)

O ver the years, I've been hospitalized 28 times and operated on so often for so many different, seemingly unrelated, reasons that it is hard to keep an accurate count. . . . I was convinced I was going to die in 1978 from this unexplainable illness. I was diagnosed with lupus in 1979.

TREATMENT OPTIONS

There is no cure for lupus. Treatment is individualized, as no two patients are alike. Some women with lupus have few symptoms and need treatment only periodically. Others need regular drug treatment, including aspirin to reduce pain and inflammation, antimalarial drugs to alleviate skin problems, and cortisone, a steroid drug used in both creams and oral drugs to reduce all symptoms. (See "Aspirin" on page 33 and "Cortisone" on page 33.) Other experimental treatments include drugs and a form of radiation therapy.

HOME REMEDIES YOU CAN TRY

• *Avoid stress and exposure to extreme sunlight.* (See suggestions for relieving stress on page 55 and "Skin Health" on page 59.)
• *Avoid excess fat, protein (especially from animal sources),* and salt, since lupus can damage kidneys. (See "How to Find Fat in Your Food" on page 29.)

• *Get enough rest* to avoid lupus-triggering infections. (See "Fatigue" on page 344.)

• *Exercise* to strengthen muscles, ease joint pain, and reduce the bone-thinning side effects of some of the drugs you may be using. (See "Exercise" on page 41.)

• *Avoid use of the drugs, including the Pill, that are known to trigger lupus.*

• *Boost your immune system.* (See "Immune System" on page 9 and "How to Stay Healthy" on page 25.)

MENOPAUSE

WHAT IT IS

Menopause signals the end of fertility and is the cessation of menstrual periods and the gradual shutdown of the ovaries' production of estrogen. (Other parts of the body will still produce estrogen, but to a lesser extent.)

It is the most obvious event in the female version of a life-cycle phase called the climacteric, which is a time of biochemical change, just as puberty is. While puberty occurs over a period of about 10 years, menopause covers a period of about 15 years from approximately age 45 to age 60. It is divided into three phases: premenopausal (still menstruating but noticing changes), menopausal (cycles definitely changing with periods becoming closer or further apart), or postmenopausal (no longer bleeding).

Just like puberty, the climacteric entails gradual changes in all body tissues for both women and men. (In men, hormones also start to decline in the late 40s, often decreasing frequency of erection and ejaculation.) About half of all women have stopped menstruating altogether by age 48, and the natural menopause range is from the late 30s to the mid-50s.

Surgical menopause is the removal of the ovaries (oophorectomy) and can occur as early as the teens, though this is rare. It nearly always accompanies the removal of the uterus (hysterectomy). Hysterectomy by itself is not surgical menopause because the ovaries are left in the body and retain their function of releasing estrogen. (See "Hysterectomy and Oophorectomy" on page 354.)

SIGNS AND SYMPTOMS

Naturally occurring menopause is characterized by the absence of menstrual periods for 12 months. It's estimated that 80 percent (though no one really knows for sure what percentage) of women experience hot flashes with perhaps night sweats and eventually vaginal dryness.

Hot flashes are harmless, sudden waves of heat that spread through the face and neck and sometimes the rest of the body, which are sometimes accompanied by heart palpitations. Hot flashes usually begin about the time your periods start to slow down, they can come and go, and they are more common during hot weather and in the evening. They can happen anywhere, anytime, and usually last from 15 seconds to two minutes. Some women barely notice them, while others find them life-disrupting. Some flashes are mild feelings of warmth; others cause a woman to turn red, break into a sweat, and then feel cold afterwards. They may occur several times a day or only once or twice a week. They usually persist for one to three years, though that will vary from woman to woman, and it's believed they are a vascular response to the body's new hormonal levels.

Women who have always perspired easily and those who exercise regularly may notice little difference between these flashes and the sweat that they've been familiar with for years. However, hot flashes are reported to be more severe among women who have had hysterectomies, particularly those who have had their ovaries removed, too. (When men have their testicles—the male version of ovaries—removed, three quarters report hot flashes as well.) Hot flashes are also commonly more severe in women who don't sweat easily and also in thin women, because they don't retain as much estrogen in their body as do women who have more fat cells. Also, women who have had more than 20 months of pregnancy generally experience far fewer hot flashes than do women with fewer or no months of pregnancy.

Vaginal dryness is another result of hormonal changes and usually doesn't occur until long after hot flashes have started. The dryness and thinness of your vaginal walls often makes intercourse painful, though your sex drive will at least likely remain the same, if not increase because of the increased role of the male hormone androgen in your body after menopause. Hormonal changes in the body at menopause speed up this vaginal change, but vaginal dryness is also associated with having little or no sex life, or at least not enough to keep the vagina moist.

The same hormonal changes that alter your vagina also cause your breast tissue to soften, and your uterus, ovaries, and fallopian tubes to get smaller.

In addition to the above symptoms, about 25 percent of women develop the bone-thinning disease *osteoporosis* after menopause. (See "Osteoporosis" on page 431.) And some women experience insomnia, which is a likely consequence of night sweats. Insomnia may cause symptoms of sleep deprivation: anxiety, irritability, depression, fatigue, sensations of breathlessness, and tingling in the extremities. Otherwise, menopausal women experience no increase in depression.

As menopause approaches, menstrual periods become shorter and perhaps lighter over at least a two-year period, though some women experience heavier periods occasionally. The ovaries cease releasing eggs and production of the hormone estrogen decreases. Typically, the ovaries gear down slowly. Periods may be skipped for a month or two and then start up again, with longer intervals between periods. It's not unusual to have several days of spotting before a period. These irregular bleeding patterns are normal. Eventually, menstruation stops altogether, though no woman can tell which period is going to be her last. A few women stop menstruating abruptly with no previous change in their cycles.

Heavy bleeding means passing more than a half cup of blood in one day. Since it's hard to actually measure the fluid, you can tell if your bleeding is heavy in one or more of the following ways: You pass many or large clots, your menstrual blood is bright red for more than a few hours, or you use a tampon plus two pads with frequent trips to the bathroom. Heavy bleeding can occur any time during your menstrual life, but it often occurs in early menopause when the time between periods is shorter and the flow is longer and heavier. Heavy bleeding is probably more common than anyone knows, and it may be perfectly normal for many women, though uncomfortable. Its causes are not clear, though it's believed by many that it is a result of a change in the balance of the hormones estrogen and progesterone (or progestin). Occasionally, heavy menstrual flow is associated with having "low" thyroid levels, too. (See "Your Body and Its Systems" on page 9 for more information on hypothyroidism.) Triggers are thought to be excessive stress, inadequate diet, and changes in exercise or daily living patterns.

Menopause, menopause. Well, it surely must have happened to me. [Pause] Of course, it did, I haven't menstruated in more than 25 years. My dear,

I've been way too busy with my own business for the last 30 years to experience whatever it is people say you're supposed to experience with menopause.

Because of my work, I travel 50,000 miles a year in my covered pick-up truck, which is my home away from home. Frankly, I miss my hot flashes because on a cold night when I climbed into the back of my truck to go to sleep, I could count on a hot flash to warm up the bed.

MAKING THE DIAGNOSIS

In order to rule out uterine fibroids or uterine cancer (which is rare) as the cause for heavy bleeding, physicians may also suggest diagnosis with an endometrial biopsy or a hysteroscope (device through which the interior of your uterus can be scanned in a doctor's office). Your physician may suggest a D & C or a hysterectomy depending in part on your age, the amount of bleeding, and the physician's point of view. (See "Uterine Fibroids" on page 522, "Uterine Cancer" on page 233, "Endometrial Biopsy" on page 369, and "Dilation and Curettage" on page 313.)

Some women have early-onset (late 30s, early 40s) or late-onset (late 50s) menopause because their mothers did, and the daughters mimic the same pattern. However, a life-style habit, such as smoking, or procedures, such as radiation therapy, chemotherapy, and occasionally even a tubal ligation, may cause an earlier menopause that has nothing to do with genetics. And for unknown reasons, women who give birth to twins start menopause early as well. On the other hand, women whose menstrual cycles over the years were on average more than 26 days or who have had children (the more children there are, the more the influence) or who are larger or taller than the norm experience menopause later. Information is not available about whether breastfeeding also causes a later menopause as well.

Researchers have found that the time in between your periods at menopause mirrors the pattern of your menstrual cycle when you started as a teenager. But few of us keep a record of our first periods, so you probably can't check that pattern similarity for yourself.

More of your periods will be anovulatory, that is, you won't be ovulating and you may not have some of your usual premenstrual symptoms, like tender breasts. This absence of symptoms can be misleading, though. For one thing, anovulatory periods can occur occasionally 20 years before menopause, and for another, you may be making lifestyle and dietary changes that reduce premenstrual symptoms like tender breasts (see "Premenstrual Syndrome" on page 408). If you've had a hysterectomy, but still have at least one ovary, you won't know you're experiencing menopause until you have a hot flash or perhaps notice that your vagina is drier.

TREATMENT OPTIONS

Estrogen Replacement Therapy (see "Estrogen Replacement Therapy" on page 337) is often prescribed to relieve hot flashes, night sweats, and vaginal dryness. Another option for vaginal dryness is estrogen cream. A traditional medical solution for heavy bleeding is a short course of Provera. It stops the bleeding usually in 24 to 48 hours. Common side effects include depression, fatigue, and appetite and weight changes.

When I went to my regular doctor because of the heavy bleeding, he suggested right away that I have a hysterectomy and take hormone pills. A friend suggested that I get a second opinion, so I did. The second doctor told me that I didn't need a hysterectomy, that it was normal for my body to do this, and why not take a wait-and-see attitude. I took Provera and iron tablets for a few days, felt much better, and eventually the bleeding episodes stopped.

If I wanted any sex life, I had to use estrogen cream. And I must say it does work.

HOME REMEDIES YOU CAN TRY

• *Eat well.* (See "The Menopause Diet" on page 32 for specific food, vitamin, and herbal suggestions.)
• *Join a menopause support group* where other women are having some of the same experiences that you are, and you can benefit from group knowledge and support. (See "Menopause" on page 618 in Recommended Reading and on page 588 in the Resource Directory.)

Specific suggestions for hot flashes and night sweats are:

• *Avoid hot flash triggers, such as spicy food, caffeine, and alcohol.*
• *Stay out of hot rooms* (and beds).
• *Exercise regularly* to improve circulation.

• *Drink cool water or juices after exercise, or when you feel a flash coming on.*

• *Learn to relax and use meditation techniques* and other stress relievers. (See suggestions for the relief of stress on page 55.)

• *Try acupuncture and Chinese herbs*, both of which are sometimes effective with hot flashes. (See "Acupuncture" on page 82.)

Specific suggestions for vaginal dryness are:

• *Have sex more often*, either intercourse or masturbation. That alone may be enough of a lubricant. Sex researchers Masters and Johnson report that if a woman remains sexually active, the vagina does not constrict significantly, and can continue to lubricate well at any age — though that's very individual. (Some women report vaginal dryness in their 20s and 30s if they have little or no sex life.)

• *Spend more time with foreplay.* That will give your vaginal juices more opportunity to flow on their own.

• *Use a water-based lubricant gel (not petroleum jelly) or vitamin E oil* while the problem exists. Vaginal dryness may be only temporary. Avoid products, such as perfumed toilet papers, that dry or irritate your vagina.

• *Do pelvic floor exercises* (see "Kegel Exercises" on page 47) to strengthen your pelvic floor and enhance vaginal lubrication.

• *Drink adequate water* daily for healthy vaginal tissues.

Specific suggestions for heavy bleeding are:

• *Avoid long hot baths and showers on heavy-flow days*, because the heat may increase the bleeding.

• *Wait it out*, while paying attention to diet and supplements to avoid anemia (see "Anemia" on page 158).

• *Exercise regularly* to help maintain your body's hormonal balance.

• *Reduce alcohol and avoid aspirin*, because it can reduce your blood's clotting ability.

Going through menopause taught me the lesson of moderation. If I ate too much, drank too much coffee or wine, or didn't get enough sleep, I would have gobs of hot flashes. When I lived my life more moderately, I wasn't bothered.

At first menopause was very difficult for me. I was waking at night with hot flashes and couldn't get back to sleep. . . . My daughter was driving me nuts, *which didn't help. My doctors said I should take estrogen pills, but they made my breasts extremely sore and gave me a funny feeling in my head. Then a friend of mine at work started taking me to her yoga class. That really turned things around for me. I guess I learned how to relax for the first time in my life. My body felt better; I stopped the estrogen and started vitamins. The hot flashes still come but they don't bother me any more. I've learned so much in that class that I think I feel healthier than when I was 30.*

I was going to an acupuncturist for shoulder pain at the time my periods stopped. When I told her that the hot flashes were driving me crazy and keeping me up at nights, she gave me some Chinese pills that I took three times a day. In a matter of days, I didn't have the flashes anymore, nor have they returned.

MENOPAUSE AND BIRTH CONTROL

General advice is to keep using birth control until you've been period-free for two years if you're less than 50 years old, and one year if you're more than 50. Be aware that natural family planning (see "Natural Family Planning" on page 212) may not be reliable during this time, and many doctors find Pill use questionable for women in their mid-40s to 50s. Barrier contraceptives may be a better option for you. (See "Barrier Contraceptives" on page 190.)

Some researchers believe that many women are sterile for several years before menopause, but this probably only applies to those who are in their 50s when they quit menstruating (though, yes, occasionally women in their 50s conceive). The so-called "change of life" baby (one who is born to a woman who thought she was menopausal because of period irregularity) is most likely born to a woman in her early 40s. If you miss a couple of periods and wonder if you may be pregnant, don't rely on home pregnancy tests because they are more likely to have a false-positive result for you (see "Making the Diagnosis" on page 447).

Check with your health care provider for lab tests, one of which measures your blood level of FSH, the hormone that makes ovarian follicles grow. Levels tend to rise dramatically around menopause. The other test is an examination of your vaginal cells to see if they have begun to get thinner. Both tests can give you indications of whether you are in menopause or not.

MENOPAUSE MYTHS

Many things happen to you at around age 50 that have nothing to do with menopause. For example, for most of you your children are leaving home and living their own lives. Research shows that only about 3 percent of women experience an "empty nest" depression resulting from being left behind as young adult children "fly" into the world. (Of course, the current avalanche of young adults returning home to live makes the prospect of an empty nest impossible for many women.) However, the woman most likely to experience empty-nest sorrow is one who doesn't work outside the home, and her focus, as well as her rewards in life, come from her family and their accomplishments.

Or perhaps your kids don't understand you. Or perhaps your parents are getting older and need more help. Many women find this depressing. Or perhaps your mate is in flux, too. It may feel like no one is stable. Friends, not just older relatives, are dying and you realize that your days are numbered, too.

You or some of your friends are newly divorced or widowed. The number of widows and divorced women increases enormously when women reach their 50s.

It has nothing to do with my body; it's my soul. I stopped menstruating this year. I expected that. I didn't expect the adults my children grew to be. I invested the best of myself in my children for 25 years, and now I see them becoming people I hadn't expected. If I'm not careful, I will think all these kids I spent so many years with are strangers.

Now I understand why my mom acted the way she did when I left home. She didn't have anything to do, and that was the 1950s when most married women didn't work outside the home. I wasn't close to her in my 20s because she always worried about me. Too heavy!

My mother is 46, and she was recently divorced. I'm afraid that she won't be able to deal with the sexual revolution. She has no idea what guys are like today. Mom says she intends to date and have all the fun she hasn't had in years. I just hope she remembers she is a grandmother and needs to set a good example for her granddaughter.

Issues with my mom had to be sorted out. She is 75 and depends upon me for many things. She will be dying soon. She has cancer and Parkinson's disease.

My oldest daughter is a senior in college. I have to work it through—this letting go of her. My husband is also evaluating his life and his work. I feel squeezed between the generations. I feel responsible for my mother, my children, everyone.

My life has been so full of changes in the last five years. The painful divorce, loss of income, finding my way at 50, surviving financially, managing the business, home, and property, social life, sex life, and concern about how to stay healthy are all possible sources for the blahs.

I became a widow at the age of 43 just when I began menopause. . . . I have been celibate since my husband's death. I cannot say with certainty my state of mind is due to my body's changes or the many adjustments I have made these past few years. However, for what it's worth, here it is: I often feel cheated because I am a widow. I was looking forward to menopause—then I could relax and enjoy having a relationship with my husband. Until that time I was always a little uneasy about having sex because of the worry of pregnancy.

To counteract some of the confusion you may be feeling:

• *Live your own life.* Quit trying to please the others in your life more than yourself.

• *Decide you are having a midlife adventure instead of a crisis.* What you do with those inevitable midlife issues is up to you. One option is to treat these midlife problems as opportunities. You'll live another 30 years or so past menopause, unlike our great-grandmothers at the turn of the last century, who often died within a decade after their last period.

• *Feel passion.* Fall in love again with your partner. Or fall in love with your work. Or decide who you want to spend the rest of your life with, and what that life will be like. But be sure to feel passion.

Our kids hated it when we sold their childhood home in Minneapolis. They thought the house and us should always be waiting for them. Here we were, just the two of us, kicking around in this 12-room house that was just right for us and six kids a dozen years ago, but not right for Jack and me now. We sold it, left our office jobs, and found work in the theater in Denver. I don't know which they found the most shocking—the move or our new careers.

I picked up my shampoo bottle and tried to spray my hair with it. I looked all over for my lipstick which was right where I had left it in front of me. I talked to myself, saying aloud, "Do you have your key? Do you know where you're going?" I was a crazy person. Then the phone rang, and it was a friend wishing me good luck. When I told her what I was doing, she laughed and said with a smile in her voice, "Maybe you're just menopausal. You know what doctors say!" "Menopausal, baloney," I said. "I'm 15 minutes away from my audition with the best regional theater in America."

When I was 50 I fell madly in love and though I had had many lovers in my life, this affair was and is now the epitome of sexual pleasure and fulfillment. When I finally realized I had hot flashes they had been going on for several months and stopped soon after. I thought those hot flashes were sexual flushes of pleasure for awhile. I had a hysterectomy at age 35, so the obvious clue for menopause of no periods didn't exist for me.

Menopause has a reputation, both good and bad, around the world. In some countries, a menopausal woman takes on her matriarchal position as tribal elder. In China, she's entitled to claim more freedom and equality with men. And in parts of Mexico, older women can get drunk and use obscene language in public, just like men can. However, in some societies, a woman's role diminishes once she is no longer fertile. Some African women are sent to nunneries, because they can't have babies anymore. And in parts of rural Ireland, a menopausal woman might take to her bed for a good part of the rest of her life because her baby days — and her value — are finished.

The U.S. menopausal culture is a combination of Margaret Mead's postmenopausal zest as the best time of your life and the medical model of menopause as a treatable disease. The good news is you get to decide where you are on the continuum.

Menstruation

What It Is

Menstruation is the periodic flow of bloody fluid (about one and one-half to six ounces) that signifies that no egg has been fertilized.

Prior to menstruation, the hormone estrogen (secreted by the ovaries) thickens the lining of the uterus. After eight to 10 days, the ovary releases an egg and begins to secrete the hormone progesterone. If the egg is not fertilized, the secretion of progesterone declines, causing the uterine lining to be sloughed off, and the menstrual flow to start.

Periods without ovulation are called anovulatory periods. They occur as women get older, though the phenomenon begins in the 20s. Although there will be blood flow, it may be less than usual, perhaps accompanied by spotting before and/or after the period and without cramping.

Menstruation commences at puberty (usually between the ages of 11 and 13 in the United States) and ceases at menopause (from about age 45 to age 52). Women at any age who have hysterectomies, however, will cease menstruating at the time of the surgery. (See "Hysterectomy and Oophorectomy" on page 354.) The average menstrual period is four and one-half days, and the average menstrual cycle is usually 30 days or more, with Pill

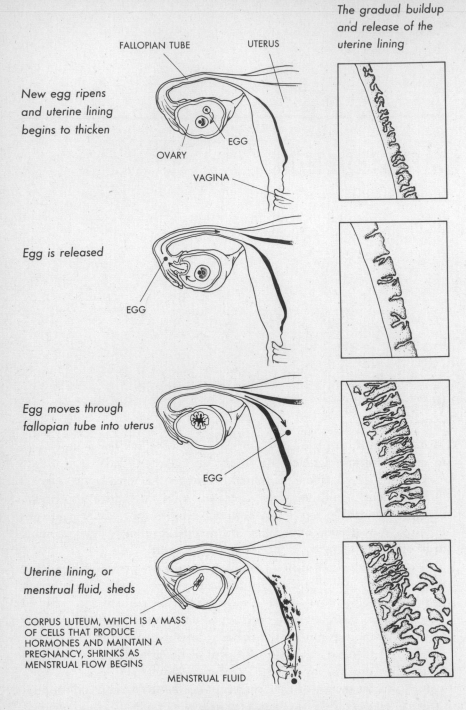

The gradual buildup and release of the uterine lining

New egg ripens and uterine lining begins to thicken

FALLOPIAN TUBE

UTERUS

EGG

OVARY

VAGINA

Egg is released

EGG

Egg moves through fallopian tube into uterus

EGG

Uterine lining, or menstrual fluid, sheds

CORPUS LUTEUM, WHICH IS A MASS OF CELLS THAT PRODUCE HORMONES AND MAINTAIN A PREGNANCY, SHRINKS AS MENSTRUAL FLOW BEGINS

MENSTRUAL FLUID

MENSTRUATION

users the most likely to have a 28-day cycle. Women in their teens, 20s, and 30s have longer periods than women in their 40s, especially those approaching menopause.

Some women who live together, like mothers and daughters, or like coeds in all-female dormitories, will occasionally experience menstrual synchrony, which is menstruation that occurs at about the same time. No one is quite sure why that occasionally happens, although it's suspected that pheromones — odorous substances released from our bodies that signal sexual interest, danger, or other emotions — are the trigger. It is also known that people who live together, whether female or male, will often develop similar hormone and monthly temperature cycles.

COMMON MENSTRUAL COMPLAINTS

DYSMENORRHEA (CRAMPS)

These are mild to severe pains in the lower abdomen, lower back, or thighs. For some women, cramps are an occasional minor annoyance. For others, they are profoundly painful. About half of all menstruating women (usually teens or women who've not had children) get cramps. Cramps sometimes start a few days before the start of menstruation and often occur on the first day or several days after your period starts. They are caused by secretions of prostaglandins (uterine chemicals) that cause uterine muscle spasms. The intensity of these spasms varies, which may be why some women experience more pain than others.

Cramps can be worsened by premenstrual bloating (water retention) and can be accompanied by nausea, vomiting, fainting, and/or diarrhea. Bladder infections can aggravate cramps, but don't cause them. (See "Urinary Tract Infections" on page 515.)

Cramps are not always due just to menstruation. They can also occur from uterine fibroids, scarring from pelvic inflammatory disease, use of an intrauterine device (IUD) for birth control, endometriosis, a tightened cervix, or be the aftermath, years later, of tubal sterilization. (See "Uterine Fibroids" on page 522, "Pelvic Inflammatory Disease" on page 441, "Intrauterine Device" on page 208, and "Endometriosis" on page 329.)

When our baby was born, we made a frantic trip to town (35 miles away) and the nurse commented that I must have had some pretty strong labor pains because she could feel the baby's head already. My reply was that I didn't know, I'd never had a baby before, but that I'd had menstrual cramps lots worse than the labor pains I'd been having. . . . The nurses and the doctor roared with laughter at my wonderful sense of humor. I wasn't joking—I had had cramps worse than that all my life.

PREMENSTRUAL SYNDROME (PMS)

PMS is a group of more than 100 symptoms, including headaches, depression, irritability, weight gain, and breast tenderness. No one really knows what causes PMS, but undoubtedly hormonal cycles are only one part of the answer. Symptoms disappear during pregnancy and after menopause (if estrogen replacement therapy is not taken—see "Estrogen Replacement Therapy" on page 337).

These symptoms, which range from mild to occasionally severe, occur in a predictable cluster. They start during the two weeks before menstruation and usually resolve with the onset of your period and are almost always gone by day two. The exception is the woman whose menstrual cycles are starting to change in the years right before her periods stop entirely at menopause. Her PMS symptoms can extend well past day two.

The hormonal changes that can trigger PMS are the onset of menstruation in the teen years and childbirth, especially following a pregnancy complicated with toxemia (high blood pressure and water retention, among other symptoms). Women with a tendency toward PMS usually love being pregnant, in particular the first three months, but they often experience fatigue, headaches, and anxiety after childbirth.

Other PMS triggers are: abortion or miscarriage, sterilization, amenorrhea (no period), going on and off the Pill (some researchers say that women who have side effects from taking the Pill are more likely to have PMS), and a hysterectomy (if the ovaries are left in).

Although PMS is common and a worldwide phenomenon, most of the time it does not interfere with women's daily functioning. No more than 5 percent of women who have PMS, however, have severe symptoms. Women in this group are more likely to commit crimes, abuse alcohol, and have accidents during their premenstrual time. PMS has been reported for centuries, but it was not labeled until the 1980s. Dr. Katharina Dalton, the British physician who studied PMS and identified it as a metabolic imbalance (as opposed to "that's what it is like to be a woman"), said that this syndrome has recognizable, predictable features, though those characteristics vary from woman to woman.

The woman most likely to have PMS in the United States today has several of the following characteristics:

• Is past age 30.
• Experiences significant emotional stress in her life.
• Has a mother and/or sisters who have PMS.
• Has poor nutritional habits (lots of refined carbohydrates and junk food) that trigger PMS.
• Lives a sedentary life (fewer than three 30-minute walks per week).
• Is married and has children.
• Has difficulty maintaining a stable weight.
• Has been diagnosed as having low blood sugar (a condition in which the blood sugar level falls either too rapidly or to too low a level).
• Was a bedwetter.
• Has an underactive thyroid. The following symptoms before your period may point to thyroid problems: dry skin, feeling cold, fatigue, sweet cravings, constipation, weight gain, and irritability.

Although reports of premenstrual syndrome go back thousands of years, there are several reasons why PMS may be more common now, or at least more commonly reported. A refined diet high in white flour, sugar, salt, and caffeine is more common today and has been demonstrated to have an effect on PMS. (The PMS symptoms of 90 percent of women are reportedly reduced or eliminated by removing these products from their diet, especially during the two weeks immediately prior to menstruation.)

In addition, women today have much more opportunity to have PMS, because they menstruate more often and for more years than women did before. U.S. women have the longest span of menstrual cycles reported in the world with approximately 37 years of monthly bleeding. They are not pregnant very often.

In the early 1800s, on the other hand, the typical U.S. woman had seven or eight children and she postponed menstruation even more if she breastfed each child 12 to 18 months, which was a common practice then. Whatever menstrual periods she had were probably welcomed in those days of little or no birth control. And by age 40, she was very close to menopause—if she lived that long. (The typical lifespan for women then was the late 40s.) Even if you have a baby (or two or three), you'll still menstruate more than 400 times, or 10 times more than your Victorian or pioneer sisters.

PMS is better known today. Millions of women never knew that common PMS symptoms (headaches, anxiety, and mood changes, for example) had anything to do with their menstrual cycles, or that those symptoms were metabolic and real—not "all in the head." Nor were they aware that there were steps they could take to avoid those symptoms in the future. Although in the popular jargon PMS means the woman becomes crazy, the reality is that the typical symptoms are commonplace, some of them occuring even in men.

PMS symptoms occur in clusters—if you have one, you'll have the others in the group, though you also may experience the symptoms in more than one cluster.

• *Group 1.* Tension, irritability, sometimes rage over minor stress, anxiety, mood swings.

• *Group 2.* Headache, food binges, increased appetite, cravings for sweets, salty food, and chocolate, heart pounding, fatigue. (Many women eat 10 to 20 percent more food overall, and after a few hours women may feel low, tired, and have a headache.)

• *Group 3.* Sore breasts (a symptom that increases with age), bloating, weight gain (usually three to five pounds).

• *Group 4.* Depression, lethargy, forgetfulness, confusion, difficulty in concentrating, crying for no apparent reason, insomnia, and chronic stress. Other common symptoms are: diminished alcohol tolerance, allergy flare-ups, and panic attacks. (See "Premenstrual Syndrome" on page 619 in Recommended Reading and on page 591 in the Resource Directory for more information.)

I am like a wound-up spring ready to let go. I feel like something is itching under my skin, and I cannot scratch it.

I can eat a jar of olives and drink the juice, and often do. . . . I binge on chocolate at times, at other times I don't care for it at all.

Sometimes this is abdominal, or it may involve my hands and feet. My rings often do not fit, and my fingers are so stiff and swollen I can hardly write. My swollen abdomen makes me look pregnant at times. This changes as soon as my period starts.

My good memory and clear mind are clouded during symptom time. I cannot think, remember, or even do simple arithmetic when experiencing PMS, yet I know I am very intelligent.

*A*lthough I do not drink often, I seem to crave alcohol before my period. However, I have a very low tolerance at that time. Even one drink may cause me to feel and appear drunk.

AMENORRHEA (ABSENCE OF PERIODS)

About 5 percent of all menstruating women experience absent or unpredictable periods not due to pregnancy, breastfeeding, menopause, or the occasional skipped period. Some women do not get their periods for a while after they quit taking the Pill, with this time period varying from a couple of months to as long as two years. Stress, weight fluctuations, thyroid imbalances, ovarian cysts, anorexia, uterine fibroids, intrauterine scarring, smoking, and athletic training can also cause amenorrhea. (See "Stress" on page 54, "Ovarian Cysts" on page 437, "Anorexia" on page 318, and "Uterine Fibroids" on page 522.)

Athletic amenorrhea is somewhat mysterious. Whatever the cause, whether it's the decreased amount of body fat, the stress of competition, or other as yet undiscovered variables, menstruation will usually return when strenuous exercise is decreased or eliminated. Athletic amenorrhea is not a good contraceptive, however. Some athletes report getting pregnant even though they hadn't menstruated for months or even years. Women athletes are less likely to experience PMS and have fewer cramps.

HOME REMEDIES YOU CAN TRY

DYSMENORRHEA (CRAMPS)

• *Exercise regularly.* The worst thing you can do is go to bed. Take a walk, or do yoga exercises that relieve cramps. (Example: Get on all fours, keep head down and hips elevated.) (See "Yoga" on page 59.)

• *Eat a calcium-rich diet.* Some physicians suggest you take calcium and magnesium supplements daily during premenstrual days if your diet is not generous in these minerals. (See "Food" on page 604 in Recommended Reading for books marked with an * for specific food supplement dosages for all vitamin and mineral suggestions in home remedies.)

• *Take hot baths or put a hot water bottle on your lower back or abdomen.*

• *Have a massage* (back massage in particular).

• *Try acupressure* (see "Acupressure" on page 56).

• *Do exercises to keep your pelvic floor strong.* (See "Kegel Exercises" on page 47.)

• *Have an orgasm*, because it can relieve pelvic congestion for some women by contracting the uterus and reducing cramping. It may also speed menstrual flow. This may not be a good practice, however, if you have endometriosis, or the women in your family have a history of it (see "Endometriosis" on page 329).

W*hen I began menstruating I also began formal dance training. As long as I kept in training I had no "physical distress." About five years ago I changed my profession. Now I'm no longer maintaining muscle tone as I did. I am suffering cramps . . . I have noticed if I indulge my craving to stuff with food, my cramps are more severe. If I stay somewhat empty my cramps are mild — more nonexistent.*

PREMENSTRUAL SYNDROME (PMS)

If you have PMS, your symptoms may not be the same each month, they will not exactly match other women's, and what gives you relief may vary, too. You need to become your own expert on what works best, particularly as there is no agreement on solutions to PMS. Following are suggestions that have worked for other women, though some are controversial:

• *Exercise regularly.* This may work all by itself to eliminate your symptoms. Exercise reduces depression and stress, while releasing endorphins, hormones that give you euphoric feelings, a sense of well-being, and an increased tolerance for pain. (See "Exercise" on page 41.)

• *Eat foods high in fiber and complex carbohydrates*, like whole grains, brown rice, nuts, fruit, vegetables, beans, and seeds to reduce moodiness, help you avoid binging, and keep your body rich in vitamins. If you know that a premenstrual "pigout" is just around the corner for you, stop before it hits you. Eat a piece of fruit, or a bowl of cereal, or a whole-wheat muffin or bagel. (See discussion of fiber on page 28.)

• *Avoid or eliminate sugar and white flour and everything made with them*, especially during the days before menstruation. This includes most fast foods and packaged snacks.

• *Use less salt* during the week before your period to reduce anxiety, depression, bloating, breast tenderness, or aching joints. That means not only table salt, but also monosodium glutamate, or MSG (found in seasonings and food cooked in Asian restaurants — see discussion of MSG on page 31), soy sauce, diet or regular soft drinks, and many canned and processed foods that are often loaded with salt.

• *Avoid caffeine* in coffee, tea, cocoa and chocolate, diet and regular cola soft drinks, and certain over-the-counter drugs. The more caffeine you have, the more intense your PMS symptoms may be.

• *Sleep eight hours at night* or as much as you need to be truly rested. (See "Fatigue" on page 344.)

• *Use your own judgment about food supplements.* Controversy continues over vitamins (B, B$_6$, E), minerals (calcium and magnesium), and other food supplements (evening primrose oil). Some women and health care professionals swear by them. Others say they don't work and there's no conclusive research to support their use.

• *Use acupressure or relaxation techniques* to reduce tension. (See "Acupressure" on page 56 and "Meditation" on page 59.)

• *Avoid cigarettes and alcohol.* They both make PMS symptoms worse.

• *Keep a diary of your symptoms* for a few months to see what is effective for you. Use your wall calendar or your appointment book. Keep it simple. Write down when your period started and ended. Fill in whatever symptoms you may have on the days they occur. It's likely that a pattern will begin to emerge, and you'll know in advance the next time what days to expect sugar craving, unexplained tears or tempers, and other symptoms. Forewarned, you'll be able to prevent or reduce those symptoms the following month by making life-style changes.

• *Enlist your family's help.* Have your partner take care of the children if they're staying up late on a night you need your sleep. Tell other family members not to bring home sugary foods, so that you're not tempted. Figure out your needs and then let them know.

We're asking these women [who come to a PMS clinic] to make major adjustments in their diet, to give up alcohol and caffeine, and to make life-style changes, too. . . . After a month or two of charting symptoms and making dietary and life-style changes, most patients rave about the improvement in their premenstrual symptoms.

AMENORRHEA

To prevent amenorrhea or reduce its consequences:

• *Eat foods rich in B vitamins* or take a B vitamin supplement, especially B_6.

• *Eat a calcium-rich diet* and/or take a supplement to prevent the bone loss that could lead to osteoporosis later (see "Osteoporosis" on page 431).

• *Maintain a normal weight.* Sometimes women who do not have anorexia, yet are very thin, will not menstruate regularly.

• *Cut back on your athletic schedule*, particularly if you want to become pregnant.

• *Try stress relievers* (see a list of stress relievers on page 55).

• *Stop any use of marijuana*, which is associated with menstrual disruption. (See "Marijuana" on page 38.)

TREATMENT OPTIONS

DYSMENORRHEA (CRAMPS)

• *Drugs.* Over-the-counter drugs like aspirin or lower-dose ibuprofen (sold as Advil, Midol, Motrin, or Nuprin) and prescription drugs like Ponstel (mefenamic acid) and Anaprox (naproxen sodium) bring relief to 80 percent of women who use them, particularly when taken two days before menstruation begins. (Some women wait until their period begins before starting the drug, because they may not know when it's two days before their period. Also, they don't want to take a drug as long as there is any possibility of pregnancy.)

• *The Pill* is also used to prevent cramps since it prevents ovulation, causing a lighter flow, and interferes with the production of prostaglandins, resulting in milder uterine cramping. (See "The Pill" on page 181.)

• *Acupuncture* (see "Acupuncture" on page 82). It can work very well to relieve cramps and other menstrual complaints.

PREMENSTRUAL SYNDROME (PMS)

Most women manage PMS with home remedies, but they are not always enough. Acupuncture along with Chinese herbs has proven to be helpful as well.

A prescription drug option is the hormone progesterone. The FDA has not approved progesterone for treating PMS, because its safety has not been established. But since this drug already has other approved uses, it's available to physicians for PMS use, too. An explanation as to why 1990 research showed that this widely used PMS treatment is ineffective (though individual women have reported that it relieved their symptoms) is that hormonal cycles are not the entire answer for what causes PMS. In addition, progesterone may cause internal blood clots, mammary nodules, and birth defects to any child conceived by a mother taking it; you'll need to have medical check-ups frequently; and the medication is expensive.

An antiobesity drug, fenfluramine, which controls food craving, may be used in the future, too. Other powerful drugs are on the horizon as well, including bromocriptine, spironolactone, and GnRH—each with their long list of potential side effects.

If you seek medical help for your symptoms, go to a health care professional who believes that there is such a thing as PMS. Look for a person with experience and success in helping women alleviate symptoms. Find someone who is able to diagnose your condition accurately to rule out other problems. And finally, find someone who is willing to work with you on your individualized treatment plan. (See Severino on page 619 in Recommended Reading for a complete review of all PMS medical options.)

AMENORRHEA (ABSENCE OF PERIODS)

Providing no underlying disorder is causing your absence of periods, there is no recommended medical treatment. If there is an underlying disorder, then the treatment will depend on the disorder.

ATTITUDES ABOUT MENSTRUATION

Menstruation has a bad name. Do you think of menstruation as "the curse," "being on the rag," *that* time of the month? Or is it more upbeat than that for you? Is it your "friend" or a "blessing"? Do you notice the surge of creative energy right before your period starts that some women have discovered? Or is getting blood on your underwear or—worse yet—on your suit at a business meeting the only thing you notice? Is it any surprise that women with few symptoms like menstruation better than women who have uncomfortable, even painful periods?

In a women's magazine survey of 100,000 women, 10 percent hated getting their periods. Another 10 percent like them and thought menstruation made them feel one with the universe. However, most women just think menstruation is a nuisance at worst, or insignificant at best, with about half saying they have PMS to some degree.

A positive attitude will not make uncomfortable symptoms go away. A negative attitude won't give you cramps or PMS. But a positive attitude always helps events pass more quickly. If you have uncomfortable menstrual symptoms, do what you can to alleviate them and know that you're entitled to your opinions about menstruation, whatever they are.

I hate my period. I always have. And I always will. I not only get terrible cramps, but I'm moody and no one can stand me, including myself. The last thing I want to hear is how great some woman's period made her feel. I not only don't believe it, but I think that's disgusting. Whoever coined the word "curse" knew what they were talking about.

The best cure for premenstrual tension is to stop calling it premenstrual tension. Call it PME—premenstrual energy—instead. "Tension" implies sickness. "Energy" suggests a gift.

DO WE REALLY HAVE RAGING HORMONES?

Women and men both have the same hormones; only the amounts are different. These chemical messengers flood the body daily traveling from your glands, including the brain, to other parts of your body and influence mental, emotional, and sexual functioning for all of us. Among the sex hormones, oxytocin, which triggers caregiving, is found in larger concentrations in women than it is in men. Testosterone, on the other hand, which triggers aggression and competitiveness, is found in amounts 20 to 40 times greater in men's bodies than in women's. However, just as most women don't have severe PMS symptoms, most men don't create mayhem.

We're all influenced by hormones, but hormonal influences are not obvious in men. Men's cycles may be more subtle and occur over longer time periods (some think even seasonally), and they don't have physical markers like menstruation and pregnancy to explain angry flare-ups, anxiety, or fatigue. A study of men on submarines, for example, showed that their feelings and behavior changed in predictable patterns, but these men attributed their feelings to outside influences — such as a supervisor who had been hard on them that day — not to a particular time of the month or seasonal cycle.

A Note to Mothers of Teens

You are likely to be your daughter's first source of information about menstruation. Regardless of your personal opinion about menstruation (no big deal, terrible, or wonderful), your daughter's menarche (her first period) is a big day in her life as a woman. Here are some suggestions on how to make her menarche a celebration:

• *Prepare her in advance*, not only with sanitary supplies but with an explanation of what's happening to her body and why. Tell her that menstruation is normal, not a disease. Although many girls naturally feel embarrassed, the more prepared she is, the more positive she'll be.

• *Give her a party*. (Be sure to take her preferences into account.) In Ghana, a girl's menarche is an occasion for a day-long party of dancing, eating, and gifts for the new woman.

• *Get rid of the negative nonsense in your head about menstruation before talking to your daughter*. (Examples are: menstrual blood is unclean or women's hormones make them less reliable than men.) You don't want your daughters growing up with these misconceptions.

When the older daughter passed her twelfth birthday, I placed a supply of sanitary napkins and a choice of belts and panties on a shelf in their closet and told both girls that the supplies were there, and if they wanted to experiment ahead of time with brands to find which was most comfortable, I would purchase any kind they wanted.

I was almost fourteen when I got my period. Even though I knew it would come some day, I was surprised. I immediately went into my mom's office and told her "I'm a woman now." But I was also very embarrassed and didn't want my brothers to know. Later my mom and dad took me out to dinner to celebrate at the restaurant of my choice. They told me I could invite anyone I wanted, but I didn't want anyone else there. My dad made a toast to me and ordered a special kind of cake.

MIGRAINE HEADACHE

WHAT IT IS

A migraine headache often is characterized by a throbbing, full feeling, usually on one side of the head. However, not all migraines occur in this manner.

SIGNS AND SYMPTOMS

About 20 percent of people who have migraines experience an aura, or a warning, that a migraine is imminent. This warning can occur immediately before a migraine or as much as a day in advance. Some common warning signs are: dizziness, numbness, language difficulties, mood changes, hyperactivity, extreme fatigue or extreme irritability, flashing lights, and micropsia (a rare condition in which all objects appear to be very small).

The most common symptom is pain on one side of the head, though the pain may switch sides during the course of the migraine. This pain may last from a few hours to a few days, although 14 to 15 hours is common. If you have migraines, your pain will establish its own pattern of locations and duration. Other symptoms are nausea, vomiting, diarrhea, nasal stuffiness and sinus pain on the painful side of the head (this can be misdiagnosed as a sinus headache), low tolerance of light and sounds, aversion to visual stripes, sleep disturbances, and mood disorders.

CAUSES

About nine million U.S. women have migraines (three times the number of men), and they're likely to be between ages 30 and 49. Migraines were once thought to be psychosomatic, but recent research has revealed that migraines stem from a biologic abnormality of nerve cells and chemical messengers deep in the brain, and there is a family link perhaps as much as 80 percent of the time.

Sixty percent of women who get migraine headaches experience menstrual migraines that develop just before and during menstruation and sometimes also at ovulation. For these women, migraines may increase or decrease during pregnancy, and they usually decrease or stop altogether after menopause.

Food sensitivities are considered culprits as well. Some physicians say migraines are caused by food allergies, while others say migraines are not an immunologic response, but rather they can be the effect of chemical compounds within food on the brain. Whichever theory is correct, some people who have migraine headaches find relief by avoiding certain common foods, including wheat, corn, and milk, or products like chocolate, caffeine, alcohol (particularly red wine, bourbon, scotch, and beer), aged cheese, and seafood. Food additives, like monosodium glutamate (MSG), nitrite, and the artificial sweetener aspartame (NutraSweet) may be triggers, too.

A common trigger is stress. In a survey of more than 3,000 people who had migraines, 68 percent said that undue stress often resulted in this headache. Other triggers are bright lights, changes in atmospheric pressure, the Pill (increases migraines 50 percent), smoking, hunger or fasting, epidural anesthesia (often used during childbirth), and environmental pollutants.

My life is so much better since menopause. I've quit having migraines, which ruled my life in many ways. I had to be careful with my eating and sleeping habits, especially around the start of my period. And I had to keep myself emotionally even. What a drag it all was.

I never, ever had headaches until my daughter was born when I was in my 30s and, in fact, was very intolerant of people with headaches. Now I get a migraine every week or so, and am on the receiving end of that attitude. Migraines have nothing to do with moral weakness, and everything to do with chemical responses within the brain.

TREATMENT OPTIONS

There are many drugs available for migraines that either prevent a migraine or offer relief from the headache.

• *Over-the-counter painkillers* include aspirin, ibuprofen, and other non-steroidal anti-inflammatory drugs that may provide relief for mild to moderate migraines.

• *Prescription painkillers* for severe migraines include ergotamine, Midrin, and sumatriptan (chemical name for Imitrex).

• *Prescription antinausea drugs* like metoclopramide may provide relief from nausea or vomiting and can be given in a suppository, too.

• *Prescription preventives* include propranolol, nadolol, and atenolol. Sometimes antidepressants are helpful, and some women with menstrual migraines have been helped with Danazol. (See "Danazol" on page 332.)

PREVENTIVE MEASURES YOU CAN TAKE

• *Keep a food diary* and note which foods seem to be associated with the onset of migraines.

• *Avoid substances that you know are migraine triggers for you.* This can be food, including dairy products, or food additives. (See "The Anti-Additive Anti-Preservative Diet" on page 30.)

• *Avoid scents that you know are migraine triggers for you*, such as tobacco smoke, perfume and other toiletries, paint, and diesel or gasoline fumes.

• *Try biofeedback.* People with headaches are taught to direct blood flow into their fingers and away from their heads. This is especially effective for children with migraines. (See "Biofeedback" on page 85.)

• *Exercise regularly* to improve circulation. This may be especially effective if you have three or more migraines a month.

• *Go to a chiropractor, or use a variety of alternative medical therapies, including massage, meditation, and acupuncture* (which can be both treatment and prevention). (See "Chiropractic Medicine" on page 81, "Meditation" on page 59, and "Acupuncture" on page 82.)

• *Try the herb feverfew.* Its effectiveness has not been proven in large clinical trials, but British research shows this herb is effective in reducing the frequency of migraines, though not necessarily the duration of each one. Typical health-food-store preparations of this herb may not be adequate, however, so you may want to consult an herbalist. (See "Migraine Headaches" on page 619 in Recommended Reading and on page 589 in the Resource Directory.)

The only help I ever received was injected ergot. Everything I tried seemed to help for a while, but the migraines returned as bad as ever. I read about feverfew in a shopper paper. . . . I had no faith that it would work but tried it anyway. Eventually I went 10 months without a headache. . . . I have never mentioned feverfew to a doctor as I assumed they would ridicule the idea.

For the past six months I have had migraines with greater frequency. . . . I am finding biofeedback very helpful. The relaxation, the imagery, and the sophisticated electronic equipment of the clinical process is teaching me to control these migraine episodes—to be able to abort the onset of a migraine.

I hated the migraines, especially when my kids were little. I would have to go into the bedroom, close the blinds, and pray that the children wouldn't make any noise. It was years before I discovered the connection with food allergies. Now my daughters avoid the same foods I do. They don't want the dreaded "mommy headache," as they used to call it.

I have been a patient of a Chinese doctor and acupuncturist for the last two years, and my migraines are much less severe and of shorter duration. With treatments twice per week I found that the reduction in severity began after two months. After six months I was able to withdraw from all prescription pain relievers. Acupuncture has not only made a difference with migraine, but my overall energy has improved.

My life has been controlled by migraines for the past 25 years. I decided that I did not want to spend the rest of my life dependent on drugs, so I tried massage therapy. I used to have three to five headaches each week. Now,

I can count on one hand the number of headaches I have experienced in the last year and a half, and none of those headaches was severe. While massage therapy may not work for everyone, it certainly has made a tremendous difference in my life.

OBESITY

WHAT IT IS

Obesity is an excess of body fat. The extra weight can be evenly distributed all over the body or centered in one or two areas. Health professionals do not agree on how many pounds are too many. The average estimate for obesity is 20 to 30 percent over normal weight. Morbid obesity is double normal body weight or 100 pounds over normal weight.

Fat women tend to have more of the hormone estrogen in their bodies. Because of that, they are likely to have fewer hot flashes during menopause than thinner women. They're also less likely to develop osteoporosis, the bone-thinning disease, or to suffer hip fractures. During pregnancy they are less likely to give birth to premature babies or those with low birth weight.

Obesity, however, has a number of disadvantages. Some are caused by the excess weight alone, and some are caused by common treatments for obesity, such as fasting. Following are conditions or diseases either caused or aggravated by obesity, especially in individuals 30 percent over normal weight: osteoarthritis of the knee; urinary incontinence and prolapsed (or falling) uterus; and adult-onset diabetes, heart disease, and other chronic conditions, especially when fat centers on the shoulders and abdomen, rather than the hips. Your body's fat distribution is genetically determined. If one of your parents had a pot belly, you likely will, too. (See "Urinary Incontinence" on page 510, "Uterine Prolapse" on page 527, and "Heart Disease" on page 348.)

Other disadvantages are varicose veins and/or leg cramps, problems with menstruation, infertility, pregnancy and childbirth, high blood pressure, and elevated cholesterol levels. (See "Varicose Veins" on page 537, "Infertility" on page 364, and "Cholesterol Test" on page 109.)

Certain forms of cancer (including cancer of the gallbladder, ovaries, uterus, and pancreas) and gallbladder disease and gallstones (the result of a low-fiber diet and severe food restriction) are also more common in women who are obese, as is sudden unexplained death in those who are morbidly obese. (See "Uterine Cancer" on page 233, "Ovarian Cancer" on page 234, and "Obesity" on page 619 in Recommended Reading.)

CAUSES

Obesity that begins either in childhood or around age 20 is likely to stay. If one of your parents is obese, your risk for obesity is 40 percent. That figure doubles to 80 percent if both parents are obese. It was once thought that obesity that ran in families was entirely due to the family's eating habits or exercise patterns, but it's now believed that there can be a genetic predisposition to fatness that plays a role.

Until recently, it was always believed that obesity was caused by overeating, perhaps, but not necessarily, in combination with too little exercise. Newer research consistently points to additional reasons:

• *Metabolism.* People who are obese burn fuel at a slower rate than do thinner people, independent of the type and amount of food that is eaten.

• *"Yo-yo" dieting.* At any one time, half of U.S. women are dieting. Repeated cycles of weight loss and gain make the metabolic rate even lower, and extra pounds harder, if not impossible, to lose, resulting in a greater accumulation of pounds in the long run. This is true of people who are of normal weight to start with, like high-school wrestlers who are trained to gain and lose weight repeatedly for athletic matches. Yo-yo dieting also accelerates the risk for heart disease and often results in an earlier death.

• *Genetics.* Heredity can determine how many fat cells your body has and how large they are, and it may also determine the way your body burns fuel. People can inherit a metabolism that burns fat slowly instead of quickly. Your genetic inheritance can also control your body's "setpoint," that is, the weight that your body is programmed to reach and maintain.

• *Cultural influences.* The Japanese consume more calories than we do, but are far less likely to be obese. However, when the Japanese move to Hawaii, and then onto the mainland United States, they become progressively fatter. Many experts say it's the result of a switch to a high-fat, high-sugar, low-fiber American diet. There are class influences, too. In the United States when women move up socially and economically, they are less likely to be obese than are poorer women with less education who are often African-American, Latina, or Native American.

TREATMENT OPTIONS

There are a number of ways to attempt to lose weight. None of the options below are totally safe, none offer permanent weight loss (90 to 95 percent of dieters regain all or most of their lost weight within five years), and some are more hazardous to your health than others.

• *Liquid diets.* Some dieters choose liquid diets or powdered formulas that dissolve in water. These diet powders are considered similar to instant breakfasts, and most experts do not think they are a problem if they are used occasionally. However, some dieters choose these options (420 to 800 calories per day for several months, then a switch to low-calorie food) to lose 50 or more pounds, and that's when problems, including gallbladder disease, may proliferate. If you choose to use these products, you should be followed carefully by a physician during the process. Avoid diet companies that offer prepackaged food or liquid without medical supervision.

• *Surgical procedures* are offered to people who are more than 100 pounds overweight, but there's been little research on these, and what has been done does not indicate that patients achieve or maintain near normal weight.

One operation is gastric-bypass surgery, or stomach stapling. The upper part of the stomach is partitioned with steel staples so that the patient's food goes into this tiny stomach, and she feels full after only a small amount of food. Side effects are: vomiting, malnutrition, unsatisfactory weight loss, obstructed intestines, infection, blood clots, and hair loss. Moreover, 40 percent of the time the operation has to be repeated.

Another surgical option is the gastric bubble, which is a deflated plastic balloon that is inserted into the stomach with an endoscope, a tube passed through the mouth into the stomach. After the balloon is blown up, and the endoscope removed, the balloon is left in for three to four months, creating the sensation of a "full" stomach. Sample side effects: stomach ulceration, intestinal obstruction, wearing-away of stomach lining, and possible need for surgery to correct these problems. And worst of all, early research shows that the gastric bubble may not be successful at all in helping women lose weight.

A procedure of the future is an appetite-switch electrode that is inserted underneath the scalp and attached to a pacemakerlike device.

A procedure performed in the past, but no longer, is intestinal bypass, the short-circuiting of the intestines to avoid the absorption of most calories. Fifty percent of the people who had the operation have serious problems, and 10 percent have died from it.

• *Diet drugs.* The new generation diet drugs are phentermine (a cousin to the high-energy appetite-depressant amphetamines of the past), fenfluramine, which kept weight off 80 percent of users in one study group but only as long as they took the drug, and orlistat, a fat-blocking agent.

Liposuction, the removal of fat by "vacuuming" it out through small incisions, is *not* an option for overweight women. It's designed for normal-weight women, and when it is performed, it removes only six to eight pounds of fat at most.

HOME REMEDIES YOU CAN TRY

Statistically, effective treatment for true obesity is rare, proving frustrating for both the obese and those who would like to help them. *The only reliable factors in permanent weight loss are exercise and a low-fat diet.* For most dieters, it's much easier to lose the weight initially than it is to keep it off over time. Following, however, are suggestions that have worked for some women and can be good health habits in general:

• *Exercise regularly.* (See "Exercise" on page 41.) Even slow walking can begin to change your metabolism, the individual rate at which your body burns fuel. But because it's easy to think we're getting more exercise than we really are, it's wise to have a plan to reduce obesity. Think about scheduling three 30-minute walks per week. (Less than this is the U.S. government's definition of sedentary.)

Exercise can also help the functioning of your hypothalamus, the gland that, when it's working correctly, sends the self-regulating messages of "I am hungry" and "I am full." A poorly functioning hypothalamus in an overweight woman will send the message, "I just don't know when to stop." Lack of exercise may also be the reason that people who view TV more than three hours a day are twice as likely to be obese as those who watch less than one hour.

• *Eat "smart" without making food your whole reason for living each day.* Forget dieting. You don't have to count calories to eat smart, but it's important to be aware that overweight people sometimes underestimate how much food they eat, particularly foods rich in fat. (See "The Anti–Breast Cancer, Healthy Heart Diet" on page 28.) If you have been fat since adolescence, you may be especially sensitive to salt and would do well to reduce your intake. (See "Fat Acceptance" on page 579 in the Resource Directory.)

• *Lose 10 percent of your total amount of excess pounds.* (For example, if you're 50 pounds overweight, lose five pounds.) It may not sound like much, but some research indicates you'll reduce your risk for high blood pressure, heart disease, and diabetes. Or if you already have one of these conditions, this loss will reduce your symptoms.

• *Join a self-help group.* These organizations provide information and emotional support to women who want to lose weight. The groups are most successful for mildly to moderately overweight individuals.

When my doctor told me to concentrate on losing just 10 percent, which in my case was 15 pounds, it sure took off lots of pressure. I wasn't so concerned with how I looked, because I thought I looked fine. I was concerned about developing heart disease.

My low-impact aerobics instructor is a stocky, vigorous, 50-year-old woman who introduces herself as someone who has lost 145 pounds. She says she lost her weight over several years by exercising regularly and eating better. She always has lots of empathy for the overweight women who come to her class, because she understands how difficult it is for them. But she reminds them that if she could do it, so can they.

When I turned 40 I decided that I was through thinking about food each day, weighing myself each day, and reading the diet columns in the women's magazines each month. That forced me to change some friends, too, when I discovered that talking about diets was all I had in common with a few of them. I wanted to find out what else life had to offer. Now five years later, I weigh about the same, but I eat better.

YOUR "RIGHT" WEIGHT

Height-and-weight charts were created by insurance companies who analyzed which policyholders lived longest. In the decades since, there's been much controversy over which chart is correct. That's because, among other issues, the data come only from people who are insured.

No chart can tell you at what weight you'll look your version of best or healthiest. That's for you to decide. But following is a chart, also based on insurance data, which shows — in terms of who lives the longest — that ideal weights are the same for both women and men, and that those ideal weights increase with age.

RECOMMENDED WEIGHTS* (IN POUNDS) FOR BOTH SEXES

20–29 yr	30–39 yr	40–49 yr	50–59 yr	60–69 yr	Height**
84–111	92–119	99–127	107–135	115–142	4'10"
87–115	95–123	103–131	111–139	119–147	4'11"
90–119	98–127	106–135	114–143	123–152	5'0"
93–123	101–131	110–140	118–148	127–157	5'1"
96–127	105–136	113–144	122–153	131–163	5'2"
99–131	108–140	117–149	126–158	135–168	5'3"
102–135	112–145	121–154	130–163	140–173	5'4"
106–140	115–149	125–159	134–168	144–179	5'5"
109–144	119–154	129–164	138–174	148–184	5'6"
112–148	122–159	133–169	143–179	153–190	5'7"
116–153	126–163	137–174	147–184	158–196	5'8"
119–157	130–168	141–179	151–190	162–201	5'9"
122–162	134–173	145–184	156–195	167–207	5'10"
126–167	137–178	149–190	160–201	172–213	5'11"
129–171	141–183	153–195	165–207	177–219	6'0"
133–176	145–188	157–200	169–213	182–225	6'1"
137–181	149–194	162–206	174–219	187–232	6'2"
141–186	153–199	166–212	179–225	192–238	6'3"
144–191	157–205	171–218	184–231	197–244	6'4"

*Without clothes
**Without shoes
(Source: Reubin Andres, Gerontology Research Center, National Institute of Aging, 1985.)

OBESITY AND PREJUDICE

Many health care professionals, reflecting our culture at large, are prejudiced against obese people and uninformed about the causes of obesity.
They often label severely overweight people self-destructive and failure
prone. This bias also shows in exaggerated comments about the consequences of obesity. ("You'll never live to see your grandchildren" or "Every
time I see you I wonder when you're going to have your heart attack.") So
in addition to whatever physical consequences that you have because of
obesity, you may also often feel depressed or have feelings of low self-
worth. (See "Emotions" on page 49.)

OOPHORECTOMY: *see* Hysterectomy

Osteoporosis

What It Is

Osteoporosis is the weakening of bones, causing them to become brittle and easily broken. It affects about one fourth of women past age 60.

Signs and Symptoms

The story of our bone strength or weakness doesn't start in our 50s. It begins decades earlier in our teens. During adolescence and our 20s we build bone mass. We start losing it by age 35 — some researchers say earlier — and the years of most intense bone loss are the five to six years following menopause.

All women and men have some bone loss over time that is considered normal. Symptoms for osteoporosis, a disease that goes on for years before symptoms become obvious, however, are: gradual loss of height, lower-back pain while standing, bending, or lifting; rounded shoulders; stooped posture (causing a protruding abdomen); and frequent bone fractures at any age, especially those that occur with little trauma. (Wrist fractures are 10

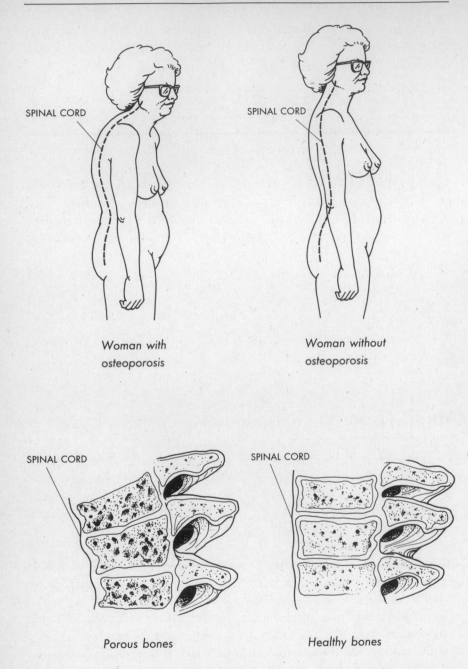

SPINAL CORD

SPINAL CORD

Woman with
osteoporosis

Woman without
osteoporosis

SPINAL CORD

SPINAL CORD

Porous bones

Healthy bones

OSTEOPOROSIS

times more common in women than in men past age 50.) Some women may lose as much as eight inches in height, all from the upper part of the body, and 75 percent lose at least four inches.

CAUSES

Osteoporosis is caused by decreased bone mass, which is the result of insufficient amounts (or poor absorption) of calcium and other vitamins and minerals, as well as absorption of undesirable elements like lead. Since estrogen helps maintain bone mass, lower estrogen levels after menopause can place women at risk for osteoporosis. An unknown number of women also have a genetic risk for osteoporosis which may result in lifelong poor absorption of estrogen.

The woman most likely to have osteoporosis has a combination of many of the following factors:

• *Family history of osteoporosis*
• *A fair complexion with blonde or red hair and freckles* (In general, the farther north of the equator one goes, the higher the bone fracture rate.)
• *Petite size, small boned, and less than five feet, six inches tall* (Obese women's bodies produce more estrogen and are less likely to have fractures.)
• *Low dietary calcium and vitamin D intake*
• *Sedentary life-style* (U.S. government definition is fewer than three one-half hour sessions of exercise per week.)
• *A diet rich in red meat and salt*
• *Smoking*
• *Consumption of excessive amounts of alcohol, soft drinks, and coffee or tea.* (Red meat and soft drinks have a high phosphorus content, which depletes calcium.)
• *Hysterectomy, including surgical removal of both ovaries with no subsequent estrogen replacement therapy* (see "Hysterectomy and Oophorectomy" on page 354 and "Estrogen Replacement Therapy" on page 337)
• *Natural menopause before age 40*
• *History of prior bone fractures*
• *No pregnancy* (If maternal diet is adequate, pregnancy and breastfeeding contribute to bone strength.)
• *Prescription drug use*, such as oral prednisone for asthma or arthritis; antiseizure medications, like Dilantin; anticoagulants; or therapeutic thyroid therapy, but only when the dose is too high from inadequate monitoring
• *Over-the-counter drug use*, such as aluminum-containing antacids like Rolaids and Di-gel

- *Periodontal (gum) disease*
- *Endometriosis* (see "Endometriosis" on page 329)
- *Scoliosis* (curvature of the spine)
- *History of anorexia* (see "Eating Disorders" on page 318)
- *Amenorrhea* (absence of menstruation), associated with weight loss or intense exercise (see "Amenorrhea" on page 411)
- *Gastrointestinal disease*, which can be a cause of poor calcium absorption

---

I think it all started 20 years ago, although I didn't know it at the time. I had aches and pains in my spine and joints and was diagnosed as having arthritis. I wasn't told anything about needing extra calcium or estrogen. Nothing was mentioned about osteoporosis. I took prednisone (a form of cortisone) for many years. It was the only thing that made the pain bearable. . . . Over the years my spine became very curved. I had terrible pains and was in and out of the hospital. My x-rays showed that I had multiple spinal fractures.

MAKING THE DIAGNOSIS

Diagnosis of osteoporosis is usually made after symptoms of bone loss are obvious. There are several ways to measure this bone loss, including single-beam and dual-beam densitometers and dual-energy x-ray absorptiometry (DEXA). (See "Bone Measurement Test" on page 109 for details about these machines and how to make the best use of them.)

Other means used to measure bone loss are computerized axial tomography (CAT) scan; bone biopsies, which are usually reserved for distinguishing between osteoporosis and osteomalacia (abnormal bone mineralization, usually associated with poor metabolism of vitamin D, or vitamin D deficiency); and dental x-rays. Some believe these may be helpful if taken periodically over many years, though loss of jaw bone doesn't always mean there's loss of bone in other parts of the body.

TREATMENT OPTIONS

If osteoporosis has been diagnosed or if you are at risk for osteoporosis, your physician may recommend drug treatment, especially estrogen replacement therapy (ERT), sometimes in combination with calcium. If you decide to take this drug, you'll need to take it for the rest of your life to avoid the bone loss due to the rebound effect once you stop taking it.

There are other drugs, some of which are still considered experimental, which are given by tablet, injection, or nasal spray. Among those are Calcimar (calcitonin) and Didronel.

Fluoride is used with calcium to enhance bone growth. However, it is not effective for one fourth to one half of users, and the new bone it generates may be more brittle than normal. Fluoride upsets stomachs and creates aching joints for many users, it may not be effective for the first year of use, and the ideal dose is unknown.

Chemically modified forms of vitamin D are used to help calcium be more effective, and rarely anabolic steroids (see "Anabolic Steroids" on page 39) are used instead of ERT.

HOME REMEDIES YOU CAN TRY

If you are already past menopause, you can probably halt any additional bone loss (unless you have genetic osteoporosis) with home remedies. If you are past age 50 and you don't take steps to preserve your bone strength, you can expect to lose about 10 percent of your bone mass per decade.

• *Exercise regularly.* This increases bone density especially when dietary absorption of vitamins and minerals is adequate, too. To avoid bone loss, exercise needs to be consistent and weight bearing, as in walking, jogging, and weight lifting. Some women benefit from regular swimming as well. (See "Exercise" on page 41.)

• *Eat a diet rich in calcium, magnesium, boron, and vitamins D and C.* When public attention was drawn to osteoporosis in the early 1980s, it seemed that adding a glass of milk each day to one's diet was all that was needed for bone strength. Since then, however, it's become clear that it's not that simple.

Calcium by itself may not prevent osteoporosis. Calcium, which varies in absorption, depending on the chemical compound, is part of an interwoven balance with many other minerals and vitamins. Vitamin D, magnesium, and vitamin C, for instance, enhance its absorption.

• *Reduce smoking, alcohol, sugar, fats, processed meats and cheeses, soft drinks, chocolate, and caffeine to enhance your body's levels of calcium.* (No more than two cups of coffee or four cups of tea per day are considered moderate use.) Emphasize soy products (including tofu), whole grains, beets, peas, green peppers, raw nuts (especially almonds), fish, bananas, apples, and nectarines. (See "How to Find Fat in Your Food" on page 29.)

Although the calcium in milk is plentiful, dairy products are also high in saturated fats (unless you use skim milk and other fat-free dairy products), and they are a source of stomach upset and allergies for millions of people. Many women can get enough calcium daily only through a combination of foods and supplements. Experts lock horns over what that ideal amount is (estimates range from 800 milligrams to 1,500 milligrams per day with a recent study showing that 1,000 mgs. per day slows bone loss). (See "Osteoporosis" on page 619 in Recommended Reading for specific dosages. Also see "Osteoporosis" on page 591 in the Resource Directory.)

• *Pay attention to your own personal health history.* If you take a drug that depletes calcium or other minerals, or if you have a history of anorexia at any age, or if you were a long-distance runner over a long period of time, don't wait until someone tells you that you may have had unusual bone loss. Adjust your diet and exercise patterns for greater bone strength.

M y mom has osteoporosis, and she's already lost four inches of height. But I'm not going to have it. While I'm still in my 30s I've made life-style changes (I run every day, and watch what I eat). She never knew that a lot of her daily habits, like smoking and drinking, would affect her bones.

I take cortisone for severe asthma. At the beginning, it made my fingernails peel and break easily. Then I read about taking calcium to replace that which the drug depleted. Now I take 2,000 milligrams of calcium each day along with magnesium, other minerals, and vitamin C. My nails have never been as strong as they are now.

OVARIAN CYSTS

WHAT THEY ARE

Ovarian cysts are fluid-filled growths that form on or near one of the two almond-sized ovaries and are the result of an underlying hormonal imbalance. Ninety-five percent of the time these cysts are harmless.

Functional cysts, the most common ovarian cysts, are small and form when an egg doesn't release properly during the monthly ovulation cycle. A *luteal cyst*, which is a type of functional cyst, delays a woman's period or makes her flow very light. A *dermoid cyst* contains bits of hair, teeth and bone, and will probably need to be removed. *Polycystic ovary syndrome* occurs when many tiny cysts form in the ovaries.

Malignant cysts are a result of cancer of the ovary. Fortunately they are rare. (See "Ovarian Cancer" on page 234.) A benefit of ovarian cysts is women who have them have a reduced risk for breast cancer. It's not clear why, but hormonal levels are suspect.

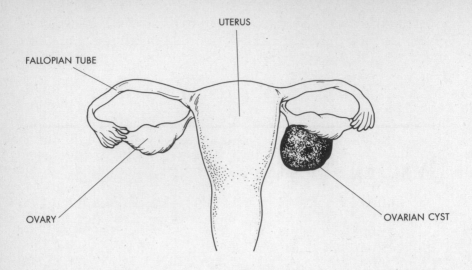

FALLOPIAN TUBE

UTERUS

OVARY

OVARIAN CYST

OVARIAN CYST

SIGNS AND SYMPTOMS

Most women do not experience any symptoms, so they may not know they have an ovarian cyst until it's diagnosed during a routine pelvic exam. Some have symptoms that can be confused with signs of other menstrual disturbances. Symptoms include one or more of the following:

- *Lower abdominal pain and/or unexplained abdominal swelling*
- *Weight gain*
- *Indigestion or bloating*
- *Delayed, irregular, or painful periods*
- *Painful intercourse*
- *Unusual growth of facial hair* (polycystic ovary syndrome)

Most ovarian cysts occur in women who are between the ages of 20 to 35. Uterine fibroids, often confused with ovarian cysts, generally occur in women past age 35. One of the causes for polycystic ovaries is the use of the drug valporate for epilepsy, particularly before the age of 20. Curiously, a newly discovered cause for some ovarian cysts, particularly those that are multiple cysts, is the eating disorder bulimia. A cyst is a symptom of a problem, like endometriosis or pelvic inflammatory disease, about 5 percent of the time. (See "Uterine Fibroids" on page 522, "Endometriosis" on page 329 and "Pelvic Inflammatory Disease" on page 441.)

MAKING THE DIAGNOSIS

In addition to a pelvic exam, the following are also used to evaluate ovarian cysts: ultrasound, x-ray, or laparoscopy, which can be also used for treatment. (See "Ultrasound" on page 476 and "Laparoscopy" on page 173.)

TREATMENT OPTIONS

Most cysts disappear on their own. If your physician has ruled out serious problems, one option is to do nothing and see if your condition improves. However, a ruptured or twisted ovarian cyst, which is rare, can cause intense pain, weakness, nausea, and vomiting and should be treated immediately.

If you have a functional cyst, taking the Pill (especially a higher-dose preparation) may shrink it and reduce symptoms. (See "The Pill" on page 181.) Acupuncture, along with Chinese herbs, also may shrink cysts. (See "Acupuncture" on page 82.)

Surgical options are a cystectomy, which removes only the cyst and is sometimes recommended for problematic cysts. Hysterectomy, removal of not only the cyst, but your entire uterus and probably your ovaries (oophorectomy) as well, is sometimes suggested, depending in part on your age and the nature of the cyst. This may be recommended to women who are finished having children, because then they won't have any more cysts. However, be sure to get a second opinion if your physician recommends this. Most physicians say a hysterectomy is too much treatment for a problem cyst unless it is cancerous. (See "Hysterectomy and Oophorectomy" on page 354 and "Get a Second Opinion" on page 95.)

I was diagnosed with an ovarian cyst in my late 20s and my gynecologist wanted to give me a hysterectomy because he said he was sure I'd have more of these in the future. I went to another surgeon who suggested that I just have the cyst removed and that's all. That's what I did, and now ten years later, I've had no more cysts.

HOME REMEDIES YOU CAN TRY

Make dietary changes, including reducing fat and dairy products, sugars of all kinds, and protein, while increasing the amount of whole grains you eat. (See "How to Find Fat in Your Food" on page 29.) Try vitamin E supplements and reduce caffeine. As with breast lumps, which are also cysts, some nutritionists have found that avoiding foods that they believe "feed" cysts (like those on the above list) can reduce the occurrence of ovarian cysts. (See "Breast Health" on page 611 and Fuchs on page 619 in Recommended Reading for specific vitamin dosages.)

Pelvic Inflammatory Disease (PID)

What It Is

Pelvic inflammatory disease is a bacterial or parasitic infection in the uterus, fallopian tubes, pelvis, and/or ovaries. Untreated PID can cause permanent damage to the reproductive organs.

Signs and Symptoms

Both women and men can carry PID-causing bacteria without showing symptoms, and can pass them on to someone else who might develop PID. When a woman has symptoms, they range from mild to severe, depending on whether the infection is chronic or acute. Chronic PID is generally less symptomatic than acute PID.

Women's PID symptoms vary enormously. Acute PID is usually associated with pain in the abdomen or back, or pain during intercourse, along with tenderness or bloating. With chronic PID, the pain may be less severe and occur midway during the menstrual cycle. The skin on your abdomen may also be sensitive. With acute PID, the fever may be high, but

Infected fallopian tube, or salpingitis

INFECTED
FALLOPIAN
TUBE

NORMAL
FALLOPIAN
TUBE

UTERUS

Infected uterus

INFECTED
UTERUS

NORMAL
FALLOPIAN
TUBE

NORMAL
OVARY

Infected fallopian tube and ovary

INFECTED
FALLOPIAN
TUBE

INFECTED
OVARY

NORMAL
UTERUS

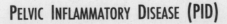

PELVIC INFLAMMATORY DISEASE (PID)

if it's chronic PID, the fever is low grade, and often goes unnoticed. Other possible symptoms are vaginal discharge or bleeding, nausea, and pain during a pelvic exam or while urinating.

About one million women each year have PID, and one quarter of the infections they have are emergency situations requiring hospitalization. PID can be a serious consequence of sexually transmitted diseases.

PID can cause scar tissue that blocks the fallopian tubes, causing infertility. That's not uncommon. PID causes infertility in 10 to 40 percent of cases, depending on the severity of the infection and the number of infections that you have had. The more often you have PID, the greater your risk of being made infertile (see "Infertility" on page 364).

If you've had PID, you're more likely to have an ectopic or tubal pregnancy, premature rupture of the membranes during pregnancy, and premature birth. PID that occurs with an intrauterine device during pregnancy usually results in miscarriage. PID can also cause difficult menstrual cramps, chronic pain, and recurrent infection. (See "Ectopic Pregnancy" on page 488, "Premature Rupture of the Membranes" on page 259, "Premature Babies" on page 259, "Intrauterine Device," on page 208, and "Dysmennorhea" on page 407.)

If you've had sexually transmitted PID, in addition to other possible consequences, it's easy to feel exploited or feel disgusted with yourself for your own behavior.

CAUSES

PID is caused by organisms that usually travel from the vagina through the cervix into internal reproductive organs. Some PID is caused by the sexually transmitted gonorrhea and chlamydia organisms. PID caused by chlamydia and transmitted through intercourse is likely to be the milder, chronic version. (See "Sexually Transmitted Diseases" on page 493.)

PID isn't always caused by a sexually transmitted bacteria, however. PID can be caused by bacteria that are normally found in the intestines that find their way into the pelvic cavity during sex, after an abortion, after a miscarriage, during childbirth, during operations such as a cesarean, dilation and curettage (D & C), or hysterectomy, or after insertion (PID risk is greatest during the first 20 days) or repositioning of an IUD. The Dalkon Shield, an IUD no longer available in the United States, was notorious for causing PID in the 1970s. This model has long since been removed from the marketplace, and the two IUDs now available in the United States have low PID risks.

MAKING THE DIAGNOSIS

The symptoms of PID can mimic those of other conditions, so PID is often misdiagnosed as endometriosis, appendicitis, urinary tract infections, ovarian cysts, or an ectopic pregnancy. (See "Endometriosis" on page 329, "Urinary Tract Infections" on page 515, and "Ovarian Cysts" on page 437.)

Since diagnosis of chronic PID from clinical symptoms alone is only about 30 percent accurate, experts suggest that if you think you may have PID, get an examination by laparoscopy, a surgical procedure. You may also be examined with ultrasound. (See "Laparoscopy" on page 173 and "Ultrasound" on page 476.)

As with any difficult-to-diagnose disease, find a physician who has a lot of experience in successfully treating this disease. (See "Pelvic Inflammatory Disease" on page 591 in the Resource Directory for a helpful organization.)

The woman most likely to have PID is sexually active, in her teens or 20s. If she's older, she is likely to have become sexually active as a teenager. She has more than one sexual partner or changes partners frequently or has a partner who has multiple partners. Often she has had PID before, and she may also be a DES-daughter (see "Diethylstilbestrol" on page 309), or she has had vaginitis recently. (See "Vaginal Infections" on page 532.)

PREVENTIVE MEASURES YOU CAN TAKE

• *Practice good hygiene.* Wipe from front to back after a bowel movement to avoid infection from intestinal bacteria, and don't have vaginal intercourse immediately following anal intercourse. Since women are especially susceptible to PID during menstruation, change tampons or pads frequently and carefully. After your cervix has been dilated for any reason (childbirth, IUD insertion, miscarriage, D & C, abortion), do not allow anything into your vagina for six weeks.

• *Don't douche.* About one third of U.S. women douche regularly. Some studies show that women who douche three to four times per month increase their risk for PID though it's not believed that douching causes PID. The theory is that it may somehow spread the infectious organisms. Douching is also a suspect for ectopic pregnancy.

• *Maintain a healthy immune system* (see "The Immune System" on page 9 and "How to Stay Healthy" on page 25 to reduce your chance of having illnesses of any kind).

• *Choose an anti-PID contraceptive.* Use barrier contraceptives with spermicides, like the condom, cervical cap, or diaphragm. This reduces your likelihood of getting PID from an infected partner. Information about the Pill and PID is mixed. There are about eight studies that show an anti-PID benefit from use of the Pill and one study that shows Pill users may be more susceptible to chlamydia-caused PID. (See "Barrier Contraceptives" on page 190 and "The Pill" on page 181.)

• *Keep track of your IUD.* If you use an IUD, become pregnant, and then miscarry, have your physician make sure the IUD is no longer in your body. If it remains, it increases your risk for PID.

• *Avoid sex with anyone who has been with another person who has had untreated PID or an untreated sexually transmitted disease.*

• *Don't smoke.* Women who smoke at least 10 cigarettes daily have a higher risk for PID.

TREATMENT OPTIONS

When you have symptoms of pelvic pain, vaginal discharge, painful sex, or a change in your menstrual flow, consider seeing your doctor to find out if your problem is PID.

The primary treatment for PID is antibiotics along with bed rest. If the infection is of the chronic variety, you probably will be given an antibiotic, although you may be given a series of different antibiotics over a three to four week period. It's believed that PID is more likely to recur if only one antibiotic is used. If the infection is acute, you may be hospitalized and given several antibiotics intravenously. Each fights several different organisms, and they may all be necessary because PID is often caused by a group of organisms, not just one.

Some women receive relief from chronic pelvic pain with acupuncture (see "Acupuncture" on page 82). Laparoscopy is used to treat PID as well as to diagnose it. Sometimes hysterectomy is recommended for severe PID, but this operation is not always effective because the infection may have spread to other internal organs, too. (See "Hysterectomy and Oophorectomy" on page 354.) If you develop PID and you use an IUD, make sure it's removed during treatment.

Another important measure in treating sexually transmitted PID is to make sure your partner is also treated for the bacteria. That's true whether he shows symptoms of PID or not. Most men don't, but if they do, it presents as a white discharge and/or pain on urination. If your partner is not treated, you could be reinfected.

I was angry when I discovered that my boyfriend had given me PID. I was in the hospital for several days and stuck with a big medical bill. We had plans to get married, but I cancelled that. My friends told me I was being hasty, but that's how I felt then, and that's how I feel now, many months later.

*W*ho would ever dream that my mom was right when she used to tell me to "save" myself for marriage. I'm 25, and I've had two bouts with this infection. My doctor told me that I've already damaged my fallopian tubes and it's possible I may never have kids, unless I'm willing to pay thousands of dollars for infertility treatment. A wonderful therapist helped me get over my disgust with myself.

PREGNANCY

WHAT IT IS

Pregnancy is the condition of having a fetus or fetuses growing in the uterus.

SIGNS AND SYMPTOMS

The most obvious symptom of pregnancy is the absence of a menstrual period, especially if your cycle is ordinarily regular and you're not of menopausal age (45 to 55).

MAKING THE DIAGNOSIS

You can find out if you're pregnant by having an examination by a health care provider or by having your blood or urine tested at a clinic or in a doctor's office. You can also use a home test kit that is available in stores, but these have mixed reports of accuracy (though they are getting better), and they will not reveal an ectopic pregnancy. Manufacturers of these kits claim they are 99 percent accurate. Research, however, shows accuracy varies from 45 to 89 percent, and the inaccurate results can be either false-positive or false-negative. (These tests are more likely to be false-positive in women approaching menopause.)

Pregnancy tests can be used the first day of a missed period. If you use a home test, follow the directions precisely to improve reliability. The accuracy in hospital laboratories is not always reliable either. Pregnancy tests detect minute traces of a hormone, human chorionic gonadotropin (HCG), that a pregnant woman produces after conception. Whatever the result of the test you use, it's probably wise to repeat the process in a few days, because each test varies in its ability to pick up the presence of HCG. That's why your doctor or midwife will also examine you.

For many women, a late period is the only symptom they notice immediately. Other women, though, notice symptoms within days of conception. Some of those are: nausea, with or without vomiting; fatigue and sleepiness; breast changes (tenderness, fullness, heaviness, tingling, sensitive nipples); and increased emotion (usually a mixture of positive and negative with added exhilaration, weepiness, and perhaps irritability) that will wax and wane throughout pregnancy.

As the weeks and months go by, other body symptoms occur. Not all women have all of them, however. Some of these are: headaches, fainting or dizziness, frequent urination, and increasing appetite. Changes in sexuality occur throughout pregnancy, such as engorgement of the vagina, heightened sensitivity of the nipples, and orgasms that become easier or more difficult. Some women have digestive disruptions, such as heartburn, indigestion, flatulence, bloating, or constipation, and some experience food aversions and/or cravings. New veins may appear on the abdomen, as well as hemorrhoids and varicose veins (see "Varicose Veins" on page 537.)

Other possible sensations and discomforts include fetal movement; lower abdominal achiness; leg cramps; increased pulse and body temperature; stuffy nose; mild swelling of the ankles and feet and occasionally of the hands and face; backache; skin changes, including color changes on the abdomen (sometimes in a line from the navel to the pubic area); itchy abdomen; difficulty sleeping; clumsiness because of added body bulk; painless contractions (which are normal); stretch marks; shortness of breath as the uterus begins crowding the lungs; and pelvic discomfort and pressure.

HOW TO HAVE A HEALTHY PREGNANCY

There are many choices you make during pregnancy that affect your health and that of your unborn baby. Following are guidelines to help you make the best decisions for you.

HOME REMEDIES YOU CAN TRY TO RELIEVE COMMON COMPLAINTS

Some of the common complaints of pregnancy can be relieved with simple measures.

• *Nausea and vomiting.* You may be able to relieve some of your symptoms with frequent small meals, mild exercise, and herbs, such as peppermint tea. You can also use pressure on the Neiguan point — the antinausea acupuncture and acupressure point on the inside of the wrist. Wrist bands (sold as MorningGarde and Sea Band) are stretchy bracelets with a button that fits over this point. These bands were originally developed to prevent motion sickness, but they have been found to reduce nausea and vomiting in 60 percent of the pregnant women who used them. When using these bands, be sure and press the button on each band every half hour or so for greatest effectiveness.

Some women find vitamin B$_6$ and ginger root capsules helpful as well. No drugs that might be helpful have been found to be safe. The good news is women who vomit are less likely to miscarry than those who don't experience nausea. (See "Acupressure" on page 56 and "Acupuncture" on page 82.)

• *Stretch marks.* About half of pregnant women develop stretch marks, which are usually a family trait. The marks are believed to be related, in part, to the level of the body's collagen, which is found in connective tissue. Various creams are marketed to prevent stretch marks, too, but none are known to be truly effective. Some women get good results (some don't) by piercing vitamin E capsules and spreading the oil on the stretch marks before and after the baby is born, while taking vitamin E internally as well. Without treatment or with treatment, these marks fade somewhat on their own after childbirth.

• *Fatigue.* This is a universal complaint of pregnant women for good reason. It's your body's message to you that you need to rest while your baby is growing inside you. Get enough sleep, eat well, take your vitamins, and exercise. (These all help prevent other discomforts as well.) Walking regularly and pregnancy yoga are especially helpful. If fatigue is a nagging problem, consider leaving your job earlier in the pregnancy than you planned or work part-time. Obviously, that's not an option for all women. (See "Yoga" on page 59, "Pregnancy and the Workplace" on page 460, and "Fatigue" on page 344.)

• *Leg cramps.* Some health care professionals recommend calcium and magnesium supplements each day to relieve leg cramps. Reduce your intake of caffeine, as caffeine overload can cause "restless leg" syndrome as you are going to sleep. (See Jimenez and Stillerman on page 620 in Recommended Reading for excellent home remedy guides.)

Exercise and Pregnancy

Women who exercise during pregnancy have less physical discomfort, including less morning sickness, less lower-back pain, fewer headaches, less fatigue, and less shortness of breath. Many also have more self-esteem, less depression, and improved heart and lung capacities, and they are in better shape after the baby is born. The second stage of labor, the pushing stage, may be shorter if you have exercised regularly during pregnancy, though that is not always true.

Standard advice from many health care providers is that you exercise moderately three times a week. Activities that are considered safe during pregnancy, in combination with common sense are: walking, golf, swimming, jogging, bicycling, racket sports, aerobic dancing, and cross-country skiing.

Your heart and lungs are more efficient during pregnancy, so that even when you're exercising intensely, your blood still reaches your baby in adequate amounts. Your baby's heart rate may be affected, but this is not considered to be harmful. Researchers caution, however, that you take a few minutes to taper off instead of abruptly stopping, especially if you're exercising vigorously.

Exercise during pregnancy is good for mothers and their babies, including diabetic women. Exceptions are women who have a heart condition, a history of preterm labor, vaginal bleeding, or who have fetuses who have fetal growth disturbances.

Pregnant women who exercise give birth without any increase in fetal complications, though these women often have gained less than nonexercising mothers-to-be and their babies weigh slightly less.

SEX DURING PREGNANCY

In both sexual arousal and pregnancy, breasts enlarge, nipples become sensitive, and both lubrication in the vagina and blood flow increase. If you're like most women when you feel tired and sick, you may prefer to do without sex altogether. Or you may feel increased arousal. In fact, masturbation is common during pregnancy for some women, even if they never experienced it before.

Whatever sexual feelings you feel or don't feel during pregnancy and birth are normal for you and they may vary from pregnancy to pregnancy. This is true for your sexual feelings after the baby is born, too.

Although many cultures have taboos against sex during pregnancy, intercourse is considered safe throughout pregnancy and does not cause premature labor or other problems. Although not all agree, some physicians believe exceptions may be women who are spotting, have a history of miscarriage, have a history of premature labor with effacement of the cervix, or who are expecting more than one child.

PREGNANCY AND RECREATIONAL DRUGS

All recreational and prescription drugs produce side effects and potentially can affect your baby. Despite that, most pregnant women use at least one prescription or over-the-counter drug (an estimated 60 percent use aspirin) during pregnancy, and more than one quarter smoke cigarettes or marijuana or drink alcohol.

Many normal babies are born to women who drink alcohol or who smoke tobacco or marijuana occasionally during pregnancy. However, no use of any of these substances, as well as cocaine and anabolic steroids, has been found to be safe during pregnancy. Ideally, pregnant women would quit all of these substances well before conception. (See "Suggestions for Users of Recreational Drugs" on page 40.)

Following is a description of the effects on your unborn child of the most common recreational drugs, listed in order of their use by U.S. women.

Alcohol

Alcohol is considered worse for your baby than smoking cigarettes or marijuana, but not as bad as using cocaine. Although not all children will show negative results, 50,000 U.S. babies, including many Native American infants, are born every year who show mild to severe side effects, resulting from their mothers' drinking. The good news is that alcohol use among pregnant women dropped significantly in the 1980s.

Severe effects, which may occur to the infants of women who drink heavily throughout the entire pregnancy, include cleft lip with or without cleft palate. Other severely affected children can have facial abnormalities, heart murmurs, ear disorders, growth and neurologic problems, and mental retardation — a cluster of abnormalities known as fetal alcohol syndrome. Daily drinks in the first two months of pregnancy, or 10 drinks a week, can result in premature birth, as well as a child who has a lower I.Q., slower reaction time, and difficulty paying attention. As there is no known level of alcohol that doesn't affect a fetus, consider stopping as soon as you know you are pregnant — or preferably before. Researchers think staying away from alcohol is good advice for breastfeeding mothers, too.

Smoking

Smoking during pregnancy is associated with the birth of babies who weigh about a half-pound less than other babies. This is especially true with mothers who are past age 35. Babies born to mothers who smoke also have a greater risk for lower scores on the Apgar test (which evaluates newborns' physical health) cleft lip or palate, and heart or lung problems. A breastfeeding mother who smokes is likely to produce less milk.

Smoking is also associated with higher rates of sudden infant death syndrome (SIDS), miscarriage, stillbirth, and a threefold increase in placenta previa (a condition in which the placenta obstructs the opening in the birth canal and often causes hemorrhage). It also may be one of the causes for ectopic, or tubal, pregnancies. However, women who quit smoking by the end of the fourth month do not give birth to lower-weight babies. Because each cigarette affects your baby's oxygen, it's never too late to quit smoking. (See "Ectopic Pregnancy" on page 488.)

Sidestream smoke or passive smoking is also harmful for your baby. As little as two hours a day of passive smoke can affect your unborn child.

Marijuana

Marijuana can cause premature birth, small-for-age baby, and problems with the placenta. It can also cause tremors, easy upsets, and disturbed sleep in the babies of mothers who smoked marijuana during pregnancy. Passive marijuana smoking (one hour, three times per week in a closed room) is suspected of affecting the fetus, too. Long-term risks are not clear, although a reduction in I.Q. is suspected with some children. Marijuana users may also have more difficulty conceiving, are more likely to miscarry, and may not produce as much milk if they breastfeed. Babies affected by either marijuana or cocaine in utero respond poorly to affection, which often makes the mother feel inadequate and can interfere with the mother-child relationship.

Cocaine

Depending on the hospital, 3 to 50 percent of pregnant U.S. women expose their fetuses to cocaine, and some of them erroneously believe that cocaine use will shorten labor. Research shows that cocaine not only doesn't shorten labor, it may make it longer. Not all exposed babies show side effects, but most do, especially those that are exposed for many months in utero, and/or in the first trimester.

It's suspected that cocaine's side effects on fetuses and newborns are probably exaggerated, but those that have been reported are: prematurity and low birth weight; miscarriage; small size; stiff limbs; either jitteriness (which may fade in 12 months) or sleepiness all the time; fragile nervous system (including chronic crying); kidney malformations and urinary tract defects; and a tenfold greater risk for SIDS.

Anabolic steroids

Not much is known about the damage to a fetus from these synthetic, body-building hormones because of scanty reports, but infertility has already been reported among steroid users who want to become pregnant.

HOW TO AVOID BIRTH DEFECTS

A birth defect is an abnormality in a baby's structure, function, or body metabolism that may result in a physical or mental handicap, may shorten life, or may be fatal. Genetic defects are present from conception and are inherited from either the mother or father, while other birth defects develop during the pregnancy.

Among the reasons for birth defects, which are the leading cause of infant deaths, are: hereditary diseases (cystic fibrosis, hemophilia, and others), environmental pollutants, drugs (prescription, over-the-counter, and recreational), nutritional deficiencies, radiation, and prolonged high fever during pregnancy.

Most women who give birth to babies with birth defects do so for unknown reasons. Three or four babies in every 100 born in the United States have major birth defects. Another four or five have less serious problems that may be easily corrected or may be barely noticeable.

Not all birth defects are avoidable, but following are suggestions for what you can do to help prevent those that are:

• *Eat a good diet during pregnancy*, especially rich in the B vitamins and folic acid in particular. There is a direct correlation between maternal diet and fetal health. In Utah, Mormons — who, like Adventists, are known for healthy diets—are far less likely to have neural tube defects than other Utah women. Take your pregnancy vitamins from the very beginning of your pregnancy, if not before, as many birth defects occur in the early weeks. According to some research, you'll have less than half the risk of having a baby with a neural tube defect. (See "The Pregnancy Diet" on page 34.)

• *Avoid drugs of all kinds*—prescription drugs, recreational drugs (marijuana, alcohol, and others), and over-the-counter drugs, including aspirin. Accutane, a prescription drug given to treat acne, is known to cause birth defects. Fathers who smoke cigarettes, use cocaine, or drink alcohol to excess increase their offspring's risk for birth defects as well.

• *Avoid environmental chemicals, herbicides, pesticides, fertilizers, pollutants, and x-rays of all kinds, including dental x-rays.* This applies not only to mothers-to-be, but also to fathers before conception. Fathers who are painters or printers have a higher risk for producing a child with anencephaly, one of the neural tube defects, and British fathers who worked at a nuclear plant had a three times higher risk for having children who developed leukemia.

• *If you're trying to get pregnant, have intercourse more than once a week*, especially near the time of ovulation. (See Down Syndrome below.)

• *Stay out of hot tubs and saunas in the first trimester*, because the heat exposure is associated with increased risk for neural tube defects.

Neural Tube Defects (NTDs)

Anencephaly (lack of a brain) and spina bifida (incompletely closed spinal cord) are the two most common NTDs. These defects occur in one or two babies in 1,000. Some researchers link NTDs to vitamin deficiencies. Spina bifida may be associated with the use of valproic acid, a drug given to some women who have epilepsy. Infants with anencephaly die at birth, but children with spina bifida or other NTDs may live through childhood or longer, depending on the severity of the NTD, often with severe disabilities requiring extensive medical and surgical care from birth. Many can't walk, and some can't control their bowels or bladder.

Down Syndrome (DS)

The focus of most prenatal testing has been on the most common cause of severe mental retardation, Down syndrome, which occurs in one in 700 U.S. babies. DS is perhaps the most feared defect for many prospective parents.

People with Down syndrome have specific facial features and retardation, which can be mild to severe. They often have heart, bowel, and eye problems, as well as increased susceptibility to infections, childhood leukemia, and Alzheimer's disease in later life. DS has been recognized since ancient times and was given its current name in 1866 by J. L. H. Down.

DS babies are born to mothers of all ages, including teens. For unknown reasons (some speculate environmental insults), younger women are having more babies who have Down syndrome than in the past in the United States and Europe.

Published lists of the incidence of Down syndrome by age group usually start at age 20. The implication is that women under 20 have even lower rates of DS. However, one study that examined the DS rate for teens found that girls 15 and under gave birth to babies with DS at the same rate as women who were 30 to 35.

About 20 to 30 percent of DS is caused by "old" sperm — that is, sperm that has been stored in the father's genital tract. The men at risk for this cause of Down syndrome are those who have sex less than once a week. The women most likely to fit that profile are women in their 30s or 40s who have been married for years (newlyweds generally have sex more often) or unmarried women, especially teens. Women who use the natural family planning method of birth control are also at greater risk of giving birth to a DS baby because this method requires infrequent intercourse prior to ovulation, the peak time for conception.

In addition to malfunctioning eggs and sperm, there is a combination of environmental factors and pregnancy-history risks that have a role in causing Down syndrome. Whatever the occurrence for DS is for your age (see "Risk for Birth Defects by Mother's Age" on page 456), that rate is not equal for all women in your age group. There are additional factors that have been found to increase the chance of having a Down syndrome baby. It's not clear though, how much each factor, alone or combined with others, increases your risk of having a baby with DS.

Exposure to ionizing radiation, which refers to medical x-rays of all kinds and gamma rays from nuclear explosions, is associated with DS babies. The damage from radiation is cumulative. It depends on the number of exposures, the dose of each, and, in the case of x-rays, the part of the body that has been exposed. Another environmental risk factor is geographical location. Occasionally, without explanation so far, the incidence of DS in one group of babies is higher than that in babies in neighboring areas. In one southern Illinois county, for instance, five times the usual number of babies with Down syndrome were born recently, and the average age of the mothers was 22.

Other pregnancy risk factors include having many illnesses before conception, drug use in the year before conception, lengthy duration of vaginal bleeding during pregnancy, and repeated miscarriages (this is especially true with women under the age of 20). Other factors are: a previous birth of a child with DS, a close relative with DS, and a grandmother on

RISK FOR BIRTH DEFECTS BY MOTHER'S AGE

Mother's Age	Risk for Down Syndrome	Total Risk for Chromosomal Abnormalities*
20	1:1,667	1:526
21	1:1,667	1:526
22	1:1,429	1:500
23	1:1,429	1:500
24	1:1,250	1:476
25	1:1,250	1:476
26	1:1,176	1:476
27	1:1,111	1:455
28	1:1,053	1:435
29	1:1,000	1:417
30	1:952	1:385
31	1:909	1:385
32	1:769	1:322
33	1:602	1:286
34	1:485	1:238
35	1:378	1:192
36	1:289	1:156
37	1:224	1:127
38	1:173	1:102
39	1:136	1:83
40	1:106	1:66
41	1:82	1:53
42	1:63	1:42
43	1:49	1:33
44	1:38	1:26
45	1:30	1:21
46	1:23	1:16
47	1:18	1:13
48	1:14	1:10
49	1:11	1:8

From *ACOG Technical Bulletin #108,* September 1987.
*These occurrences of abnormalities range from very mild or near normal to severe.

the mother's side who was at least 30 years old when she gave birth to the mother of the child with DS. (This does not apply to the paternal grandmother, however.) The final factor is having a positive antibody to the herpes virus, which means the mother has been exposed to herpes, but she may or may not have active signs of the disease. Not all women who give birth to babies with DS report these conditions, nor will women who have these situations necessarily give birth to a baby with DS.

Having a child with Down syndrome is not always the tragedy many parents fear. Many appreciate their child's individuality.

Some children with DS are seriously retarded and have physical problems requiring frequent surgery. But some are mildly retarded and live near-normal lives if they receive early stimulation and education. The treatment of these children has changed enormously in the 1980s, due to greater understanding of the capability of people with DS. Some say that the greatest disadvantage these children face is discrimination from others.

---

*N*o one wants a child with a handicap . . . but Greg is our son and there is no way we think of him as second best. Every time he learns a new word or understands a new concept, his eyes light up and he is full of joy.

*S*omeone told me [a woman with DS and also a recent graduate with a two-year associate degree in early childhood education] that a person with Down syndrome couldn't graduate from college. . . . I think that society should never underestimate us, and I don't feel they should put a label on us, either. Because once we've got that label, it's on us for the rest of our lives.

A note about father's age. Men 40 years of age and over have a 20 percent greater risk of fathering a baby with a birth defect than do younger men, although paternal age is not associated with Down syndrome.

ILLNESSES DURING PREGNANCY

Sometimes during pregnancy diseases that are ordinarily harmless can cause birth defects. Not all health care providers routinely screen for these infections, so if you think you may be at risk for one of them, request screening.

• *Rubella (German measles)* is a usually mild disease that causes a rash and fever. If contracted in the first 10 weeks of pregnancy, more than half of affected fetuses are born with birth defects such as cataracts, deafness, and heart defects. If you have rubella later in pregnancy, your child may be born with the illness. If you've not had rubella, consider immunization *before* pregnancy.

• *Chickenpox (varicella)* is contracted in childhood more than 90 percent of the time. If it's contracted during pregnancy, birth defects occur in about 3 percent of exposed fetuses and include pock-like skin scarring (which will fade), eye problems, or motor or growth retardation.

• *Cytomegalovirus*, which causes flulike symptoms and is more common among women who have children in daycare, can cause birth defects such as blindness, seizures, anemia, and neurologic disorders.

• *Hepatitis B* is a liver infection that your baby can contract from you during pregnancy. The virus can also cause liver failure in a newborn, but more commonly it is associated with premature birth.

• *Sexually transmitted diseases (STDs)*, including herpes, AIDS, syphilis, gonorrhea, and chlamydia can also damage unborn babies (see "STDs and Babies" on page 499.)

• *Toxoplasmosis* is known as "cat-box disease" and can cause birth defects. The parasite *Toxoplasma gondii* is carried by many animals, especially cats, and is present in their feces in the form of eggs. You can contract toxoplasmosis by handling a cat or cat box and not washing your hands afterwards, by eating rare or raw meat (as in steak tartare), or by handling raw meat (for example, when you cut up raw chicken) and not washing your hands afterward.

Mild symptoms of toxoplasmosis are easily confused with flu and can include feeling blah, with a slight rash, some achiness, low-grade fever, headaches, sore throat, swollen lymph nodes, and eye infections. Every year hundreds of U.S. babies are born who have been infected with toxoplasmosis during pregnancy, though few pregnant U.S. women are tested for it or have been diagnosed with it.

The chances of passing on the disease to the fetus are 15 to 20 percent if you contract the disease in the first trimester and up to 60 percent if you contract it in the last trimester. However, effects on the baby are likely to be more severe with a first-trimester infection. Toxoplasmosis can cause stillbirth or miscarriage. Most babies who are affected by the disease show no symptoms at birth, although a few may be small and/or show signs of damage to the brain, eyes, or other organs. Often the damage appears weeks, months, or years later in the form of poor vision, epilepsy, or psychomotor or mental retardation, among other problems.

Screening for toxoplasmosis involves several tests, starting with a blood test, because one test is not always accurate. If your results are questionable and you're not at risk for the disease, consider having other tests performed at a different lab. Find a health care provider who has a lot of experience with diagnosing and evaluating this disease.

The treatment of choice for those women who test positive and who have those results confirmed several times is the drug spiramycin. Although it's controversial, it's believed to be the safest drug for toxoplasmosis to use during pregnancy, and it reduces your baby's risk of contracting the disease by 50 percent. Possible drug side effects for you are stomach upset, headaches, and a bad taste in the mouth. This drug will cross the placenta to the baby.

To avoid contracting toxoplasmosis during pregnancy, let someone else take care of the cat litter if you have a cat, especially if your cat goes outdoors. If that's not possible, wash your hands before and after changing the cat litter and/or wear rubber gloves. Change the litter daily. Avoid other people's cats and stray cats, and avoid sandboxes or gardens where cats may have deposited feces, because the moist soil can hold the infectious potential for toxoplasmosis for up to one year.

Have your veterinarian check to see if your cat has an active toxoplasmosis infection. If the cat does, then consider boarding it in a kennel for at least six weeks, or have a friend care for it. Wash your hands before and after handling raw meat and don't eat rare or raw meat during your pregnancy.

A friend and I were pregnant at the same time, and we both had cats. We had heard about toxoplasmosis, so we had blood tests several times. Each time the results were negative; we had never had the disease. Because of that we were extremely careful in handling our cats, and I gave up eating rare meat.

During my first pregnancy I was told that I tested positive for toxoplasmosis, though I had no cats and didn't eat or handle raw meat. It took several tests to show that the first test was wrong. It's easy now to say that someone made a mistake, but at the time I thought I might have a retarded child.

We don't have a cat, but our neighbors have several. My daughter saw them around the sandbox several times, so we decided that the easiest solution was to empty the sandbox for the duration of my pregnancy, and we bought Sarah a swingset as a substitute. I didn't want to be worrying about *whether or not she would be carrying the parasite into the house and giving it to me.*

PREGNANCY AND THE WORKPLACE

Most U.S. pregnant women work outside the home, and almost half are on the job into their ninth month. U.S. law protects the rights of pregnant workers so they can't be treated differently from other workers with a temporary disability. (See "Occupational Health" on page 589 in the Resource Directory.) Research in the United States and Europe shows that women who work at outside jobs (especially those who have early prenatal care) have fewer pregnancy-related problems than other pregnant women.

Exceptions are women who mostly stand on their feet while working, women who work 40 or more hours per week (they have higher risk for low-birth-weight baby), women who work night shifts (they are more prone to miscarriage), and also working women who smoke, who have high blood pressure, who eat a poor diet, and who have other young children. The other exceptions are women who work in industries where there is a known higher rate for certain pregnancy-related problems, like miscarriage. Health care workers who are exposed to radiation, migrant workers and other agricultural workers who are exposed to pesticides, and plant workers who assemble semiconductor chips are the women most frequently affected.

Another possible cause for increased miscarriages is video display terminals (VDTs). Research on this is mixed, so the subject is controversial. VDTs are considered a potential workplace risk for pregnant women because some research shows that pregnant women who use a VDT with a strong magnetic field for at least 20 hours a week have a threefold increased risk for miscarriages. It's estimated that at least 25 percent of U.S. computers have strong magnetic fields. If you work at a computer, ask to have its magnetic field evaluated. The issue is complicated by the many other reasons for miscarriage — use of drugs, poor diet, and multiple pregnancy, among others. (See "Miscarriage" on page 487.)

Women comprise most of the 25 million VDT users in the world. Known VDT risks are eyestrain, eye irritation, blurred vision, and chronic headaches. To reduce your possible risk from VDT use if you are pregnant, you can request a non-VDT job. Some states are now considering legislation that would require companies to give a pregnant worker that choice. Other pregnant women have asked for a guarantee in writing that VDT use is safe for them, and when the employer realistically cannot provide such written assurance, it makes job transfer easier.

If a transfer is not possible, rest for 15 minutes for every two hours of VDT use, and use a VDT during only 50 percent of your work day. Sit at least three feet away from the back of a terminal to avoid the low-level radiation. Avoid sitting to the back or side of anyone else's terminal, if possible, and turn off your VDT when not in use. Consider installing a filtering device for your screen and/or an antiglare screen, especially if your VDT was produced before 1980. Both will help block your VDT's electronic fields.

No increase in miscarriage rates has been shown in women who use the machines 20 hours or less per week, nor is there an increase in the rate for administrative-level pregnant women who use a VDT more than 20 hours per week. (Perhaps that's due to these women using terminals away from large typing pools of workers.)

TESTS PERFORMED DURING PREGNANCY

PRENATAL TESTING

Women who have chronic health problems or unusual health histories will have more tests than most women, although not all health care providers use the same tests and procedures.

In addition to checking your baby's growth and position at each visit, common procedures include:

• *Complete physical and medical history* (including pelvic exam, urine test, blood pressure, and weight check)
• *Tests for sexually transmitted diseases* (see "Sexually Transmitted Diseases" on page 493)
• *Complete blood count* to look for anemia or iron deficiency (see "Anemia" on page 158)
• *Blood typing*
• *Blood glucose tests to screen for diabetes.* It's thought that gestational diabetes is found most often in nonwhite low-income women and occurs in about 3 percent of pregnancies, though some researchers think this figure is overstated. The use of this test is controversial because there is no universally accepted rule of who should take the test, nor what a safe blood level is — that is, what is a troublesome number in some laboratories across the country is not in others. What's worse is that based on this test, only 25 percent of those women who are told they are at risk for diabetes ever develop this disease.
• *Hepatitis B antibody test*

A variety of prenatal tests and procedures can be used to determine fetal health, including amniocentesis, alpha-fetoprotein screening (AFP), chorionic villi sampling (CVS), ultrasound, and electronic fetal monitoring (EFM). Amniocentesis and CVS are used to determine whether or not your baby has any one of about 200 to 300 metabolic and chromosomal disorders out of 3,000 known genetic defects. AFP is used primarily to screen for neural tube defects (see "Neural Tube Defects" on page 454).

At least three fourths of amniocentesis and CVS tests are given to women because they are age 35 or older. These tests may also be performed when a woman has a previous child with a birth defect or when there is a family history of birth defects, including Down syndrome, Duchenne muscular dystrophy, hemophilia, cystic fibrosis, or neural tube defects, among others. Prenatal testing is also often recommended if the pregnant woman has a history of miscarriage, if her mate's previous wife had a history of miscarriages, or if she or her mate has a known chromosomal abnormality.

None of these tests is 100 percent accurate. You will only know the outcome for sure after your baby is born. Sometimes an inaccurate test result or misinterpretation has led parents to abort a normal baby who was believed to have a defect, or to give birth to a baby with a defect who was believed to be normal.

Many of the four million U.S. women who have babies every year have one or more of these tests. No one method of testing is best suited for all women who want it. Nor is prenatal testing welcomed by all women. However, many women appreciate prenatal testing, and many governments, along with most doctors, encourage its use. In California, where one ninth of the U.S. population resides, all prenatal care providers are required to give information about alpha-fetoprotein screening (AFP) to pregnant women who are less than 20 weeks pregnant, although these women are not required to have the screening. In most developed countries prenatal testing is standard for certain age groups.

From the beginning of amniocentesis use in the 1970s, there's been concern that it would result in the abortions of children of an unwanted gender. Since prenatal tests do not have to be reported, no one knows for sure how many are performed or for what reasons. In one amniocentesis study of more than 3,000 U.S. women, however, it was suspected, but not proven, that less than 1 percent of fetuses were aborted based on sex selection.

Prenatal tests can be very reassuring if the news is good. If the news is not, many parents appreciate having time to prepare for the birth of a baby with a known defect (or, alternatively, to terminate pregnancy).

The disadvantages of amniocentesis, CVS, and AFP are the anxiety while you wait for results, the less than 100 percent reliability of any of the tests, and the risks to the fetus.

Different procedures entail different risks to the fetus, but complications of amniocentesis and chorionic villi sampling include fetal death, fetal puncture wounds, premature rupture of the membranes, premature birth, a low-birth-weight baby, and maternal bleeding or leaking of amniotic fluid. There may be unknown side effects as well because studies have not been performed to determine long-term side effects of either procedure. The risks for AFP are a possible misinterpretation of test results and your consequent anxiety.

Even when prenatal tests are 100 percent accurate, they cannot determine all possible defects. Women can have accurate prenatal testing and still bear a child who has birth defects. It is impossible to engineer the "perfect" baby.

I love my unborn child for who she or he is—not for who I want that baby to be. Genetic testing would not be right for me.

Genetic testing gave me confidence that all was well, and it told me that my baby was the longed-for "Sarah."

I discovered that this baby would be severely retarded and handicapped. As an ex-nun and ex-Catholic, the decision to abort might have been relatively simple, but it was not. Our doctor reached us with the final results. . . . "We made a mistake on the first tests. Your baby is fine—a healthy boy."

How to Decide

A woman who is willing to have an abortion based on prenatal test results is among those who benefits the most. Although no one woman probably has all of the following characteristics, surveys indicate that the best candidate for prenatal testing is likely to have some college education, believes a small number of children is ideal, has perhaps had an abortion previously, is not much of a church-goer, and does not believe that the

Bible is the literal word of God. She may also believe a child with a severe defect would not have a good life.

Another woman who especially benefits from prenatal testing is the one who already has a child with a severe birth defect. She often feels intensely that she would not have another child with a birth defect, and she faces the consequences of prenatal testing with the assurance of that knowledge. For example, a couple with a child who has Tay-Sachs disease faces in each pregnancy a one-in-four chance of having another child with Tay-Sachs who will be blind, deaf, retarded, and who will die young.

Another woman who especially benefits is one who has ingested and/or been exposed to teratogens, substances that can cause harm to her baby in utero. These are drugs like the anti-acne drug Accutane, and the anti-convulsant drugs Dilantin and valproic acid; chemicals, like Agent Orange (dioxin); and environmental agents, like lead.

---

*I*f I knowingly brought a handicapped child into this less-than-compassionate world, with no guarantee of the permanent presence of loving parents, my conscience would plague me with that, not the more merciful abortion. And if the child knew, would it not be justified in saying, "You did this to me?"

*O*nce parents experience the statistically unlikely event of a major birth defect, it is impossible to go into a subsequent pregnancy with the usual faith that all will be well. For my current pregnancy, we have opted for a full battery of prenatal tests. Without the availability of these tests, I'm not sure I would have had the courage to attempt another pregnancy.

How to Make the Best Use of Prenatal Testing

• *Know yourself.* If you are not willing to have an abortion, then prenatal testing will not change the outcome of your pregnancy. So why do it?

• *Choose the prenatal testing method that's best for you.* Amniocentesis is slightly more accurate than CVS. On the other hand, CVS is performed earlier in the pregnancy, which makes it preferable for many women. AFP is noninvasive, but is reliable only for detecting neural tube defects.

• *Choose an experienced physician to perform the procedure whom you are comfortable with and who will explain everything in a helpful way.* The effectiveness and safety of each procedure varies according to who performs the test and who interprets the results. Research shows again and again that the success of prenatal testing depends most of all on the experience of the person performing the test. It's okay to ask how many procedures your physician has performed. Many doctors who perform these procedures themselves suggest that you comparison-shop.

• *Have your prenatal testing performed where counseling is part of the package.* The typical genetic counselor has more training in and understanding of genetics than the typical doctor does. That person may also be particularly helpful in letting you know what you can expect during the procedure and immediately after. A genetic counselor will interview you regarding your family history and help you understand your risk for all birth defects.

• *Have someone with you*, whether your partner or a friend.

• *Decide what it is that you want to know.* It's a good idea to go in prepared with a knowledge of your family's genetic history and that of your partner's. Although amniocentesis and CVS can determine whether your baby has any of hundreds of disorders, typically your combined genetic history determines which abnormalities, along with Down syndrome (DS), for which you will likely be tested.

If you only want to know about DS, however, say so. If you don't want to know the rest, including your baby's gender, tell them that, too. Prenatal testing can determine chromosomal abnormalities that might never show up as a problem. Information sometimes leads to inappropriate or unnecessary labeling. You can end up worrying about an issue that is not a problem and never will be.

I feel besieged—by an increasingly cavalier attitude toward abortion as a simple technical procedure and by a pervasive disregard for the fact that although my baby is still in utero, I am already as attached and committed and in love as if I were holding it in my arms.

My sister was in a wheelchair all of her life. She couldn't talk or use a bathroom. It ruined my parents' marriage and didn't help the rest of us kids. Would I get an abortion to avoid that? Of course I would—with great relief.

My second child was born with Down syndrome, so amnio was expected when I again became pregnant. I chose to have the procedure so that we would know what to expect and try to prepare for, not to abort, an imperfect baby. . . . Our son did require extra attention and visits to the pediatrician, but his differences greatly enriched the lives and awareness of our family, friends, and neighborhood.

*A*fter weeks of agonizing, should we or shouldn't we have amnio, I had it. And it was great! First we spoke to a genetic counselor. Then we viewed a video of the procedure which included a thorough explanation of Down's. Next we spoke with the doctor, who had performed thousands of these procedures. He enthusiastically told us everything that he would do before he performed the amnio.

I learned with my last pregnancy always to have my husband with me when I went to see the doctor or had any procedure done at the hospital. I was treated with more respect when he was with me, my questions were answered more fully, and he brought new insights into the situations.

Waiting for Test Results

As with other medical tests, you may experience both pretest jitters and the after-it's-all-over fear that the test will reveal something seriously wrong. Some people prefer to gather all the facts that they can. Others want to avoid thinking about it.

Here are suggestions on how to cope with the waiting time:

• *Remember that more than 95 percent of those tested receive good news,* so expect good news and enjoy your pregnancy.

• *Understand how the procedure is performed, and why you had it.* Women who say they received adequate counseling feel more secure during the waiting period.

• *Take brisk walks to reduce anxiety, and find ways to relax.* (See suggestions for relieving stress on page 55.)

• *Share your concerns with a caring person.* Talking through your fears often helps put them into perspective.

AMNIOCENTESIS

Amniocentesis ("amnio" for short) is a procedure in which a physician inserts a thin, four-inch needle through your abdomen into your uterus. About one to two tablespoons of amniotic fluid are withdrawn from the amniotic sac that surrounds the baby. It's believed that the amniotic fluid that's removed is quickly replaced in the womb, but its replacement time is actually unknown. After removal, the fluid is transferred to test tubes and sent to a laboratory for chromosomal analysis. This fluid contains fetal cells, and each cell contains the baby's chromosomal structure. When the cells are cultured in a laboratory, a picture of that structure, known as a *karyotype*, can be obtained at the moment of cell division.

Amniocentesis is performed during both the second and third trimesters. It's used during the second trimester for the determination of fetal flaws. Third-trimester amnio is used to evaluate the maturity of the baby's lungs and is sometimes used before planned cesareans to avoid the birth of a premature baby.

Amniocentesis is performed when there's enough amniotic fluid, ideally between the 14th and 18th week of pregnancy, although with newer experimental techniques amnio may be performed as early as eleven weeks.

The Procedure

Amniocentesis is a common procedure. It is also very accurate, because it has been in use long enough for errors in the procedure to be identified and corrected and for physicians to become familiar with it.

Some physicians, but not all, recommend that immediately before an amnio, you first get down on your hands and knees and bounce up and down to stir up some of the fetal cells in the amniotic fluid for better sampling.

Usually amniocentesis is performed using continuous ultrasound, which allows a constant view of the path of the needle to avoid injuring the fetus or placenta. This reduces mistakes, repeat procedures, and accidental miscarriages.

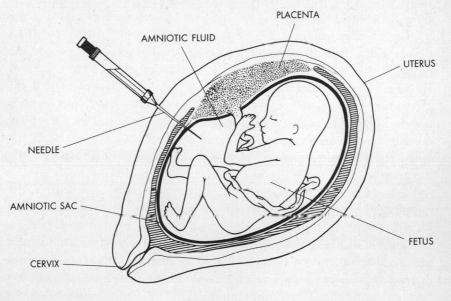

AMNIOCENTESIS

You will lie on your back with your upper body slightly elevated. Your abdomen will be cleansed with an antiseptic solution and covered with sterile drapes. A small amount of local anesthetic may be injected into the skin. The needle is gently inserted and the fluid withdrawn. Pressure is placed over the puncture site for a minute or so to stop any bleeding.

If an anesthetic is injected, you will feel a sharp stinging or burning sensation for a few seconds. During the insertion of the needle you will feel only pressure or a sharp pain lasting a few seconds, similar to having your blood drawn. Ideally, only one needle insertion is needed, but occasionally more are required — particularly with less experienced physicians. Some physicians suggest you stop at two needle insertions and wait for a week or ten days to repeat the procedure.

When the fluid is withdrawn, some women describe a "pulling" sensation or pressure in the lower abdomen. You may be more comfortable if you breathe slowly and let your abdominal muscles remain soft and relaxed.

After the procedure you may experience some mild lower abdominal cramping. About 7 percent of women who have amniocentesis require bed rest afterward. If you notice significant abdominal pain or cramping, chills, fever, dizziness, or a leakage of fluid or blood from the vagina or puncture site, notify your doctor immediately.

How to Decide

The advantages of amniocentesis are that it will give you information about your baby, and it's more reliable than chorionic villi sampling or alpha-fetoprotein testing.

One disadvantage is that some women remain emotionally aloof from the pregnancy until the laboratory results are in, though this may not be the problem it once was when results took about a month. Today, a week to 10 days is more typical, and occasionally only two days is needed for preliminary results on Down syndrome. Anxiety until test results are in is higher for women past age 35 than it is in younger women. Also, if you are considering terminating pregnancy based on the amniocentesis results, the longer the wait, the further you are into your pregnancy and the more costly the abortion will be emotionally, physically, and financially.

Other rare disadvantages are that sometimes there is an error in the sampling, the reading of the sample and the verdict is wrong, or the label on your sample gets switched with someone else's. (If your sample will be evaluated in a lab in the same building where you have your amnio, consider delivering the sample yourself to avoid this rare mix up.) This can work either way: a normal baby gets worrisome results, or a baby with a defect gets perfect results. Also, bear in mind that amniocentesis does not detect all chromosomal defects.

Damage to the baby is uncommon, but possible, during the procedure. About 1 to 3 percent of babies are left with a slight dimpling of the skin where the baby was poked during an amniocentesis procedure. Some babies' legs have been damaged during amniocentesis for prenatal testing, and very rarely, a baby dies during amniocentesis.

In about 0.5 to 1.5 percent of cases, amniocentesis causes the woman to miscarry within three to four weeks. The rate for your physician, however, could be higher or lower, since there is a direct correlation between the rate of miscarriage from amniocentesis and the physician's experience. More experience and the most effective techniques for amniocentesis mean fewer needle insertions. (See "Miscarriage" on page 487.)

Fewer needle insertions mean less likelihood of discolored or meconium-stained amniotic fluid. (Meconium is a dark, greenish mass that accumulates in the bowel during fetal life and is discharged shortly after birth. Meconium in the amniotic fluid, however, is considered a sign of a potential problem.) In addition, fewer needle insertions also lessen the risk of a blood-stained needle (caused by puncturing the placenta, the baby, or you), a perforated placenta, needle puncture scars, and a miscarriage.

The rate of miscarriage after amniocentesis sometimes ranges as high as 17 percent in twin pregnancies. This is related to the difficulty of doing the procedure on two amniotic sacs, and like amniocentesis performed on singleton babies, the level of risk involved is related to the experience of the person performing the procedure. Although it may seem difficult to determine whether a miscarriage is due to amniocentesis or normal chance (about one in three pregnancies miscarry in the first trimester), in fact amniocentesis usually is performed during the second trimester when miscarriages are rare.

A history of previous miscarriage is apparently *not* a reason for miscarriage after amniocentesis, although prior bleeding in this particular pregnancy may increase the chance for a miscarriage after amniocentesis.

Amniocentesis is sometimes used in the last trimester to determine the maturity of fetal lungs in cases where the baby is believed to be in danger, such as when the mother shows signs of toxemia or has diabetes. It's also used to indicate infection, or Rh incompatibility. Amniocentesis at this stage is not to be confused with its use earlier in pregnancy for prenatal testing. Needle puncture scars are a risk, because the baby is bigger and harder to avoid. Also, leaking amniotic fluid is possible, and one in five procedures causes premature rupture of the membranes and premature birth.

Whether you choose to have an amnio depends on many factors that make up your particular story. No one can dictate your beliefs or fears or tell you if amnio is right or wrong for you. Since people tend to be opinionated about amniocentesis, take time to make your decision, and then know you made the best choice for you, whatever you decide.

---

*B*y this time I [43 years old] was becoming so attached to the being within me that I really didn't see how I could end its life even if it did have Down syndrome. I moped around and tentatively tried to bring this up to different people, but the struggle was internal. No one really could see how I felt. . . . The call finally came after 25 days. They said the results of the test were negative and that the baby was a boy. . . . It took me several weeks before I really started to relax, gain weight, and really enjoy my pregnancy. . . . As of today I feel that if I were to get pregnant again I would not get an amniocentesis, but would accept the child I bore without conditions.

*S*ure, I was anxious during my pregnancy. I waited nearly a month to get the amniocentesis results. Even though my belly was getting big, I didn't want to talk about the pregnancy because what if. . . . But if I have another baby, I'll do exactly the same thing. Amnio gave me some reassurance.

I had amniocentesis when I was pregnant. The results came back just fine. Four months later I gave birth to my son, who had a birth defect known as radial aplasia. He has a very short arm and a hand with only three fingers. There are also potentially serious problems with his spine.

*W*hen I miscarried a week after amniocentesis, and we knew it was from the procedure, I knew I would eventually get over it. All I would have to do is remember our neighbor when I was growing up. That woman raised kids all of her life, and one of them was severely retarded. She never had a moment to herself, it seemed to me, and I'm sure she worried on her deathbed about her retarded child. The risk of the miscarriage was worth it for me to avoid that.

I got my amnio results in about ten days with my second child. That wait was much more tolerable than with the first child when I didn't know for almost a month.

CHORIONIC VILLI SAMPLING (CVS)

The chorion is a layer of tissue surrounding the amniotic sac and the fetus. This tissue contains cells with a genetic composition like that of the

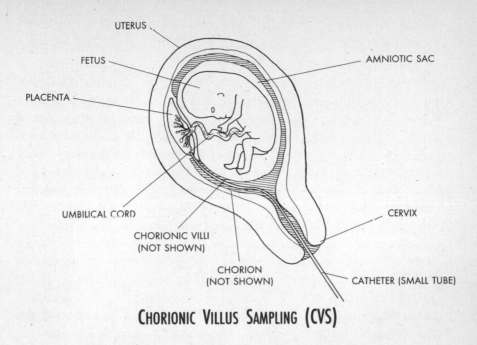

UTERUS

FETUS

PLACENTA

AMNIOTIC SAC

UMBILICAL CORD

CHORIONIC VILLI
(NOT SHOWN)

CHORION
(NOT SHOWN)

CERVIX

CATHETER (SMALL TUBE)

Chorionic Villus Sampling (CVS)

fetus. The villi, a sample of which are snipped and removed for this test, are small hairlike projections in the chorion.

CVS is ideally performed at 10 or 11 weeks of gestation and can detect about 200 genetic disorders. European research suggests that waiting until after 10 weeks is best both to obtain more accurate results and to avoid fetal limb damage.

The Procedure

CVS is performed by either of two methods. Both require guidance via ultrasound. The most common one is to pass a flexible plastic hollow tube through the opening of the cervix to collect a small amount of chorionic tissue. A newer, more experimental method is to insert a needle into the abdomen to remove a small amount of tissue and is more commonly used when CVS is performed past 14 weeks gestation.

There may be cramping and/or fluid leakage for a few days afterward as well as spotting or bleeding. Bed rest is required for one third of the women who have had CVS. Infection, occasionally severe, is also possible.

Fetal defects show up in laboratory analysis of these cells within three days for a preliminary report, which is usually faster than most amnio lab results.

How to Decide

Women who have active herpes or other infections, who are Rh-negative and sensitized to Rh-positive fetal blood (CVS may make the problem worse), who have a placenta located in a low position (this makes the procedure difficult to perform accurately and safely), or who have uterine fibroids are not good candidates for CVS. Some physicians would add women who are pregnant with more than one child to this list as well.

The big advantage of CVS is that the procedure determines some chromosomal defects in the fetus, including Down syndrome, earlier in the pregnancy than will amniocentesis. If a woman chooses to have an abortion because of results that indicate that the fetus has birth defects, it is usually easier on her physically, emotionally, and financially if she has the abortion in the first trimester. On the other hand, if the results are good, the pregnant woman can "get on" with her pregnancy with confidence that much sooner.

The disadvantages of CVS include the possibility of inaccurate test results, miscarriage, maternal infections, a higher rate of fetal limb damage than with amniocentesis, and depleted amniotic fluid, which can cause a miscarriage or a premature birth. Occasionally results may not be conclusive and amniocentesis must be performed as well.

The inaccuracy rate is slightly higher with CVS than it is with amniocentesis. This may have less to do with the procedure than with the experience of the physician performing the test.

The miscarriage rate from the procedure itself is slightly higher (1 to 3 percent) for CVS than it is for amniocentesis (0.5 to 1.5 percent). Whether a woman has a miscarriage that is caused by CVS depends on several factors. The most significant one is the number of catheter insertions. The least risk occurs when there is only one insertion. However, when three to four insertion attempts are made, the miscarriage rate is 11 percent. Multiple insertions occur because it is not always possible to obtain enough of a sample with the first insertion or the physician does not have enough skill to obtain a sample in one insertion. (In one study, only half of the first CVS procedures was performed with one insertion. By the time 500 procedures had been performed, however, 96 percent had only one insertion.) Another cause for a higher CVS miscarriage rate is performing this procedure before 10 weeks.

I went with a friend when she had a 20-week abortion after amniocentesis. On the one hand, she was relieved that she would not give birth to a baby with *severe defects, but on the other hand, the labor was hard. It's not like an early abortion that only takes minutes.*

My doctor wanted me to have chorionic villi sampling, but after he explained the miscarriage rate, I said no. I've waited too long to have this baby to risk it for a minuscule risk for a birth defect.

ALPHA-FETOPROTEIN (AFP)

Alpha-fetoprotein (AFP) is a protein produced by the liver cells of all unborn babies that is found in the amniotic fluid and in the mother's blood.

AFP screening uses a blood sample taken from the mother between the sixteenth and eighteenth week of pregnancy, and results are known in a few days. Blood may be drawn in a doctor's office, clinic, laboratory, or hospital. As prenatal testing procedures go, this one is relatively routine. It's also the most used—an estimated 40 percent of pregnant women use AFP every year.

An elevated level of AFP in the mother's blood can be an indicator of neural tube defects (NTDs) in the fetus. (See "Neural Tube Defects" on page 454.)

AFP can also spot Down syndrome (DS). As a DS indicator, AFP is more accurate if levels of two other proteins, estriol and chorionic gondadotropin, which are also present in fetal cells, are analyzed in blood samples as well. If Down syndrome is suspected, amniocentesis will be offered for confirmation. (See "Down Syndrome" on page 454.)

Sometimes an elevated AFP level is not an indicator of problems. It can mean that the mother is carrying twins or triplets, that the fetus is older than it was thought to be, or that there is an irregularity in the placenta. It's also possible that the mother normally has a high AFP level. Whether an AFP level is too high or too low is an estimate. There is no exact measurement. African-American women normally have AFP levels 10 percent higher than white, Asian or Latina women.

If test results indicate that your AFP levels are two and one-half times to three times higher than the estimated normal level, then the AFP test will be repeated. If the second test also shows an elevated level, then ultrasound and amniocentesis will be suggested for final diagnosis.

About 3 to 5 percent of tested women will have elevated AFP levels the first time. Of this group, about 3 percent will still have elevated levels on a repeat AFP screening. These women will be offered amniocentesis, and 10 percent of that group will have a fetus with a neural tube defect that will range from mild to severe.

How to Decide

The advantage to AFP testing, if the results are accurate, is that you will know if your baby does *not* have a neural tube defect. (You'll need more tests to confirm an NTD.)

The disadvantage of AFP testing is that it is not always accurate. Out of 1,000 AFP tests, 20 to 50 will show elevated AFP levels indicating that the fetus may have a defect. Actually, only one or two babies in that group will have a defect.

AFP testing puts some women on a testing treadmill. First, they find they have elevated AFP levels, so they do another AFP test. If their AFP levels are still high, they will most likely have further tests to confirm or negate the early tests. If subsequent tests reveal that the baby has no known birth defect, they may still have lingering doubts about their child's well-being — who knows which test is right? If you're one of the 48 out of 1,000 women tested for AFP who receive inaccurate test results, a disadvantage for you may be all that unnecessary anxiety and grief. However, in child-birth there are no guarantees. If you are one of the two whose test results were accurate, you at least learned of the problem at a relatively early point in your pregnancy.

WHAT TO DO IF YOU'RE TOLD THAT YOUR BABY HAS A BIRTH DEFECT

Speak to a genetic counselor. If counseling was not part of your testing, find a genetic counselor now. Get a reference from your doctor or midwife, or look in the Yellow Pages under "Physicians and Surgeons — Genetics," or call your local university medical center. A genetic counselor will help you and your mate think through the possible personal, religious, family, and human factors involved. (If you're single, bring a friend.)

This counselor can help you evaluate the accuracy of the particular kind of testing that you used, and discuss whether it would be helpful to get a second opinion. The counselor can often explain the mildness or severity of the defect and give you information that helps in your decision-making.

When you're told that your baby has a birth defect, you're faced with the decision of what to do next. Whatever you decide — whether you keep a pregnancy with a child who has a defect or whether you abort — there is grief and families are affected. Individual reactions will vary and your reaction, whatever it is, is valid. The burden of that decision-making responsibility may cause great strain, especially if you're halfway through the pregnancy, have felt movement, and may be wearing maternity clothes — the universal sign to the world that you're pregnant.

If You Decide to Have the Baby:

• *Get help and support from an organization that represents the birth defect your child has.* A genetic counselor can give you an idea of what the future would hold with that child, and the counselor may be able to arrange for you to meet a family who has a child with that birth defect. Visit a school or educational center for children who have the defect your child has and get acquainted with what to expect. (See "Birth Defects" on page 559 in the Resource Directory.)

• *Tell friends and family.* Let them know what they can do for you. Maintain your contact with people so that they don't fade from your life because they are overwhelmed by your situation.

Those most likely to choose to keep the baby are older mothers and older fathers, parents who have previous children, and people who perceive the birth defect as not severe.

If You Decide to Abort:

• *Get help and support.* Then decide what your timetable is. No matter what you choose — whether to have the abortion within hours of the news or to wait for a few days — it is not likely to be easy. A few women who became pregnant with twins, of whom one is normal and the other has a birth defect, have the option of aborting the fetus with the birth defect. This, too, is a difficult decision.

The woman having an abortion because of the results of prenatal testing is likely to feel she's losing something. She feels attached to the baby and must now give up her dream. This is a very different experience from having an early abortion to take care of an unwanted pregnancy. When asked, the overwhelming majority of women say that women have a right to abort a defective fetus. But that doesn't make it easy when you're the one facing the abortion.

• *Get your abortion at a clinic or hospital that is experienced with second-trimester abortions.* As with prenatal testing, there are fewer errors, less trauma, and better outcomes with doctors who've done many, not just a few, 18- to 20-week abortions (see "Abortion" on page 127).

• *Decide what you're going to tell others*, including your other children, family members, and friends. Some women who abort babies because of birth defects tell people that the baby died, but they don't say how. That protects the woman's privacy and may reduce potential anxiety in children. But it still allows you to grieve and be helped through that process by family and friends. Other women, however, choose to tell the full story.

I received a birth announcement from a couple who had twins. In it, they explained that one of the twins had Down syndrome and the other didn't. They asked their friends not to feel sorry for them, because there hadn't been a tragedy, and invited everyone to come and visit.

Maybe it gives you time to think about it—but at the time, you feel a baby, you become attached to the baby, and every time it moves it reminds you that you're going to put an end to its life and it's very hard to imagine taking more time. It really is. Maybe theoretically it sounds like you should, but in reality it's very difficult. You imagine your baby. This is your baby. Hard to think of it as a fetus—you say fetus, but you imagine a baby. It moves and you become attached to it. Every time it moved those three days, I said, "Please don't move."

The results were the dreaded ones: trisomy 21. I have since then had the grim second-trimester abortion. . . . After our bad result, my husband and I did tell everyone. Sympathy and support from our friends, family, and colleagues have helped us to survive the ordeal of aborting a wanted pregnancy.

ULTRASOUND

Ultrasound, or sonography, is a procedure used to reveal the body's soft tissue by means of sound waves emitted by an electronic device. The procedure gets its name from the sound waves involved, which travel at ultrahigh frequencies (greater than 20,000 cycles per second) beyond the range of human hearing. When an ultrasound device directs sound waves into the body, some of those waves are reflected back and then translated

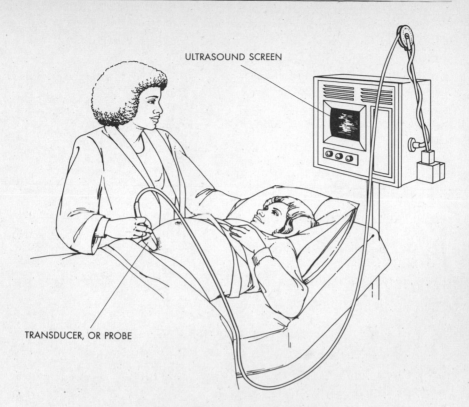

ULTRASOUND SCREEN

TRANSDUCER, OR PROBE

ULTRASOUND SCAN OR SONOGRAM

electronically into patterns on a video display screen and/or on paper, usually in shades of grey.

Ultrasound is most commonly used in the following devices:

1. An *ultrasound scanner* with a video display screen is often used in a physician's office, clinic, hospital, or radiology office.

2. *Doptone* or *Doppler* is a hand-held fetal stethoscope used to detect your baby's heartbeat. Virtually all doctors and some nurse-midwives use it routinely in monthly prenatal visits. Direct entry midwives who attend homebirths either don't use this device at all or use it sparingly.

3. An *electronic fetal monitor (EFM)* has a Doppler ultrasound device contained in a belt that goes around the mother's abdomen. Some hospitals use the new *EFM telemetry unit*, which allows the mother to walk around while carrying a small transmitter in her pocket. (EFM is discussed on page 484.)

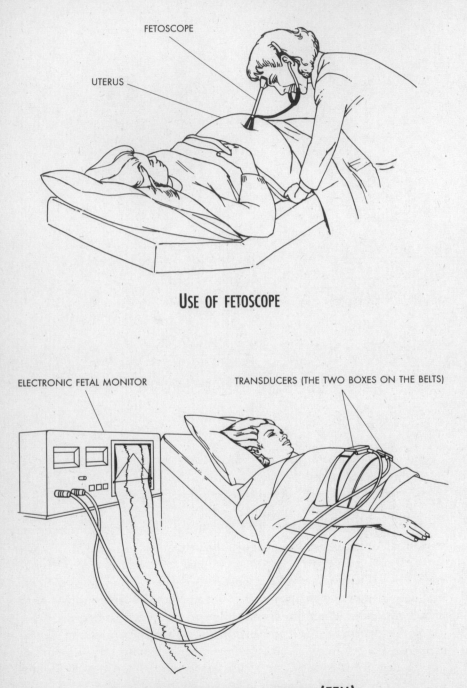

FETOSCOPE

UTERUS

USE OF FETOSCOPE

ELECTRONIC FETAL MONITOR

TRANSDUCERS (THE TWO BOXES ON THE BELTS)

EXTERNAL ELECTRONIC FETAL MONITOR (EFM)

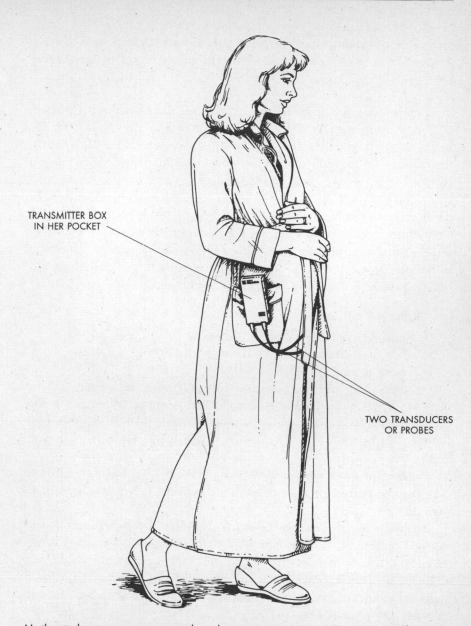

TRANSMITTER BOX
IN HER POCKET

TWO TRANSDUCERS
OR PROBES

Mother-to-be wears two external probes, one to monitor contractions and one to monitor the fetus. The fetal monitor located at the nurses station traces the signals from the box, so the laboring woman can move around.

Telemetry EFM

4. The *vaginosonographic scan* or *endovaginal probe* is a newer version of prenatal ultrasound that can be used as early as the sixth week of pregnancy. A wandlike device called a vaginosonographic transducer is inserted into the vagina.

Before using any of the first three methods, your health care provider will apply a lubricant to your abdomen that acts as a conductor for the sound waves. The transducer — the tip of the device, which has a microphone in it — is moved back and forth over your lubricated skin while you lie motionless on your back. That's because the scan is easier to interpret if you don't move. That is also why you are asked not to move during labor when you wear an external EFM.

Before an ultrasound scan, you'll be asked to drink several glasses of water so that your bladder will be full, which makes it easier for the fetus to be seen on the screen. This aspect of the procedure is uncomfortable, but easily remedied as soon as the scan is complete.

Ultrasound's Uses

Ultrasound can can be used to determine or evaluate:

- *Fetal heartbeat*
- *Position of the fetus during amniocentesis and chorionic villi sampling.*
- *Age of the fetus*, if there is some question about when conception occurred. However, ultrasound is no more accurate than dating from your last menstrual period. (See "Determining Your Baby's Due Date" on page 258.)
- *Twins, triplets, or more*, but even with ultrasound it is not always easy to diagnose the correct number of babies, especially if there are more than two.
- *Larger-than-expected pregnant uterus.* Multiple births can be ruled out, and unusual conditions, such as uterine fibroids, can be diagnosed. (Uterine fibroids are usually harmless uterine growths, but they can cause your uterus to be larger. They are more likely to occur in a mother who is at least 35 years old and occasionally will cause a preterm or longer labor. See "Uterine Fibroids" on page 522.)
- *Unexplained vaginal bleeding*, which is a common occurence during the first three months of pregnancy and does not always lead to miscarriage.
- *Ectopic pregnancy*, which is a pregnancy in one of your fallopian tubes (see "Ectopic Pregnancy" on page 488).
- *Fetal abnormality.* Neural tube defects can sometimes be diagnosed by ultrasound, and Down syndrome can be determined in the second trimester by very experienced ultrasonographers with about 75 percent accuracy.

• *Fetal death*. Ultrasound used for this purpose before eight weeks gestation, however, is associated with inaccurate diagnoses.

• *Faster or slower than normal fetal growth*. This can be helpful for women with chronic diseases, such as diabetes or hypertension. Doctors are on the lookout for the postdate baby or the small-for-gestational-age baby. (See "Postdate Babies" on page 260.) In order to ensure an accurate diagnosis, however, these conditions require many scans, especially for the small-for-gestational-age baby. Moreover, babies grow at different rates in the womb, just as they do after they are born. A baby labeled one month as a slow grower in the uterus may catch up the next.

You are most likely to have several ultrasound scans if you are over 35 and if other ultrasound tests have yielded unusual or inconclusive results. Ultrasound is common for women who have a chronic problem or a multiple pregnancy, who have been labeled high risk, or who may have been exposed to DES in utero (see "Diethylstilbestrol" on page 309). Some physicians like to use ultrasound routinely, although research doesn't show that babies are any better off for it. According to 1992 research, doctors who own their own ultrasound machines prescribe scans four times more often than other doctors. The woman who receives the least ultrasound is a woman who chooses a midwife.

Ultrasound's Safety

Most doctors believe that ultrasound use during pregnancy is safe. But in 1982 the American Medical Association and the U.S. Department of Health and Human Services warned against ultrasound's routine use for pregnant women. Although their message hasn't changed since then, ultrasound use has at least doubled.

No one can claim that ultrasound is 100 percent safe because no comprehensive studies have been done comparing the outcomes of children who received all forms of ultrasound versus the outcomes of children who received no ultrasound at all. Nor have enough years passed to establish long-term side effects. Another reason is that many researchers claim that most of the completed studies are flawed by poor design and execution.

There may be no side effects from ultrasound. But if there are, it's suspected they would be subtle and could easily escape detection. In addition to being subtle, the suspected side effects for your baby (such as cell changes, impaired immune system, and shortened attention span) are considered more likely if there's been lengthy and intense exposure. In fact, recent Australian research showed that babies who were scanned five times during pregnancy, along with regular Doppler use as well, had slower fetal growth than the babies who were scanned only once.

Theoretically, the more time your baby is exposed to ultrasound, the greater the risk. The lowest exposure is found in a pulsed ultrasound scan, even though it uses a higher dose than continuous-wave instruments like the Doptone. This is because the scan's picture of your uterus and your baby is obtained in fewer minutes.

The greatest exposure is found in continuous-wave ultrasound, as in the hand-held Doptone in your doctor's office and the external electronic fetal monitor. They have both been used, however, for about two decades without known visible effects. Possible ultrasound damage is also related to the point in the baby's development when the ultrasound was used (earlier is potentially more damaging than later in the pregnancy), the quality and calibration of the machinery used, the skill of the operator, and your particular baby's and your body's vulnerability.

How to Decide

Many women are thrilled to see their baby in early pregnancy, and many doctors believe that mothers bond earlier with their babies if they see them on the ultrasound screen. Some research shows that women who use ultrasound may be motivated to quit smoking or alter other undesirable behavior after viewing their babies. It also appears to help make the baby seem more "real" to fathers.

Ultrasound is undeniably helpful when it's being used to guide prenatal testing instruments (for example, the needle used during amniocentesis), or to find a wayward IUD. It can also be helpful in determining the condition and overall health of the baby, while many parents are thrilled to know their baby's gender before birth. Another advantage is that ultrasound doesn't have the documented, long-term risks of prenatal x-rays.

Ultrasound's biggest disadvantage isn't that it hurts the baby, but that as a diagnostic procedure it is subject to interpretation with no one claiming 100 percent accuracy. That's why many procedures are repeated. When ultrasound is repeated for clarification of birth defects or other problems, some women worry during the rest of the pregnancy because they don't know which ultrasound is correct. A scan that seems positive is no guarantee of a normal baby, because it does not have the capacity to determine all aspects of fetal health.

Another disadvantage of ultrasound is that it may reduce your contact with your doctor. Some women report that fewer questions are asked of them about how they feel or what they think is happening with the baby when ultrasound is used routinely to evaluate the condition of the fetus.

Some women have mixed emotions about ultrasound. Yes, many women are thrilled to see their baby in early pregnancy, and this thrill is often their initial response. No wonder many doctors believe mothers bond earlier with their babies if they "see" them on the ultrasound screen and know their gender. But according to British research, later there can be ambivalence and sometimes even worry. (Is my baby's head too large or too small? What didn't the ultrasound see?) Of course, a case could be made for the fact that pregnant women will worry with or without ultrasound.

When you're deciding about ultrasound, ask yourself and your health care provider how an ultrasound scan might affect the course of your pregnancy, particularly now that research overwhelmingly shows there is no advantage to routine ultrasound use. If you believe it serves no useful purpose, then are you sure you want it? On the other hand, if you just want to "see" your baby, that's probably reason enough for you.

Embrace whatever decision you make about ultrasound as the best one possible for you. Then find a doctor or midwife who shares your philosophy about ultrasound use, whatever that might be.

I had ultrasound with my first pregnancy and knew the gender of that baby before she was born. With my later pregnancies I decided not to have ultrasound. I wanted the magic and mystery of not knowing.

I had an ultrasound scan to "prevent" an amnio. I really didn't want to do AFP, or CVS, or amnio, or any of that stuff my doctor was pushing for. So I took myself to a different doctor to see how things looked. Happily, they looked fine, so I felt better about turning down the other tests.

How to Get the Most Helpful Ultrasound Scan

Have the procedure performed by someone who can interpret the results and who is authorized to explain them to you on the spot. Get as much immediate feedback as possible. View the ultrasound screen, if possible, and have the details of the scan, including your baby's size, shape, and movements, explained to you and whoever accompanies you. You will feel less anxious about the procedure if the results are made clear immediately. Conversely, you will feel highly anxious if your scan is performed by someone who only tells you "to discuss it with your doctor," with no other details given. A poorly handled ultrasound procedure can put otherwise calm women into a panic.

Get your ultrasound from people who are very experienced in using and interpreting it. Inexperienced sonographers are more likely to make an incorrect diagnosis. For example, they may see what appears to be an abnormality in the first trimester that further scans in the second trimester show does not exist.

Radiologists are required to have special training in ultrasound, obstetricians are not. Some ob/gyns have special training, others do not. Currently, there are no licensing requirements for interpreting ultrasound, and the changing technology of ultrasound machinery makes continuing education essential.

Ask that your ultrasound, including the photograph and the interpretations of the findings, be made a part of your permanent record. Ask for your own copy, too. This avoids unnecessary repetitions of the procedure if you change physicians or if there's a question later on.

ELECTRONIC FETAL MONITORS (EFMs)

Electronic fetal monitors — there are different types — are used to record the fetal heartbeat during labor. Newer models register fetal movement as well.

EFMs are often used during labor as follows:

• The *external EFM* is an ultrasound device attached to a laboring woman via one or two belts around her abdomen. The laboring woman must lie still for best results while it is used.

• The *EFM telemetry* unit also uses ultrasound but allows the mother to walk around while carrying a small transmitter in her pocket.

• The *internal EFM* measures the fetal heart rate with an electrode inserted into the baby's scalp and measures the mother's uterine contractions by means of a catheter placed just inside the uterus.

EFMs are also used in two ways before labor begins:

• During a *nonstress test*, the pregnant woman lies down part way for about 20 minutes while the EFM is strapped on her to detect fetal movement. A nonstress test is used to evaluate the function of the placenta and overall status of the infant.

• During an *oxytocin stress test*, the pregnant woman is given Pitocin (the synthetic form of oxytocin which is used to start or speed up labor) while an EFM is strapped on her abdomen.

Perhaps the most studied of all labor interventions, the EFM has been a disappointment. It was believed since the early 1970s that the EFM would provide information that could prevent death, brain or neurologic damage, and cerebral palsy. Unfortunately, that's not been true. EFMs generate lots of information, but—as with ultrasound—the interpretation is as much an art as a science.

Worldwide research shows that the EFM doesn't improve the outcomes for babies, whether full-term or premature, and that its use increases the incidence of cesareans. Nonetheless, EFMs are here to stay. The American College of Obstetricians and Gynecologists (ACOG) recommends that the EFM be used for all women in labor even though in 1989 they said that the appropriate use of the fetoscope, a hand-held stethoscope that magnifies the sound of the fetal heartbeat, is as reliable in monitoring labor as an EFM.

The medical profession's reluctance to give up the EFM, which is used in about 75 percent of all U.S. labors, is due in part to the nursing shortage. In many hospitals there are too few nurses to monitor women's labors by fetoscope. Both doctors and nurses have become accustomed to the convenience of EFM, too. Neither the nurse, who often has to care for five or six women in labor, nor the doctor needs to spend as much time with a woman if she is attached to an EFM. (EFMs don't get sick or go on vacation either.) This is particularly true if EFM screens are duplicated in the nurses' station so that many labors can be "watched" at one time. Another convenience is that some EFMs are connected to computer systems that include all patient records.

Other reasons for the widespread use of EFMs are a fear of malpractice, lack of training in the use of a fetoscope, and a belief in the superiority of technology. (See "Be Aware of Your Doctor's Malpractice Fears" on page 76 and "Don't be Seduced by Medical Technology" on page 71.)

As for the use of the EFM before labor in "stress" tests, research findings usually show no improved infant outcome. Yet both tests may cause unknown consequences to fetuses, particularly the oxytocin stress test (because of the stimulation of labor while it's still too early for the baby to be born) and misdiagnoses.

EFMs may be here to stay, but you can decide how they're used. That is, unless you use Pitocin or have an epidural for pain relief. Then you'll likely be required to use the EFM for the rest of your labor. If you want to eliminate the EFM from your labor, or limit its use, you can:

• *Choose a doctor or midwife, birth center or hospital, where all are comfortable with a fetoscope.* The best way to get what you want is to find people who *already* are doing it. Proper use of the fetoscope equivalent to the EFM, according to the American College of Obstetricians and Gynecologists (ACOG), is listening to the fetal heart tones every 15 minutes in early labor for high-risk patients and every five minutes in the pushing stage. (EFM read-outs are supposed to be checked that often as well.) The ACOG also points out that checking intervals of 30 minutes in early labor and every 15 minutes in the pushing stage is standard practice for low-risk patients.

But don't count on a cheaper bill if you avoid the EFM. It costs more than $350 per woman, and it is usually not a line item on your bill. Its use is often part of the hospital obstetrics package or general overhead.

• *Do what you can to make your labor as smooth as possible and soften the negative side effects of EFMs by having a labor companion with you who's had a baby herself.* (Her presence will also cut your cesarean risk in half, shorten your labor, and reduce your need for pain medication.) And, no, husbands and hospital nurses are generally not going to be enough help for you. Husbands, particularly with the first child, are frightened and inexperienced, and the nurse won't be able to stay with you because she has other women in labor to care for as well.

• *Know what you can expect.* EFMs are a part of accepted routine in hospitals, where 99.1 percent of U.S. births occur. In most hospitals all laboring women are required to use external EFMs for up to 30 minutes to see if labor appears to be progressing normally, and so that there's a printed record of the birth, which is kept on file for possible future legal action. However, chances are that the nurse who attached you to the machine is not watching the clock, so it's up to you to ask the nurse to disconnect the EFM or have someone else do it for you.

• *Request an EFM that functions when you walk, sit, stand, or squat, if you are required to have an EFM.*

• *Ask questions*, such as: Why do you want me to use the EFM now? What would happen if I didn't use it? If I use it, what are the risks for my baby?

• *Refuse the EFM.* You have the legal right to refuse any procedure in a hospital, including EFMs, by signing a waiver if you don't want to use it or if you want to use it less than the staff prefers. Some women do that, though social pressure often makes that difficult.

PREGNANCY LOSS

The events that are considered pregnancy losses are miscarriage (the most common), ectopic pregnancy, and stillbirth. Others are a birth defect, especially one that is severe, as is the death of a newborn. Also, some birth mothers and surrogate mothers who gave up their babies for adoption, and some women who've had abortions experience pregnancy loss.

MISCARRIAGE

A miscarriage, medically called a *spontaneous abortion*, is the expulsion from the womb of a fetus not yet able to survive on its own. About one third of all pregnancies end in miscarriage, most often before a woman even knows she's pregnant.

Most miscarriages occur in the first three months of pregnancy. Only 1 percent occur after 20 weeks gestation. Women who don't have "morning sickness" during pregnancy are more likely to miscarry for unknown reasons believed to be related in part to hormonal levels. Of course, many women who don't have morning sickness do not miscarry.

Many studies report that women past age 35 miscarry at twice the rate of younger women. However, that rate is not the same for all women in that age group. Research usually does not distinguish between healthy women with their first or second pregnancy and those women who have chronic health or infertility problems and/or a history of repeated pregnancy loss.

Symptoms of a miscarriage are bleeding, which progresses from light to heavy, and usually cramps. The process may take one day or several days. Some women experience pain and others don't.

If you think you're having a miscarriage, contact your doctor or midwife. You'll have a physical exam, perhaps an ultrasound scan as well. An injection of Rhogam is given if you are Rh negative. If the miscarriage is complete and the uterus is clear, then no further treatment is usually required. Occasionally, the uterus is not completely evacuated and a dilation and curettage (D & C) or a simpler office procedure is performed to remove any remaining tissue. (See "Dilation and Curettage" on page 313.)

Causes and Prevention

About half of the miscarriages that occur are caused by genetic abnormalities, which may be hereditary or spontaneous, in the father's sperm or the mother's egg. The other half are caused by a variety of known and unknown factors, including infection (mumps, for instance, in the first trimester increases the risk for miscarriage) and exposure to environmental and workplace hazards: pesticides, Agent Orange (dioxin), tap water near industrial sites, using a video display terminal (VDT) more than 20 hours a week, and regular exposure to nitrous oxide (laughing gas), used most commonly in dentists' offices. (See a discussion of video display terminals on page 460.)

Other factors behind miscarriage are hormonal irregularities, uterine abnormalities, radiation, and drugs, including the acne drug Accutane and others — whether recreational (including alcohol), over-the-counter, or prescription. Severe malnutrition can cause a miscarriage, as can an elevated blood sugar level in women with diabetes. If dietary problems are the culprit, then an improved diet sometimes helps prevent miscarriage. Induced ovulation with fertility drugs sometimes results in miscarriages, as does in vitro fertilization. Two prenatal tests, amniocentesis and chorionic villi sampling, are also associated with miscarriages.

To prevent miscarriage, some women are treated with the hormone progesterone, which is needed for implantation in the uterus. Although this treatment is frequently recommended, according to the Food and Drug Administration, progesterone or progesterone-like drugs have not been proven to be either safe or effective in pregnancy. Further, it's thought that their use may be associated with a risk for congenital abnormalities in both female and male babies.

Despite this, and though some infertility specialists agree that the drug is overused, they consider it to be a valid treatment for women who have a menstrual irregularity called luteal phase inadequacy in which the body doesn't produce enough progesterone. This drug is also routinely used with in vitro fertilization. (See "Infertility" on page 364 and "In Vitro" on page 373.)

Repeated Miscarriages

Most women who have miscarriages have subsequent normal pregnancies and births. But about 1 percent of pregnant women have repeated (three or more) miscarriages, usually without a history of any normal births. Some researchers believe that this is an autoimmune disorder (see "Immune System" on page 9). Early (before age 11) or late (after 16) menarche (the start of menstruation) is associated with multiple miscarriages as are ovaries with many cysts. Women who have repeated miscarriages are four times more likely to have multiple ovarian cysts. (See "Ovarian Cysts" on page 437.) Another link to repeated miscarriages is an "allergy" to the mate's sperm. Many women with repeated miscarriages are successfully treated today with experimental immunological tools, including infusions of gamma globulin. And some women go on to have normal pregnancies and births after they change partners.

ECTOPIC PREGNANCY

An ectopic pregnancy is one located outside the uterus, usually in one of the fallopian tubes. If a tube is damaged in any way, the fertilized egg may never complete its journey to the uterus. Ectopic pregnancies rarely last past eight weeks but will occasionally go to 12 to 16 weeks.

Common symptoms are: lower abdominal pain, often on one side at the beginning, light bleeding, nausea and vomiting, dizziness or weakness, and/or pain in the shoulder or rectum. If the fallopian tube ruptures, the pain and/or internal bleeding can be severe, enough to cause fainting. Ectopic pregnancy is a life-threatening condition.

Although recognized by physicians from at least the tenth century, ectopic pregnancies can be difficult to diagnose, and sometimes evaluation is made with ultrasound or laparoscopy (see "Ultrasound" on page 476 and "Laparoscopy" on page 173). If you suspect that you have an ectopic pregnancy, go *immediately* to your doctor's office or an emergency room, since this problem goes from bad to worse quickly. Treatment varies from drugs to surgery.

The rate of ectopic pregnancy increased more than fourfold between 1970 and 1990, in part because of damage to women's reproductive systems caused by sexually transmitted diseases (STDs), in particular chlamydia and gonorrhea, as well as pelvic inflammatory disease (PID), which is often, but not always, sexually transmitted. (See "Sexually Transmitted Diseases" on page 493 and "Pelvic Inflammatory Disease" on page 441.)

Other causes of ectopic pregnancy include a previous ectopic pregnancy, the use of an intrauterine device (IUD), especially the Progestasert, congenital abnormality of the fallopian tubes, the Pill (minipills, progestogen-only oral contraceptives), prior pelvic or abdominal surgery, and a failed tubal sterilization. Other risk factors associated with ectopic pregnancy are smoking, regular douching, and fertility drugs, in vitro fertilization, and/or GIFT (gamete intrafallopian tube transfer). (See "Birth Control" on page 162 and "Infertility" on page 364.) Maternal age, number of children, and abortion and miscarriage history are not factors, although for unexplained reasons, African-Americans and other minority women are three times more likely to have an ectopic pregnancy than are white women.

The consequences of an ectopic pregnancy depend on many factors and range from no damage to your reproductive organs to the complete removal of a ruptured fallopian tube. Overall, women who have had one ectopic pregnancy have a greater chance of a subsequent ectopic pregnancy, and a 20 to 40 percent chance of infertility. Although less than 2 percent of pregnant women have an ectopic pregnancy, it is the leading cause of death for pregnant women in the first three months.

STILLBIRTH

A stillbirth is the birth of a fully formed baby who is dead. The death of the baby in the uterus may have occurred weeks or hours before labor or during labor.

For many stillbirths, the cause is never clear, and a stillbirth is not likely to occur in a subsequent birth. When a cause can be identified, it is often traced to defects in the baby, especially chromosomal, lack of oxygen, or the position of the umbilical cord. Smoking, cocaine use, and high blood pressure may all be risk factors.

A few women who have given birth to stillborn infants suspect that interventions used during their births contributed to the death of their newborn. Although it's become common to blame doctors when there's a problem with pregnancy or birth, there is no research that supports the theory that birth interventions cause stillbirths.

Women are less likely to have a stillbirth if they eat well, get early prenatal care, and avoid cocaine and all recreational drugs during pregnancy. (See "The Pregnancy Diet" on page 34.)

Some physicians have suggested that pregnant women count fetal movements several times a day during the last weeks of pregnancy to prevent stillbirths. It's believed that if the baby moves less often than is perceived as normal (one estimate is 10 movements within two hours) that intervention — often with induced labor or a cesarean — will prevent a possible stillbirth. However, research findings are mixed, and it isn't certain that counting fetal movements and intervening reduces the number of stillbirths.

---

*T*welve days before the due date, the umbilical cord tore. Our daughter was born soon after — dead. I cannot describe the disappointment and heartache. These terrible losses happen more often than we know. One out of every 100 babies is stillborn, often to women like me, in apparent good health, who do not drink, smoke, or take drugs.

*M*y twin girls were born 30 years ago, and I still remember it all clearly. One was alive and healthy, the other stillborn. They told me the dead baby was a girl, but they wouldn't let me see it. My doctor said it was for the best. Later when I was crying to see that baby, the nurses said I should be ashamed of myself because I had a healthy baby to take home.

PREGNANCY LOSS AND BODY GRIEF

Years ago a woman was not supposed to grieve after a pregnancy loss.

If you have a pregnancy loss, you are entitled to whatever feelings you have, whether they are mild or intense, mixed or very clear. Some women feel as if they're in shock, or depressed and guilty. They may feel that way for many weeks or months. If you are told that you're "overreacting" or "exaggerating your feelings," know that this is not true. On the other hand, some women feel sad for a few days at the most and that's all. You don't have to believe those who say you are "repressing" or "denying your feelings." Your feelings will vary depending on many factors, including whether this was a planned pregnancy.

Another factor in pregnancy grief is how far advanced the pregnancy was. Were you six weeks pregnant, or did you go through labor and give birth to a perfectly formed baby who was dead? Often, but not always, the intensity of feeling increases the more real the baby seems.

Be aware that your body "grieves," too. It suddenly has to adjust hormonal levels and make other bodily changes. The further along you are, the more adjustments your body has to make. This "body grief" affects a woman who gives up a baby for adoption or has an abortion, too. (Breasts leak and other body changes occur.)

If you have a miscarriage, ectopic pregnancy, stillbirth or newborn death, ask your health care provider to explain to you as much as possible what happened. Ask what may have caused the loss and also clarify what *didn't* cause it (that glass of wine you had six months ago or the chocolate bars you ate last week). Ask what the chances are of it happening again. The more you know of the details, the more likely it is that you will resolve your grief and move on.

It's normal to want to talk about a pregnancy, whether it ended happily or unhappily. Talking about it helps put it into perspective. If you want to talk to other women who also have had a pregnancy loss, contact one of the "Miscarriage" organizations on page 565 in the Resource Directory. These organizations can also give you information on what other parents do when babies die, including holding the baby, taking pictures, and funeral arrangements.

My miscarriage was frightening and devastating. I had been treated for infertility. I was 37 years old and didn't know how many more chances I had.

I was so relieved when I miscarried. I was 43 and dreaded the thought of having another baby. My children were all in high school and I didn't want to start over now.

I had an early miscarriage several years ago, but it was not a big deal. But this time, it was different. I had felt the baby move, I was in maternity clothes, and

I went through labor. I gave birth to a dead baby, but my body didn't seem to know that. It produced milk and reminded me daily for weeks that I had had a baby.

I have dealt with Michael's [the baby's] surrender in a number of vastly different ways. For 10 years I blotted out everything, then remembered, and acknowledged. I'm not sure that I regret the basic concept of adoption; it is, rather, that I regret that there is so little place for me within it.

After the autopsy of my baby was performed, my doctor wouldn't talk to me about it. All he would say is how sorry he was. Why wouldn't they tell me? Was it something that I did? My husband wants another baby, but I don't. I'm afraid.

At our first meeting it was as if someone had physically removed a great heavy burden that was bearing down on my shoulders. We all shared our feelings about our losses. . . . From this kind of sharing comes a sense of hope, fragile and sometimes elusive, but hope nonetheless.

Sexually Transmitted Diseases (STDs)

What They Are

Sexually transmitted diseases, formerly known as venereal diseases or VD, are those contagious infections that enter your body through close personal contact, including vaginal or anal intercourse, oral sex, or occasionally kissing. There are dozens of STDs. The five most common STDs in women are chlamydia, herpes, gonorrhea, syphilis, and genital warts. Acquired immune deficiency syndrome (AIDS) is an STD, but until the early 1990s, it was transmitted to women mostly through other means. (See "Acquired Immune Deficiency Syndrome" on page 138.)

It's possible to contract any STD with one contact. If you are told that you've been exposed to an STD or if you have sores or blisters on your genitals or mouth, go to a clinic or a doctor's office as soon as possible. It's best to be evaluated and treated early. Don't wait for symptoms to appear or to worsen. If you have been raped, go to an emergency room, ideally one designated as a rape crisis center, so evidence can be handled appropriately, and you can be tested for STDs.

If you have an STD, your doctor or clinic will ask you to tell your sexual partner(s). It's important that both you and your partner be treated, so that you don't become reinfected and/or pass the STD to someone else. In addition, some states require you to report your partner's name.

Some STDs can be completely cured, but others never leave the body once they are contracted. This is one reason why preventive measures are so important.

WHO GETS STDS

The incidence of STDs has risen more in the past 25 years than in all the years before then. Part of the increase is due to a greater number of STD viruses, as well as a greater number of young people, the most susceptible age group for STDs. The known rate continues to climb, and no one knows how many cases have not been diagnosed.

Once associated only with prostitutes and sailors, STDs are second only to the common cold in number of infections, and many women have more than one STD at a time, including formerly rare versions. An estimated 20 to 30 million people in the United States now have herpes and millions more have the other STDs.

Today the U.S. woman most likely to have an STD is sexually active and does not use a condom each and every time she has sex. If she has only one partner, that person has multiple sexual partners, is bisexual, or uses IV drugs. Or she may have multiple partners and uses the Pill without any barrier contraceptive.

She is a teenager, or she became sexually active as a teenager (when her cervical cells were especially susceptible to STDs, especially chlamydia). Or she may live in a big city and/or is inner-city African-American or Latina, although white women are more likely to have chlamydia. Lesbians don't usually have STDs, but when they do, it's likely to be herpes. If a lesbian has gonorrhea or syphilis, it's associated with prior heterosexual activity.

SIGNS AND SYMPTOMS

• *Chlamydia.* A woman may have a yellowish vaginal discharge, spotting between periods or after sex, and occasionally abdominal pain. These symptoms may appear within weeks after contact or they may not show up until months have passed.

• *Herpes* (herpes simplex type 2). A woman may have blisters, which turn into small ulcers and then crust over, in or around her vagina or, as a result of oral sex, on her mouth, gums, or throat. (Sores on the mouth, or "cold sores," can also be caused by a herpes virus, herpes simplex type 1, which is often transmitted by kissing.) These symptoms will appear two to 20 days after contact. Other symptoms may include a slight fever, headaches, unusual vaginal discharge, and general discomfort. Without treatment, symptoms disappear in a week or two, but may flare up later.

Once it is contracted, the herpes virus never leaves the body, though only about 50 percent of those with herpes have a recurrence of symptoms. Women are more likely than men to have flare-ups, which are often associated with stress or menstruation. Another flare-up trigger, though probably rare, is epidural anesthesia when used for cesarean childbirth. Herpes flare-ups are usually preceded by warning signs, such as tingling or burning in the genitals. People who have herpes are contagious for several days *before* flare-ups become symptomatic and whenever there are visible herpes lesions. In addition, some people are contagious at other unpredictable times.

• *Gonorrhea*, also known as the "clap" or GC. A woman may have a burning sensation during urination, thick yellow or greenish-yellow vaginal discharge, and fever or stomach pain. Symptoms appear two to eight days after contact.

• *Syphilis.* A woman may have a hard, painless lesion or chancre on her mouth, vagina, or anus, which will appear between 10 and 90 days after contact. Without treatment, the sore will slowly disappear, but a low fever, sore throat, and sores or rashes can appear several weeks later. These symptoms may come and go until treatment is obtained.

• *Genital warts.* A woman will have itchy small growths, or bumps, that look like tiny cauliflowers, on the vulva or cervix between 20 and 90 days after contact.

Some STDs can cause pelvic inflammatory disease (PID), which in turn can cause infertility and ectopic (tubal) pregnancy. STDs are responsible for one half to one third of the increase in infertility. Untreated gonorrhea or syphilis brings increased risks for arthritis and infected eyes, and untreated syphilis leads to central nervous system degeneration, hearing loss, and brain damage. Herpes and genital warts are associated with an increased risk for cervical cancer. The virus that has been implicated as a cause of cervical cancer is a cousin to the viruses that cause genital warts and herpes.

Often an STD, especially syphilis, which is rapidly increasing among U.S. women and occasionally resists antibiotics, is the first symptom of AIDS in women. STDs weaken a woman's resistance to other diseases, including AIDS, and sores or open lesions caused by STDs allow the AIDS virus to enter her body more easily. That's because blood is the best transmitter of the AIDS virus, not semen.

In young women in particular, untreated chlamydia can lead to pneumonia as well as endometritis, an infection of the uterus (not to be confused with endometriosis — see "Endometriosis" on page 329).

MAKING THE DIAGNOSIS

Each STD is diagnosed with a different test. The tests for gonorrhea and herpes use a sample of material from the sore (if there is one) that is then examined under a microscope. If there are no lesions, other tests are used. A blood test is most often used for syphilis, and an immunofluorescent antibody test is used for chlamydia along with a newer, more reliable culture test. A Pap smear is used for genital warts, and occasionally a blood test and newer DNA probes are used as well. (See "Pap Smear" on page 105.)

None of the tests is 100 percent accurate, so you may want to get at least two to verify a diagnosis. And if you continue to have problematic symptoms, seek other testing. A herpes diagnosis, for instance, is often missed if you do not have any telltale herpes lesions. Syphilis is difficult to diagnose when you are pregnant, or if you have lupus or arthritis. Tests for gonorrhea can be false-negative, as well as false-positive. Sometimes a Pap smear is used for chlamydia, but it's not reliable for that, though it is for genital warts. (See "Sexually Transmitted Diseases" on page 595 in the Resource Directory.)

PREVENTIVE MEASURES YOU CAN TAKE

There are no vaccines for the five most common STDs, nor will taking antibiotics in advance "just in case" help you. (No one drug is effective against every STD.) You can prevent or reduce your risk for STDs in the following ways:

- *Be monogamous with a monogamous partner.*
- *Be celibate* (which, of course, is not a permanent option for everyone).
- *Choose your sex partner(s) carefully.*
- *Reduce the number of people with whom you are sexually intimate.* Your risk for STDs increases with the number of your partners, not just the number of times you have sex. It's the exposure to the organisms that causes STDs. Your risk increases with each additional sex partner you have and each sex partner he or she has had. (In 1992, typical female college students had more than five sexual partners — male college students had eleven — before graduating with an undergraduate degree.)
- *Get to know your partner(s) well, and discuss STDs.* Remember that not

everyone is informed or honest, especially about sex. STDs affect women far more than they do men, so you may have more reason to be careful than many men.

• *Note (and stop what you're doing) if your partner complains of genital pain or has a sore, rash, discharge, unusual odor, or redness in the genital areas.*

• *Use a male condom that has spermicide or the Reality female condom,* even if you're already on the Pill, have an IUD, or are sterilized. None of these protect you against an STD, and the IUD increases your risk for pelvic inflammatory disease. Other barrier contraceptives, such as diaphragms and sponges, offer some protection against STDs, although they do not offer protection from AIDS. Be aware that male condoms may not offer 100 percent protection against genital warts when there are lesions outside of the area covered by the condom. Female condoms offer more protection for this because they fit over the outer lips or labia. (See "How to Use a Male Condom with Pleasure" on page 194, "How to Use a Female Condom" on page 198, "Diaphragm" on page 200, and "TODAY Sponge" on page 203.)

• *Get annual STD tests if you do not use condoms and have multiple sex partners.*

• *Boost your immune system to avoid all STDs.* (See "How to Stay Healthy" on page 25.)

• *Be aware that if your resistance is low because you already have another illness, like a cold or the flu, you will more easily become infected with an STD.* Recreational drugs, including alcohol, reduce your resistance to disease, too.

• *Exercise regularly to reduce depression,* which may be a trigger for flare-ups of herpes and genital warts. (See "Exercise" on page 41.)

• *Use relaxation techniques to reduce negative stress that might trigger recurrences of herpes.* (See suggestions for relieving stress on page 55.)

• *Get lots of the B vitamin folic acid in your diet to avoid genital warts.* Studies show you'll reduce your risk for genital warts by having an adequate intake of folic acid. (See "The Anti–Breast Cancer, Healthy Heart Diet" on page 28 for suggestions on how to include this vitamin in your diet.)

• *Make dietary changes to reduce outbreaks of herpes.* These changes include eating foods high in the amino acid lysine (eggs, brewer's yeast, fish, potatoes), while avoiding foods high in the amino acid arginine (peanuts, nuts, chocolate, seeds, beans, peas, untoasted grains). (See Fuchs on page 604 in Recommended Reading for more information about dietary measures for herpes.)

I don't pick up guys anymore because I don't want to get a disease. Some of my girlfriends have gotten herpes, and two have chlamydia. I am unwilling to *carry condoms in my purse, and the thought of checking some guy over to look for sores is gross. Now I'm looking for a regular boyfriend.*

A *boyfriend gave me herpes. I was furious. When I called him and told him, he said he was sorry. He told me that he hadn't mentioned that he had herpes, because he didn't think that he was contagious.*

A *fter I was diagnosed with warts, my boyfriend told me that neither of the doctors who treated him for his warts told him that he should wear a condom or warn his sex partners to have an exam.*

TREATMENT OPTIONS

Treatment for STDs depends on the particular disease and whether you're pregnant. Gonorrhea, chlamydia and syphilis, especially if caught early, are easy to treat. Herpes, however, requires more treatment over a longer period of time because its viruses stay in your body.

In general, treatments are antibiotics for gonorrhea, chlamydia, and syphilis. There has been a fivefold increase in penicillin-resistant STDs in the 1980s, resulting in the use of newer and more expensive antibiotics.

Genital warts are treated with laser therapy (see "Surgery" on page 596 in the Resource Directory), Podophyllin, trichloracetic acid, and cryosurgery (the application of frozen carbon dioxide). Newer treatments are interferon, an expensive immune system—stimulating drug, and the drug fluorouracil.

Herpes flare-ups are often checked by the daily use of acyclovir, though this drug is not recommended for pregnant women.

Acupuncture may relieve the pain of all STDs and reduce the reoccurrence of herpes. (See "Acupuncture" on page 82.)

HOME REMEDIES YOU CAN TRY

There are no home remedies to cure STDs, so go to your health care provider if you suspect a problem. For herpes flare-ups, spread a mixture of vitamin E ointment and powdered vitamin C on the lesions. This may relieve pain and redness in 24 hours and reduce the total number of days that you have lesions. These two vitamins can also be taken orally.

STDs AND BABIES

As STDs have increased, so have the consequences to babies. A pregnant woman with any STD can pass it on to her infant either during pregnancy (AIDS, syphilis, herpes) or during the birth process (AIDS, herpes, gonorrhea, chlamydia, genital warts). That's true whether she's had any STD symptoms or not.

However, all STDs are not equally infectious for infants. There's a greater chance that chlamydial and gonorrheal infections will be passed on to the baby than herpes or genital warts. Some babies will get an STD while in the hospital, but not from their mothers. Chlamydia has been reported in newborns who picked up the infection while in the hospital nursery, probably from a nurse who failed to wash her hands between babies. (See "The Hospital Stay" on page 92 for more on handwashing.)

Babies who are diagnosed with an STD are treated with drugs. Eyedrops for newborns are mandated by many states and are to be administered within the first 24 hours after birth as a first-line defense against sexually transmitted infections, regardless of whether the mother has an STD. Some STD-free mothers avoid this controversial practice by signing a waiver.

The effects of STDs on newborns are reduced when treatment is successful. However, possible consequences of gonorrhea include eye infections and sometimes blindness, heart defect, and bone deformity. Syphilis may cause stillbirth, problems with vocal cords, sometimes requiring several operations, and breathing difficulty. Chlamydia may cause premature birth and low birth weight; eye infections, starting in the second week of life, along with pneumonia within two or three months; impaired breathing for as long as eight years and a susceptibility to asthma; and middle-ear abnormalities. Herpes may cause birth defects, miscarriage, premature birth, and eye infections.

A NOTE ABOUT HERPES AND CESAREAN BIRTH

Herpes can affect the baby as it comes through the birth canal. That's why many women with a history of herpes have had cesareans during the 1980s. Now that more research has been done, it's been discovered that some babies have the herpes infection in spite of being born by cesarean, and many babies born to mothers with active lesions do not get the infection. In fact, about 70 percent of the babies who are born with a herpes infection have mothers who have no history of genital lesions.

Although many pregnant women with a herpes history are tested during the weeks before birth, research has shown that these cultures are not reliable predictors of the infant's exposure to and risk for herpes. (It's just as important to test the father of the baby for herpes.) If the mother has a flare-up—not a primary (first-time) case—of herpes during labor, the baby's risk for herpes is only 5 percent.

There's still much confusion about the best way to manage a birth with a mother who has a history of herpes. The same is true of a mother who has genital warts, though cesareans are usually not recommended for that reason unless the warts are very severe. If you're told that you must have a cesarean because of an STD and you're not convinced, get a second opinion. (See "Get a Second Opinion" on page 95 and/or contact one of the "Cesarean Birth" organizations in the Resource Directory on page 562 for a physician referral.)

A NOTE ABOUT AIDS BABIES

About 2,000 U.S. women with the HIV virus give birth every year, though that number is increasing steadily. Many of these women discover that they have the HIV virus after their child has been diagnosed with AIDS. Of those women who do show AIDS symptoms during pregnancy, some have viral diseases, sometimes severely, because their immune system has been compromised by the disease. This means their children can be doubly affected. It's believed that babies are infected either during the pregnancy by transmission through the placenta or at the time of birth. Because the HIV virus has been found a few times in breast milk, it is also suspected (though unproven) as a transmitter of the HIV virus. Babies may also contract the virus through a transfusion, but that's unlikely in the United States, as fewer than 1 percent of U.S. children receive transfusions.

Each baby of a woman who tests HIV-positive has an estimated overall 20 to 30 percent chance of being infected. (For unknown reasons the transmission rate is lower in Europe than in the United States and varies from region to region in this country.) Research shows that uninfected babies have antibodies that prevent transmission of the virus. And for some reason, about half of those who do test HIV-positive at birth are free of AIDS antibodies and any sign of the illness by the age of nine months.

Babies with full-blown AIDS usually sicken and die sooner than do adults with the disease. Many AIDS-infected children die by age two or three; some die as early as six months; some as late as twelve years. These babies suffer many illnesses, including fevers, weight loss, and recurrent diarrhea. If their mothers were in poor health at the beginning of the pregnancy and/or were IV-drug users, these babies are likely to be born prematurely with low birth weight. In addition, they have severe forms of childhood illnesses, like chicken pox, strep, and ear infections. They also often have neurologic abnormalities and developmental delays in sitting up, crawling, or walking.

Like adults, babies who have AIDS are often treated with the drugs AZT or DDI. (See "Treatment Options" for AIDS on page 142.) What's considered best care for these children varies from hospital to hospital, city to city. Many AIDS babies are abandoned by their parents. Caregivers of these children are often foster mothers, who find that other adults are usually afraid of getting AIDS from these children, though there have been no reported cases of transmission of the AIDS virus from a baby to another person in the household.

I chose to keep my pregnancy even though I have AIDS, because I believe abortion is murder. But I didn't understand really how much pain my baby would be in. I feel terrible that my baby is sicker than I am.

I just didn't know what to do. If I kept the baby, my life would have probably ended. If I had the baby, there was the possibility that the baby wouldn't last very long.

Temporomandibular Joint (TMJ) Syndrome

What It Is

The TMJ syndrome occurs when the temporomandibular joints, which connect the upper and lower jaw, are not in their proper position, causing the head to be thrown off balance and the muscles in the head, neck, and shoulders to be strained.

Signs and Symptoms

Symptoms of TMJ syndrome are limited jaw movement (for example, difficulty biting and chewing) and facial pain, including in front of the ears. This pain may occur on just one side of the face, and it may last for days and then go away and reappear months later. Occasionally, there is jaw locking. (Ordinarily, your jaw can be opened to the width of your first three fingers.)

There can also be clicking and popping in the jaw joint when opening or closing your mouth, particularly when it's painful to do so; headaches;

toothaches not caused by decay or infection; and tooth clenching or grinding during sleep of which you may be unaware. Other symptoms are earaches with perhaps ringing in the ear; burning sensation or tingling of the tongue or in the mouth or throat; sensitive teeth; aches in the neck, shoulder, or back; and facial tenderness and/or swelling.

CAUSES

- *Ill-fitting crowns, fillings, or dentures*
- *Malocclusion, or a "bad bite,"* often caused by crooked, missing, or worn teeth
- *Blow to the head or to the TM joint*
- *Muscle tension and stress*, particularly if they cause you to clench or grind your teeth (most people who do this don't have TMJ)
- *Arthritis*
- *Bad posture*, when combined with some of the other causes

MAKING THE DIAGNOSIS

Millions of Americans, most of them women between the ages of 15 and 44, have TMJ syndrome, although many are affected only mildly. If TMJ symptoms are mild, they may disappear without treatment.

In addition to a thorough history, the following may also be suggested to diagnose TMJ syndrome: dental x-rays, arthography (an x-ray of the TM joint after injection of a dye), or newer technologies like computed tomography and magnetic resonance imaging.

Diagnosis is difficult, because the symptoms can point to other problems, not only TMJ syndrome. It's also hard to find practitioners who know much about it. Dentists are the most likely to be helpful. If you have a severe problem, you may also need the help of a physical therapist or surgeon, among others. You may be told that your symptoms are all in your head, as are many women with other difficult-to-diagnose conditions, or perhaps you'll be given treatment that doesn't work.

PREVENTIVE MEASURES YOU CAN TAKE

- *Avoid excessive amounts of chewing gum and chewy foods*, biting your fingernails, or clenching your teeth, all of which put stress on the jaw joints. When you become aware of tension in your jaws, just let go of the tightness. After a while, the releasing of tension may become as habitual as the tension once was.

• *Release tension in general* through exercise, meditation and other relaxation techniques. (See "Exercise" on page 41 and "Meditation" on page 59.)

• *Be aware of correct posture.* Stand with your weight slightly on the balls of your feet, not back on your heels. Avoid lying on your back with your head propped up, or positioning a phone between your shoulder and chin.

• *Have your jaw checked if you receive head or neck injuries.*

• *Get a new filling or crown checked if it doesn't feel right after a day or two.*

TREATMENT OPTIONS

The first treatment approaches are likely to be relaxation exercises, including biofeedback (see "Biofeedback" on page 85); applying heat or cold, whichever feels better; and dental appliances, including jaw splinting, bite plates, and nightguards.

Other options are painkillers, from aspirin to tranquilizers. If these measures don't help, surgery may be indicated, including arthroscopy, a procedure in which a thin telescopic tube is inserted through an incision in the jaw and debris is then washed out and the jaw disk repositioned, if necessary. Surgery may not work, should be used with extreme caution, can be involved, expensive, and may require having the jaws wired shut during recovery. (It's reported that this operation may leave a mark about the size of a freckle in front of your ear.)

A shortcut to helpful treatment is to call your local dental school and ask for the name of someone who specializes in and has much experience with TMJ. You could also contact a TMJ support group (see "Temporomandibular Joint Pain" on page 596 in the Resource Directory and on page 620 in Recommended Reading) for information and referrals in your city.

Many of the two dozen treatments for TMJ are experimental, so you may want to get several opinions before deciding on surgery or high-dosage drug therapy.

M y gynecologist sent me to an allergist for the headaches and the pain. The allergist said I wasn't allergic and sent me to a psychiatrist. She said I should take tranquilizers. It was my dentist who diagnosed TMJ and helped me get relief.

TRICHOMONIASIS: *see* Vaginal Infections

Toxic Shock Syndrome (TSS)

What It Is

TSS is a flulike disease that is caused by a poison produced by a common strain of bacteria that spreads to the bloodstream.

Signs and Symptoms

The symptoms of TSS appear quickly and are often severe. All cases are not alike, but among the symptoms are: sudden high fever (usually 101 degrees or more), vomiting, fainting or near fainting, dizziness, diarrhea, flulike symptoms, sunburnlike skin rash, and a drop in blood pressure.

The skin of the palms and soles of the feet may start to peel one to two weeks after onset of TSS. Sometimes this peeling will occur after a mild episode of TSS and will serve as a warning, since a mild episode may be followed by a more severe case. Other symptoms may be aching muscles, bloodshot eyes, or a sore throat. Severe symptoms include shock, kidney failure, and liver failure.

CAUSES

A high-absorbency tampon used by a menstruating woman with heavy bleeding is a factor in nearly all cases of TSS. Tampons, especially when kept in place for many hours, mixed with warm menstrual fluid, offer an ideal environment for the the bacteria, *Staphylococcus aureus*, which is always present with TSS, to grow. No one knows the exact cause of TSS, which is an ancient disease, nor is there just one contributing factor. TSS, for instance, has appeared in geographic clusters separate from known risk factors.

The known risk factors for contracting TSS are: the use of high-absorbency tampons and, occasionally, the use of the TODAY birth control sponge or, rarely, the diaphragm. TSS also occurs, uncommonly, in postoperative patients, including women who have had cesareans.

Tampons are now used by 70 percent of U.S. menstruating women. A 1985 survey showed that the TSS scare of the early 1980s — associated with the Rely superabsorbent brand of tampon subsequently taken off the market — caused many women to either switch to pads or to change tampons more frequently and avoid them at night altogether.

Of those known women who have contracted TSS after using the TODAY sponge, most had just had a baby, had left the sponge in for days, or had difficulty removing it. There have also been 18 cases of TSS reported with diaphragm use. (It is theoretically possible that a woman could contract TSS using a cervical cap, too, but no cases have been reported.)

The danger of contracting TSS while using these barrier contraceptives is not great and, therefore, not a good reason to avoid using them, unless you've had TSS in the past. The issue is to use the barrier wisely, just as you use a tampon wisely, to avoid TSS.

MAKING THE DIAGNOSIS

TSS is a rare illness and its occurrence has declined sharply since 1980, probably due to the improvement of tampon ingredients and better education about the correct use of tampons.

TSS can be confused with other illnesses and therefore misdiagnosed, and physicians are not required to report it to public health agencies. TSS occurs mostly in women younger than 30, though it's been reported in men and children, too. In women, seven of 10 TSS cases are menstrual, and nine in 10 cases of menstrual TSS are due to a tampon.

PREVENTIVE MEASURES YOU CAN TAKE

• *Use sanitary pads instead of tampons*, especially if you already have had TSS, as you have a 30 percent chance of having it again. (You may also want to avoid tampons if you have frequent urinary tract infections. Use of tampons may spread bacteria from the vagina to the urethral opening, and moreover, the inserted tampon may put pressure on the urethra, making it difficult to empty one's bladder completely. (See "Urinary Tract Infections" on page 515.) Tampon fibers are also made with chemicals and dyes which may irritate delicate vaginal walls.

• *If you use tampons, use less absorbent tampons*—"regular" instead of "super"—as that will reduce your risk for TSS. (The meaning of the terms "regular," "super," and "super plus" became uniform for all tampon brands in early 1990.) Change tampons at least every four to six hours or so, or alternate with sanitary pads. Use tampons that have an applicator included to avoid carrying extra germs into your vagina with your fingers. Insert tampons carefully to avoid scratching vaginal walls (some women can't use tampons when their flow is scant, because the vaginal walls are too dry), and avoid using tampons that you've dropped before inserting, especially if you're in a public bathroom. Avoid tampons if you have a chronic vaginal infection, and remove a tampon immediately if you develop TSS symptoms. Don't wait. Call your physician or clinic immediately.

• *Do not leave the TODAY sponge or diaphragm in for more than 24 hours* to avoid the possibility of triggering TSS. Do not use them at all during menstruation. Also, do not use these devices for a few months after having a baby, if you have an abnormal vaginal discharge, or if you have ever had TSS. Remove these devices immediately if you develop TSS symptoms. Don't wait. Call your physician or clinic immediately. (See "TODAY Sponge" on page 203 and "Diaphragm" on page 200.)

TREATMENT OPTIONS

Go to a hospital immediately. Usual treatment includes large amounts of intravenous fluids to replace lost body fluid, drugs to raise blood pressure and lower temperature, and antibiotics to reduce the risk of recurrence. A newer option is intravenous immunoglobulin, which helps neutralize the toxins responsible for TSS. Recovery occurs within two to three weeks and death is rare if TSS is treated immediately. Most women get well without any side effects, though in some of the cases reported in the early 1980s, nerve damage occurred.

Urinary Incontinence

What It Is

Urinary incontinence is the involuntary leaking of urine, and it ranges from mild to severe. The most common form is stress incontinence, which, because of structural differences, almost always affects only women.

Signs and Symptoms

The symptom of stress incontinence is leaking urine with the "stress" of coughing, sneezing, laughing, jumping, running, jogging, or lifting.

Nearly all women have had an episode or two of stress incontinence, but it is not an ongoing problem for most women. For those who do have it on a regular basis, however, the condition does grow worse with age, if not at least treated with preventive measures (see below), and that's especially true for women who are past menopause. (Incontinence is the major reason for admission to nursing homes.) Sometimes stress incontinence, when severe, includes fecal incontinence, too.

Although most women don't seek help, virtually all forms of incontinence are treatable with a 90 percent success rate. Treatment options depend on the type and severity of incontinence and range from pelvic exercises and biofeedback to medication and surgery.

CAUSES

The cause of urinary incontinence is most often a weakness in the muscles of the pelvic floor. Some experts believe this is directly due to damage from a vaginal birth. Others believe, in a controversial finding, that this weakness is more a result of lack of proper use of these muscles rather than the result of damage. However, there is no question damage occurs during childbirth, especially a traumatic birth, and that can weaken the pelvic floor muscles. Stress incontinence is associated with damage to the pelvic floor, especially to the pudendal nerves; a forceps (tonglike instrument that pulls the baby down the birth canal) delivery; rapid second-stage labor or prolonged pushing; a third-degree perineal tear; and/or a large baby.

Not all women who have given birth, however, have stress incontinence. That's especially true for women who perform pelvic floor exercises. Research shows that the regular performing of those exercises on a daily basis may influence the health of your pelvic floor muscles more than whether you've had four or more children and/or a traumatic childbirth.

About one third of women who exercise, including those who've never had children, experience urine leakage. This is especially true for those who do repetitive bouncing, such as running and aerobics.

Other reasons for incontinence are the shrinking of the bladder and urethral sphincter weakness, especially after menopause, which also results in more frequent urination. A prolapsed or fallen bladder that, like a fallen uterus, begins to descend into the vagina may result in incontinence because it forms a *cystocele*, a protrusion of the bladder that holds urine. A cystocele aggravates incontinence by pulling on and weakening the neck of the bladder. If you put your fingers in your vagina and then purposely cough or strain and something comes down and touches your fingers near the opening of the vagina, you probably have a cystocele.

Obesity puts pressure on internal organs and intensifies incontinence. Urinary tract infections can be a temporary cause of incontinence, which usually stops when the infection is healed. Other reasons include drug side effects, chronic constipation, hysterectomy (because it may cause internal damage that results in incontinence), and the genetic factor. This is the explanation for young, childless women who have stress incontinence. It's believed that they have inherited weak muscle structure.

In addition to the pelvic muscle weaknesses that cause stress incontinence, other reasons for incontinence may be: disease, like multiple sclerosis or cancer; damaged spinal cord; congenital defects; or a weakened sphincter muscle around the opening of the bladder.

MAKING THE DIAGNOSIS

Although stress incontinence is the most common form of incontinence for women, there are several others with their own causes and solutions. That's why you need to find out which kind you have before you select a treatment or undergo surgery. The diagnostic tests used for more severe urinary incontinence include ultrasound, cystometrogram (which measures how well the bladder is functioning), and cystourethrogram (which uses x-rays for the same purpose). Many women can be diagnosed, however, with a detailed personal history and careful physical exam.

OTHER FORMS OF INCONTINENCE

Several other less common forms of incontinence are:

• *Overflow incontinence* occurs when a person doesn't feel the urge to void or isn't able to urinate the usual amount, so the bladder overfills and spills urine. This is most common with women who have neurologic problems, diabetes, or lower back problems, and medication is the solution.

• *Urge incontinence* occurs when a person feels a strong desire to urinate but can't get to a toilet before the bladder empties. This is most common with women who have had back injuries, strokes, or a disease like multiple sclerosis. Treatment is drugs and occasionally surgery, though surgery is usually ineffective with this kind of incontinence.

• *Reflex incontinence* occurs when the bladder fills and empties, but the person is unaware of the need to urinate because the brain does not get the signal that the bladder is full. This is most common with women who have a damaged spinal cord, congenital defects like spina bifida (see "Neural Tube Defects" on page 454), or paralyzed bladder muscles. One solution is the implantation of a pump to create an artificial bladder sphincter that allows for manual control of the emptying of the bladder. (See "Urinary Incontinence" on page 621 in Recommended Reading and also on page 597 in the Resource Directory for helpful organizations.)

• *Surgical incontinence* can occur after cesareans or hysterectomies and is usually temporary.

TREATMENT OPTIONS

• *Estrogen replacement therapy* (ERT). When applied vaginally or taken orally, ERT thickens the lining of the vagina and the urinary tract in women who are past menopause. Obese women are the least likely to be helped with ERT for this. (See "Estrogen Replacement Therapy" on page 337.)

• *Drugs.* There are some that increase bladder capacity.

• *Biofeedback.* This is a technique that gives the person moment-to-moment information on how well the sphincter muscle is functioning. Complete control was regained by 20 to 25 percent of women in studies who used this technique, and another 30 percent showed improvement. (See "Biofeedback" on page 85.)

• *Surgery.* There are several procedures that can be used to realign a fallen bladder, and which is best depends on your anatomy and your specific problem. These operations tighten vaginal tissue underneath the bladder. Stress incontinence may return in time after all of them, so try nonsurgical options first. Possible complications are scar tissue, pelvic infection, or a prolapse, or falling down, of internal organs with resulting problems during sexual intercourse.

• *Collagen or teflon injections.* These experimental injections into the neck of the bladder would probably work best with women who have mild stress incontinence. No one knows how long these injections last nor how safe they are, because the procedures are still new. In 1992 the Food and Drug Administration began to more closely examine all uses of collagen, due to problems with this product in breast implants. (See "Breast Implants" on page 302 for more information about collagen.)

HOME REMEDIES YOU CAN TRY

• *Urinate more often*, which is often the solution for women who have mild stress incontinence. (For women past 55, according to a 1991 study, bladder training that included education about the body parts involved and a strict urination schedule reduced incontinence 57 percent.)

• *Do Kegel exercises*, the tighten-and-release exercises of the pelvic floor used to enhance sexual pleasure and prevent the prolapse, or the falling or slipping out of place, of internal organs like the uterus and bladder. (See "Kegel Exercises" on page 47.) In many Asian and African countries, where mothers often teach their daughters how to use and exercise their pelvic-floor muscles, far less stress incontinence is reported. These exercises, once known only by a minority of childbearing women in the United States, are now helping women of all ages, including some in nursing homes. Kegels are most helpful with mild to moderate stress incontinence.

• *Try to lose weight.* Stress incontinence decreases fivefold when obese women lose at least 50 percent of their excess weight. However, this amount of weight loss is probably impossible for nearly everyone. You may lose some stress incontinence by losing far less. (See "Obesity" on page 424.)

• *Eat a fiber-rich diet to avoid constipation.* (See discussion of fiber on page 28.)

• *Exercise regularly to help keep your internal organs in place.*

• *Give birth in the best position* for your perineal muscles. That position is upright, because with the help of gravity, this position puts the least amount of stress on the vagina, reduces the likelihood of tearing or the need for an episiotomy, and may avoid the use of forceps.

• *Consider acupuncture and Chinese herbs,* which help some women. (See "Acupuncture" on page 82.)

---

*E*very time we started jumping in my aerobics class, I knew I better go to the bathroom. Now I avoid that by tightening my perineal muscles before we start bouncing and not drinking anything for several hours before class.

I gained 50 pounds with both pregnancies and ended up 30 pounds overweight. After I started eating less and walking more, I lost the weight and gained control of my bladder as a bonus.

Urinary Tract Infections (UTIs)

What They Are

Urinary tract infections (UTIs), also known as bladder infections or simple cystitis, are bacterial infections of the bladder and urinary tract.

Signs and Symptoms

Symptoms of a UTI are burning pain during urination and an urgent need to urinate with scant flow, increased frequency of urination, painful pressure in the lower abdomen or back pain, and fever. When a woman has a high fever along with other symptoms, she may have a kidney infection. If that happens to you, or if you have blood or pus in your urine, see a doctor right away.

UTIs typically last about one week, although with treatment severe symptoms are usually present only for a day or two. However, for 20 percent of women with UTIs, these infections become chronic and return periodically, often in a predictable pattern (for instance, on the third day of your menstrual period or when you've left your diaphragm in too long.)

Chronic UTIs are bacterial in origin, which distinguishes them from interstitial cystitis (see "Interstitial Cystitis" on page 387), a condition with similar symptoms that are not associated with the presence of bacteria.

MAKING THE DIAGNOSIS

Irregularities in urinating can be caused by other medical conditions as well as by stress, caffeine, alcohol, and certain medications. UTIs are always bacterial, however, so correct diagnosis depends upon testing the urine for bacteria.

Your health care provider will get your urologic history and take a sample of your urine (clean voided specimen) to confirm that you have an infection. Some women have false-negative results to the test, which means that the test says that you don't have an infection, but in fact you do. This can happen when your urine sample is not handled well or is overly dilute. Be sure to let your health care provider know if you've been drinking lots of water since the first sign of an infection. Ideally, the sample is your first void for the day.

CAUSES

A UTI, especially a first infection, is usually caused by a species of bacteria called *Escherichia coli*, or *E. coli*. These bacteria travel up the urethra, the narrow tube which is located between your vagina and your clitoris, and which is the exit path for urine from your body. These bacteria are harmless in the bowel, and even harmless if they are "flushed out" of the bladder on urinating, but they are not harmless if they remain in the bladder. The situations that cause UTIs are rarely anatomical, such as a shorter-than-usual urethra. They are usually the result of everyday living habits, such as how much fluid you drink in a day, how often you urinate, how you make love, and your choice of birth control.

Although men have UTIs, too, they are more common in women and rival the common cold in frequency for some women.

Frequent sexual intercourse or a sudden increase in sexual activity can result in so-called "honeymoon" cystitis. This infection usually occurs within a day or two after sexual intercourse, but not always. It may occur because your urethra became traumatized, either because the penis had been inserted before you were fully lubricated or entry had been especially forceful. (Nuns and celibate college women have far fewer UTIs than do sexually active college women. However, the problem may not be frequency of sex, but sexual habits and contraceptive choices.)

Types of birth control associated with UTIs include:

• *A too-tight diaphragm.* Many doctors believe that a diaphragm is supposed to be a tight fit if it's going to be effective, but that's not necessarily so. The spermicide does most of the birth-control work. The diaphragm is not just a barrier, it's a receptacle for spermicide. Diaphragms, especially those with a too-tight fit, or a diaphragm rim that rubs, may press on the bladder and become an irritant. Also, sometimes a diaphragm may cause reduced urinary flow because when the device is in the proper position, you may not feel the urge to urinate as soon as you might if the diaphragm weren't there. You also may have to consciously squeeze out the last of your urine, because the diaphragm obstructs the neck of the bladder. (This is an unnecessary step if you're not wearing a diaphragm.)

Other forms of birth control, like those listed below, may also cause UTIs, but an ill-fitting diaphragm is implicated more often than other contraceptives.

• *Contraceptive foams or vaginal suppositories,* because they may irritate the urethra.

• *Nonlubricated condoms,* because they may put pressure on the urethra.

About 10 percent of pregnant women have UTIs, and many of them also had UTIs before they were pregnant. There are several theories about why UTIs occur in pregnant women. One is that these women release more estrogen in their bodies and estrogen makes the urinary tract a friendlier place for bacteria. A second hypothesis is that the pressure of the growing fetus may cause some urine to be retained in the bladder, which allows bacteria to grow. Another theory is that some pregnant women with UTIs have a history of not going to the bathroom very often and they continue that practice during pregnancy, a time when your body requires more fluid and more frequent urination. It's especially important for pregnant women with severe and/or chronic UTIs to see their physicians for treatment, because untreated UTIs are a risk factor for premature labor.

Menopause is also associated with UTIs. The bladder and urethra of some, but not all, postmenopausal women shrink and become more fragile. These changes may allow bacteria to travel more easily up the urethra to the bladder. Some researchers suggest that a change in vaginal flora may also be a reason for postmenopausal UTIs. And for those women who have a cystocele (see a discussion of cystocele on page 511), all of the urine doesn't always leave the bladder, creating a breeding area for bacteria.

Use of a urinary catheter, a long plastic tube inserted into your urinary tract to drain the bladder, after hospital surgery often causes a UTI. Sexual activity with a partner who has a genital tract infection can give you a UTI, too.

Diabetic women are two to four times more likely to have UTIs, and women under stress are more likely to develop a UTI. For some women, when they become run down or anxious and prey to infections, their body's area of least resistance is their bladder. These particular women then get UTIs. With other women, their area of least resistance may lead to colds, flu, or allergies.

PREVENTIVE MEASURES YOU CAN TAKE

If you become aware of any of the typical UTI symptoms coming on, you may be able to take steps to prevent a full-blown infection. You will find out by trial and error what measures work for you. Pay attention to what triggers your UTIs, whether they're on this list or not. If preventive measures fail, contact your health care provider promptly. Most of these home remedies have not been confirmed as helpful (or harmful) through research, mostly because these suggestions have not been examined in that way.

• *Urinate often* to prevent your bladder from becoming overfull. Go when the urge strikes. Typically, women need to urinate more often than men.

• *Drink eight or more glasses of fluid daily.* This helps to flush bacteria from the bladder and to keep the bacteria from multiplying. This is especially helpful if you have an active infection or you're aware of one starting. Drinking lots of water also dilutes the effect of caffeine, alcohol, or soft drinks on your bladder. Soft drinks change the composition of urine, making it more hospitable to bacteria. Dilute fruit juices with water, too.

• *Drink an herb tea* that relaxes your urinary tract.

• *Choose hygiene products carefully.* Avoid douches, bubble bath products, feminine deodorant sprays, perfumed toilet paper, soap, and talcum powders since these products can trigger an infection. (Frequent douches are also a risk factor for ectopic pregnancy and pelvic inflammatory disease. See "Ectopic Pregnancy" on page 488 and "Pelvic Inflammatory Disease" on page 441.)

• *Soak in a tub of plain hot water* several times a day.

• *Keep your vaginal and anal areas clean.* Wipe from front to back after a bowel movement to avoid spreading bacteria.

• *Change tampons or sanitary napkins frequently*, preferably every time you go to the bathroom. This discourages bacteria from traveling up your urethra, and in the case of tampons, you'll avoid blocking the neck of the bladder when you urinate.

• *Wear cotton underpants* or pantyhose with cotton panels to keep this area drier.

• *Avoid tight jeans.*

• *Avoid any activity that might put pressure on your urethra* (bicycling, horseback riding).

• *Boost your immune system.* Keep up your resistance to infections of all kinds by eating and sleeping well. (See "How to Stay Healthy" on page 25 and "Fatigue" on page 344.)

• *Do exercises, like yoga*, that strengthen your lower back. (See "Yoga" on page 59.)

• *Drink cranberry juice* (preferably sweetened only with apple juice). Folk wisdom has often suggested that you take either 500 milligrams of vitamin C (a known infection fighter) daily or drink cranberry juice, unless it increases the burning sensation. It was believed that they both change the urine to make it less friendly toward undesirable bacteria. However, Israeli researchers found another reason for the success of cranberry juice. It has compounds that coat the urinary tract cells, making it difficult for the problem bacteria to stick to the sides. (Concentrated cranberry products are available at many health food stores.)

If intercourse is a UTI trigger for you, have sex in a position that allows the penis to enter your vagina at a lower angle than the straight-up-and-down missionary position. This avoids dragging on the urethra, and it also enhances contact with your clitoris. Urinate after intercourse, and before, too, if possible. This helps flush out unfriendly bacteria. If you drink fluids before lovemaking, you'll have enough urine to cleanse your urinary tract when you void. If you didn't drink fluids before, then do it after. Keep anything that touches the anal area during lovemaking away from the vagina. Use lubricants such as K-Y jelly sparingly, because they can provide transportation of bacteria.

If you can feel your diaphragm, have it refitted. You cannot feel a properly fitted diaphragm once it is in place. Don't keep your diaphragm in place for more than six to eight hours after intercourse. While the diaphragm is in place, be sure to urinate frequently. (See "Diaphragm" on page 200.)

Switch to lubricated condoms, if you currently use dry ones, or change the brand of your contraceptive foam. When it comes to birth control, you have the option of alternating contraceptive methods.

I thought I had a bladder infection, because my urine was cloudy and occasionally I had a burning sensation when I went to the bathroom. My doctor examined me, though, and said I didn't have an infection. She suggested that I drink more water each day, and I do. I've never been bothered again.

Every time I get the symptoms of a bladder infection I know that my body is telling me to pay attention. I slow down, take time to drink lots of water, and soak in my bathtub while reading a good book.

TREATMENT OPTIONS

Antibiotics are prescribed if you have a UTI that is caused by excess bacteria in your urine. However, antibiotics in the absence of bacterial infection are useless and potentially harmful because of side effects. Another reason it's important to be sure of the diagnosis is UTIs are often confused with vaginitis, yeast infections, and chlamydial infections. If you do have a confirmed UTI, you'll receive the drugs usually for three days, occasionally for seven days. Drug treatment for fewer days is generally associated with a greater chance of relapse, and treatment for a greater number of days is associated with more drug side effects. Contact your physician if you have side effects from your antibiotic, such as nausea, a rash, yeast infection, diarrhea, or vaginitis. (See "Vaginal Infections" on page 532.)

What kind of antibiotic your physician prescribes will depend on the kind of infection that you have, whether it's your first or a repeat infection, and what your particular history with antibiotics has been. If you are taking other drugs, be sure and tell your physician, so that you can avoid the potential side effects that sometimes occur when two drugs are mixed. For instance, sometimes the Pill loses its contraceptive effect when taken with antibiotics. (See "How to Use the Pill Wisely" on page 188.)

Estrogen cream is sometimes helpful in treating UTIs for women who are past menopause and who are troubled with urinary tract problems, because of too little estrogen in the vagina or the urethra. Acupuncture, often along with Chinese herbs, may be helpful with chronic UTIs. (See "Estrogen Replacement Therapy" on page 337 and "Acupuncture" on page 82.)

An approach that doesn't work (and is still used) in treating UTIs is urethral dilation. This is a usually painful procedure that stretches the urethra with the intent of reducing both the opportunity for UTIs and frequency of voiding. Instead, it often makes the condition worse.

If you have chronic UTIs, you may want to discuss the use of a home testing kit for urine with your health care provider. (See "Home Testing Kits" on page 112.)

UTERINE FIBROIDS

WHAT THEY ARE

Uterine fibroids are lumps of muscle tissue, usually located in the wall of the uterus, and they are nearly always benign. They come in all sizes from as small as a pea to (rarely) as large as a grapefruit or even a basketball. You may have one fibroid or many. More than 99 percent of them are not cancerous.

Large fibroids can distort the shape of the uterus and the position of internal organs. With larger fibroids, a woman's uterus might grow to the size of a 12-week-plus pregnancy.

MAKING THE DIAGNOSIS

Some women with fibroids experience pelvic pressure, heavy bleeding during periods, and pain, but many women who have fibroids do not have any symptoms, so they may not know about them until they are diagnosed

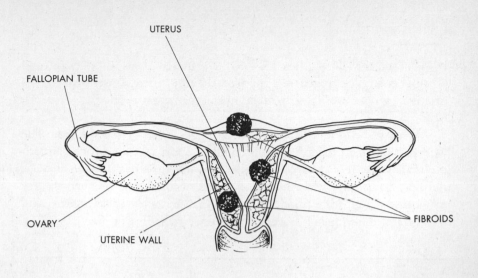

UTERUS

FALLOPIAN TUBE

FIBROIDS

OVARY

UTERINE WALL

UTERINE FIBROIDS

during routine pelvic exams. If necessary (for example, when fibroids occur during pregnancy), they are verified by ultrasound. (See "Ultrasound" on page 476.)

SIGNS AND SYMPTOMS

Women who do have symptoms may experience the following: abdominal swelling (if it's a large fibroid) and heavier menstrual bleeding or bleeding between periods (if the fibroids push against the endometrium, the lining of the uterus). Anemia from extra blood loss is also possible, as is pain, including backache, painful sex, and painful periods due to the fibroid's pressure on any one of several internal organs. (See "Anemia" on page 158.)

Other symptoms are frequent urination from pressure on the bladder; chronic constipation from pressure on the rectum; infertility due to blockage of the fallopian tubes, interference with sperm movement, or distortion of the uterus; and inability to have an orgasm caused by fibroid interference with uterine contractions. (See "Infertility" on page 364.)

CAUSES

It's believed that fibroids are affected by estrogen levels in the body, and postmenopausal estrogen replacement therapy often causes existing fibroids to grow. The Pill may cause fibroid growth, too, but the evidence is not clear.

At least one in four U.S. women past age 35 has uterine fibroids. The woman most likely to have them is childless, more often is African-American than white, and often has a mother or other close relative who also has fibroids. Sometimes when uterine fibroids occur during pregnancy, they may cause a premature labor. After menopause, they gradually shrink and disappear if the woman is not taking estrogen replacement therapy (ERT).

When I was three months pregnant, my midwife's measurements indicated that I was around five months pregnant! She didn't think I had twins and suggested that I have an ultrasound. The scan showed that I had several uterine fibroids. We were aware that the fibroids might affect my labor or cause me to come into labor early. As it turned out, I gave birth vaginally the day before my due date.

PREVENTIVE MEASURES YOU CAN TAKE

- *Reduce fat and sugar and increase whole grains* in your diet. (See "How to Find Fat In Your Food" on page 29.)
- *Avoid red meat and poultry unless they are hormone-free.* (The hormones used in animal feed are generally derivatives of estrogen.)
- *Eat foods rich in those factors that help the liver function well:* beets, garlic, and foods rich in vitamin B_6, inositol, choline, and magnesium.
- *Keep alcohol to a minimum*, since it tends to be harmful to the liver and the liver detoxifies excess estrogen.
- *Reduce caffeine.*
- *Avoid estrogen replacement therapy (ERT)* because it can cause fibroids to grow. (See "Estrogen Replacement Therapy" on page 337.)
- *Exercise regularly* to reduce your body's fat and estrogen levels.
- *Maintain a normal weight*, because it's likely that the heavier you are, the more estrogen there is in your body that in turn encourages your fibroids to grow.

TREATMENT OPTIONS

Most women do not have to have fibroids treated because usually they are small, harmless, and painless. But some women find that their fibroids cause heavy bleeding and/or pain and require some treatment.

• *Myomectomy*, an operation in which the surgeon cuts the fibroid out of the uterine wall, while preserving the rest of the uterus is an option particularly preferred by women who want to have children. It is considered a difficult operation and, like all surgery, is best performed by a surgeon with much experience. This operation is more popular in Western European countries than it is in the United States, because culturally there's more interest there in preserving women's childbearing abilities. (See Payer on page 617 in Recommended Reading for more information on the European use of myomectomy.)

Possible complications of this surgery include profuse bleeding, infection, and scar adhesions, which may cause chronic pain and infertility. Even if all of the fibroids have been removed, some women find that they return eventually. If this occurs, some decide to have the operation repeated.

• *Laser myomectomy* involves burning the fibroids instead of cutting them. This results in less bleeding while preserving more of the normal tissue. (See "Surgery" on page 596 in the Resource Directory.)

• *Dilation and curettage (D & C)*, an operation that does not require an incision through the abdomen, is occasionally used for very small fibroids. (See "Dilation and Curettage" on page 313.)

• *Hysterectomy*. This operation may be necessary for severe bleeding that does not respond to other treatment and, rarely, for a very large fibroid. Regardless of the size of fibroids, if a woman wants no more children, many doctors will recommend a hysterectomy, since the fibroids will not reoccur then. (See "Hysterectomy and Oophorectomy" on page 354.)

The American College of Obstetricians and Gynecologists recommends a hysterectomy for uterine fibroids the size of a 12-week fetus, even if the woman is experiencing no symptoms. It's believed that surgical complications are more severe with larger fibroids and that these benign growths — if left in the uterus — make detection of ovarian or endometrial cancer more difficult. Research shows these conclusions are not true, however. A second opinion may be especially helpful for those of you considering surgery, as there is much controversy about the appropriate use of surgery in general for fibroids. Many insurance plans now require second opinions for surgery to treat uterine fibroids. (See "Get a Second Opinion" on page 95.)

• *Drugs.* These are expensive and their effects are only temporary. They may cause fibroids to shrink, but side effects create a menopausal state, including no periods, hot flashes, and vaginal dryness, among other symptoms.

M y doctor suggested that I have a hysterectomy for my fibroids, because I would be going through menopause soon and would be taking estrogen therapy, and that would make the fibroids grow even faster. My mother had a hysterectomy for the same reason and it made sense to me. I had my operation the next week.

W hen my gynecologist recommended a hysterectomy for my fibroids, I put on my clothes and left her office for the last time. Since then, I've changed my diet, exercise more, and pay more attention to my body. My fibroids have stopped growing, and I feel good about what I've done.

Uterine Prolapse

What It Is

Uterine prolapse is the falling or slipping out of place of the uterus from its usual position in your body.

Signs and Symptoms

• *A feeling of heaviness and discomfort in the vagina*, especially if you feel a lump or bulge there. When you are standing, you may have a feeling that something is falling out.

• *Constant backache or back pressure*, especially after straining your muscles.

• *Urine-flow change*, depending on the location of the prolapse, which results in either stress incontinence or difficult urination, which may lead to frequent urinary tract infections. (See "Urinary Incontinence" on page 510 and "Urinary Tract Infections" on page 515.)

• *Constipation.* Constipation can also be one of the causes, not just a symptom, of a prolapsed uterus.

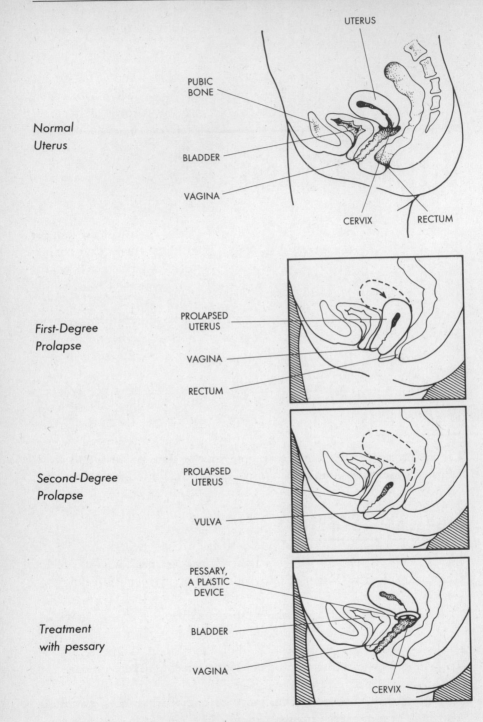

Normal
Uterus

UTERUS

PUBIC
BONE

BLADDER

VAGINA

CERVIX   RECTUM

First-Degree
Prolapse

PROLAPSED
UTERUS

VAGINA

RECTUM

Second-Degree
Prolapse

PROLAPSED
UTERUS

VULVA

Treatment
with pessary

PESSARY,
A PLASTIC
DEVICE

BLADDER

VAGINA

CERVIX

UTERINE PROLAPSE

• *Difficult penetration or painful intercourse*, if the tip of the uterus has moved down into the vagina.

In some women, the uterus falls only slightly into the upper vagina and poses no health problems. In others, the uterus moves down into the vagina in degrees. Rarely, the cervix (the tip of the uterus) protrudes from the vagina. This is not only uncomfortable, but it can lead to infections of the cervix and uterus.

CAUSES

Uterine prolapse affects women past age 60 more than it does younger women. For many, the symptoms begin after menopause. That's when some women's bodies begin to show the side effects of a lack of estrogen, including the loss of some of the strength and elasticity of the ligaments that hold the internal organs in place.

Causes of uterine prolapse may be present alone or in combination and include constipation, obesity (which puts pressure on internal organs), and the presence of a large fibroid tumor, which may interfere with internal organs. (See "Uterine Fibroids" on page 522.)

Pregnancy and birth, especially a traumatic childbirth, may put undue pressure on the birth canal and can result in damage to the vaginal walls, the anus and rectum, and the uterus and bladder. This is most likely to occur after a very quick labor or the birth of a large baby. Women who have had many children can also experience uterine prolapse, though not all women who have had many children and/or traumatic births have prolapsed uteruses. Some women who are childless experience uterine prolapse as well, because of genetically associated (mother or other close relative) weakness in the internal organ-support structure.

MAKING THE DIAGNOSIS

Uterine prolapse is diagnosed during a pelvic exam.

PREVENTIVE MEASURES YOU CAN TAKE

• *Do Kegel exercises*, the tighten-and-release exercises of the pelvic floor. These can be used to prevent uterine prolapse and urinary incontinence and to enhance sexual pleasure. These are helpful only as prevention or when started in the early stages of a prolapse (see "Kegel Exercises" on page 47). Don't feel like a failure if Kegel exercises aren't enough for you. They can't fix a severe prolapse.

• *Maintain a normal weight.* (Any excess pounds put pressure on internal organs.)

• *Eat a high-fiber diet to avoid constipation.* (See discussion of fiber on page 28.)

• *Exercise regularly.* Any kind of regular exercise, not just the Kegels, helps keep internal organs in their right place.

• *Use acupuncture or yoga.* These are helpful if started in the early stages. However, yoga, especially the plough pose, is sometimes helpful with a more advanced prolapse. (See "Acupuncture" on page 82 and "Yoga" on page 59.)

• *Give birth in the best position for your perineal muscles.* That position is upright, because with the help of gravity this position puts the least amount of stress on the vagina and avoids the use of forceps, a tonglike instrument that pulls the baby down the birth canal.

For decades, U.S. doctors have given an episiotomy, the surgical widening of the birth canal, to most women right before their babies are born to prevent uterine prolapse. Yet research shows that an episiotomy does not prevent uterine prolapse. Many doctors also believe that a cesarean, especially a scheduled one in which a woman never experiences labor, will also help prevent uterine prolapse as well as stress incontinence. International studies dispute that finding, too, perhaps because whatever stress is placed on internal organs occurs during pregnancy, not just during birth.

A bout the time of my period I felt a pressure in my vagina that didn't seem right and was painful sometimes. After reading several books, I decided it sounded like the beginning of a uterine prolapse. Since I don't like doctors and the thought of surgery even less, I tried yoga as a first choice. Now several months later, I feel the pressure far less often.

TREATMENT OPTIONS

What treatment options you choose will depend on your preference, your age, whether you want to have children, and the severity of the prolapse.

A pessary is a rubber or plastic device used to hold the uterus and/or vaginal walls in place to prevent the prolapse from worsening. The kind of pessary used depends on your anatomy, age, and whether you are sexually active. Pessaries have to be removed and cleaned, and occasionally, they cause problems because of a poor fit.

A surgical option is one in which a wedge of vaginal tissue is removed. Possible complications are excessive bleeding, damage to bowel or bladder, and painful intercourse due to vaginal scar tissue. Another surgical option is surgical realignment of the uterus, which resuspends this organ in its proper place. Possible complications include a reoccurrence of prolapse.

The final surgical option is a hysterectomy (see "Hysterectomy and Oophorectomy" on page 354). This is often your doctor's first choice. Yes, this would solve the problem of a prolapsed uterus, because you wouldn't have a uterus anymore. Sometimes this is the best solution, especially when the prolapse is severe. Many experts, however, say that this is too much treatment when the prolapse is mild, because the problem can be solved with less surgery, or none at all. Also, a possible side effect of a hysterectomy within two years is the prolapse of your bladder, rectum, and vagina.

Vaginal Infections

What They Are

The three most common vaginal infections are *vaginosis* (which half of all U.S. women have at least once in their lives), *yeast infections*, and *trichomoniasis*. They have different causes, but all three are diagnosed through a careful history and a wet-smear examination (mixing a sample of your discharge with a drop of either salt water or potassium hydroxide solution and examining it under a microscope). Diagnosis by means of culturing may be more accurate. These three infections are treated differently, and accurate diagnosis is important to avoid confusion and incorrect treatment.

Misdiagnosis is common for all vaginal infections. In one study, more than one fourth of the women diagnosed with yeast infections actually had other vaginal infections, including trichomoniasis, gonorrhea, chlamydia, and herpes. (See "Sexually Transmitted Diseases" on page 493.)

VAGINOSIS

Vaginosis is also known as nonspecific vaginitis and is sometimes sexually transmitted.

Symptoms are: thick or watery, white or gray discharge with a disagreeable "fishy" odor. Itching and redness are mild or nonexistent, but pain with urination or intercourse is common. Unlike yeast infections, vaginosis is treated with oral antibiotics, and prompt treatment usually clears up vaginosis within a few days. (Remember that antibiotic use can interfere with absorption of the Pill. See "How to Use the Pill Wisely" on page 188.)

YEAST INFECTIONS

Yeast infection is also known as monilia, candida, or fungus infection. Unlike vaginosis and trichomoniasis, which are caused by "invader" organisms, yeast infections are caused by excessive growth of a fungus that is normally present in harmless quantities in the vagina.

Symptoms are: itching (usually quite severe); thick, white, yeasty-smelling, curdy discharge from the vagina; burning and soreness in the vulva (the outer lips of the vagina); and a vagina that is bright red rather than the usual pink. A burning sensation with urination is also common.

It's important to be clear about the diagnosis, because a burning sensation is the primary symptom for urinary tract infections, which are usually treated with antibiotics. Antibiotics not only do not help a yeast infection, they will likely make it worse.

Some women have yeast infections rarely; others have them regularly, for instance, every month at the time of the menstrual period or early in a pregnancy. (Babies born to women with active yeast infections often have thrush, a yeast infection in the mouth.) Recurring yeast infections are common.

The common drug preparations for a yeast infection are Nystatin, miconazole, clotrimazole (available over the counter), and/or terconazole, and butoconazole, which all can be used in creams applied topically to the vulva and/or in vaginal suppositories. Gentian violet leaves a purple stain, and boric acid powder may not be safe. If you are pregnant or breastfeeding, be sure to check with your doctor about the safety of any drug you've been given.

I've learned to avoid yeast infections by combining good food and reducing stress. One of the first signs of a yeast infection for me is crankiness. Of course, it took several bouts before I figured that out. Now when my kids ask me why I'm crabby, I'll say to myself, "Oh-oh, time to relax and eat better."

THE CHRONIC CANDIDA CONTROVERSY

Nearly all people carry *Candida albicans*, the organism that causes yeast infections, in their bodies, and the overgrowth of this organism is far more common in women.

The controversy over candida centers on exactly what diseases and disorders are caused by this ubiquitous organism. Some health care providers say that candida affects one third of the population and that its overgrowth causes far more than yeast infections. They say it causes chronic heartburn, bloating, belching, gas, abdominal pain, indigestion, headaches, fatigue, depression, menstrual irregularities, allergies, migraine headaches, bladder infections, arthritis, and endometriosis.

The cures for some people are lactobacillus (found in some yogurts), garlic supplements, caprylic acid (derived from coconut oil), oleic acid (found in olive oil), and other dietary changes.

Meanwhile, other health care providers say that candida is overrated and unproven as a troublemaker on such a grand scale. As there is not much data either way, chronic candida will remain controversial. But there certainly have been many anecdotal stories in which women say that their symptoms have left since they've made the recommended changes. (See Calbon on page 604 in Recommended Reading. See also "Yeast Infections" on page 621 in Recommended Reading and on page 599 in the Resource Directory.)

Within one week of beginning the program, starting with the cessation of urinary tract problems, my health began improving. I have been on the program for four months, and still each week or so seems to bring relief from another long-standing physical problem.

TRICHOMONIASIS

Trichomoniasis (trich) is a protozoan infection that is usually, although not always, sexually transmitted. It's caused by the parasite *Trichomonas vaginalis*. Sometimes this parasite will remain dormant in the vagina for many years before flaring up.

Some women do not have symptoms, but most do. Some women become aware of trich as a result of a Pap smear that appears to be abnormal. Common symptoms are vaginal itching, pain, and a watery, foamy greenish or yellowish discharge, which often worsen following menstruation, and "strawberry marks," small red dots, on the cervix. Several bouts of trich are associated with infertility.

The most effective medication, given to both partners, is the prescription antibiotic metronidazole (Flagyl), prescribed for either one or two days or seven. Side effects may be: unpleasant stomach symptoms, headache, and a sharp, metallic taste in the mouth. Don't drink alcohol while taking this drug, as the combination causes severe illness.

PREVENTIVE MEASURES YOU CAN TAKE

Here is an all-purpose list of suggestions for avoiding all three of these vaginal infections:

• *Understand the role of contraceptives.* To prevent the development of vaginosis, avoid leaving contraceptive sponges and diaphragms (tampons, too) in the vagina longer than the recommended six to eight hours. Objects left in too long encourage the growth of unfriendly bacteria (vaginosis and trichomoniasis). Have an IUD removed if you have repeated bouts of vaginosis, since its presence in your body may be triggering the infection. Avoid spermicides if they are an irritant, or change brands and see if there's an improvement. Use condoms to avoid the vaginosis or trichomoniasis that are transmitted sexually, or if you know you're allergic to any properties in your partner's semen. Avoid using the Pill if you have recurrent yeast infections. In fact, you may want to avoid intercourse altogether during a yeast infection (unless you use the female condom), because it may spread the infection and make you itch even more. (See "TODAY Sponge" on page 203, "Diaphragm" on page 200, discussion of tampons on page 507, "Intrauterine Device" on page 208, "Spermicide" on page 207, "Male Condom" on page 193, "The Pill" on page 181, and "Female Condom" on page 197.)

• *Eat well* to keep up your resistance to all of these infections. (See "Food" on page 26.) If you have a yeast infection, include an eight-ounce serving of yogurt (make sure the label indicates live cultures) every day to help restore your body's natural bacterial defenses against yeast (if you are allergic to dairy products, and not a fan of soy-based yogurt, purchase acidophilus in liquid, tablet, or powdered form); avoid sugar, since that causes yeast to grow more rapidly; and use herbs, including golden seal, comfrey, and bayberry bark (see "Medicinal Herbs" on page 610 in Recommended Reading).

• *Avoid becoming overtired or unduly stressed.* When many women get too much stress, for whatever reasons (poor eating habits, too little sleep, use of recreational drugs, among others), their bodies respond by developing their own "standard-brand" illness. That can be a cold, the flu, allergy flare-ups, or for some, a vaginal infection.

• *Practice good hygiene.* Wipe from front to back, wash regularly, and make sure anything introduced into your vagina is scrupulously clean.

• *Avoid perfumed, colored, or deodorant soaps and colored or printed toilet paper* and encourage your partner to avoid them, too.

• *Avoid douches, hygiene sprays, deodorant pads, and deodorant tampons, as well as other people's damp towels and sheets.* Douching is a good thing to avoid in general. It increases your risk for both pelvic inflammatory disease and ectopic pregnancy. (See "Pelvic Inflammatory Disease" on page 441 and "Ectopic Pregnancy" on page 488.)

• *Wear all-cotton underpants* (or don't wear any), and avoid tight-fitting pants.

• *Make sure your partner is checked and treated to avoid reinfection.*

• *Avoid the use of antibiotics if you have a yeast infection,* unless you're positive their use is necessary. They may trigger a yeast infection by impairing your immune system. If you must be on antibiotics, talk with your health care provider about taking yeast medication at the same time to prevent another infection. (See "The Over-the-Counter and Prescription Drug Diet" on page 33.)

Varicose Veins

What They Are

Varicose (Latin for *enlarged*) veins are usually those in the legs that are distended or swollen. Varicose veins in the legs are five times more common in women. Varicose veins located in the anus are called hemorrhoids and are more common in men (but not unusual in women, particularly when they are pregnant).

Varicose veins in the legs become obvious as bluish marks, while larger varicose veins look like bumpy, purplish ropes, sometimes as large around as a finger.

Spider veins are the tiny, swollen veins in your thighs that often show up during pregnancy. They are not varicose veins and are harmless, but they are cosmetically undesirable. Many women who have varicose veins have spider veins, too.

537

SIGNS AND SYMPTOMS

Symptoms are: muscle cramps in the middle of the night, swollen ankles, general feeling of leg soreness or fatigue, itching and skin flaking on your legs (caused by oxygen shortage to the skin), and, in severe cases, swollen or perhaps ulcerated legs.

These veins do not go away on their own, except perhaps after pregnancy, and usually become worse over time. The rate at which they worsen depends on your genetic history, general health, weight, and number of pregnancies.

CAUSES

Varicose veins are caused by weakened valves in the veins that allow some blood to pump the wrong way and go back into superficial veins.

These veins may show up in your 20s, or as late as your 70s, and may be more troublesome near menstruation. The woman most likely to have varicose veins has relatives who have them, too. It's believed that what's inherited is a defect in the venous valve or a vein with a weak or absent wall. A woman who is obese, who is frequently pregnant, or who has pregnancies close together is also more likely to have varicose veins, perhaps because of the added weight from the pregnant uterus as well as hormonal changes that affect the veins. Others causes are too much sun, Pill use, and standing at a job for six or more hours per day. (See "Who Shouldn't Take The Pill" on page 182 and "Varicose Veins" on page 621 in Recommended Reading.)

PREVENTIVE MEASURES YOU CAN TRY

To avoid varicose veins, or their worsening:

- *Maintain a normal weight and exercise regularly.*
- *Avoid alcohol, cigarettes, and the Pill.*
- *Eat high-fiber foods* (to avoid constipation) and foods rich in vitamins E and C, as well as bioflavonoids found in citrus. (See discussion of fiber on page 28.)
- *Avoid crossing your legs and wearing garters or girdles* to have good circulation. Wear support stockings instead.

TREATMENT OPTIONS

For most women with varicose veins, the worst problem is cosmetic. Many of these mildly affected women are satisfied to use a cosmetic cover cream on their veins. The makeup is usually not visible when worn with stockings.

There are three medical solutions to consider when your condition has become both acutely bothersome and painful. One procedure is surgical removal, also called vein stripping, an operation that eliminates the varicose veins by tying off and removing the main vein to which they're connected.

Another is injection therapy, an office procedure that uses a chemical solution that causes the walls of the vein to become inflamed and mat together.

The third is laser treatment, another office procedure that uses a powerful beam of high energy light instead of a chemical injection. (See "Surgery" on page 596 in the Resource Directory. See also "Get a Second Opinion" on page 95 as insurance companies often require another opinion for these surgeries.)

In our family all the women have varicose veins. The veins don't show up at the same age for all of us, and they have only been a real problem with one sister who is quite overweight and has had several children.

In my business of selling real estate, I always have to look well dressed and professional. After spending hundreds of dollars on suits, I'm not about to have my veiny legs ruin the effect. I put base makeup on my legs to cover the worst veins, and then wear colorful support stockings that match my outfits.

YEAST INFECTION: *see* Vaginal Infection

PART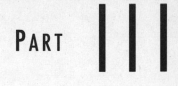

RESOURCE DIRECTORY

This section is organized alphabetically by topic (groups with toll-free and hot line numbers listed first) and provides you with a list of suggested organizations that you may contact about a particular women's health issue (for example, childbirth, endometriosis, or battering) or about an illness that affects you or someone in your family (such as cancer, heart disease, or Alzheimer's disease).

These organizations are mostly national, occasionally regional, and a few are located in Canada and England. Some organizations provide help over the phone and publications in Spanish as well. Each listing has been confirmed by mail or phone at least once, but contact names, addresses, and phone numbers change frequently, particularly in volunteer organizations. In addition, some organizations provide only phone numbers, while others provide only addresses.

Many of the listings belong to self-help, often volunteer organizations (rather than only governmental offices, for example), because they often are the source of immediate help. Perhaps reflecting our American pioneer spirit, the United States has more self-help organizations per capita than any other country.

The listing of any person or organization in this directory is not an endorsement by me, however, as I'm not familiar with all of the published material and services each one provides. If you know of an organization I missed, or you have new addresses or phone numbers for existing listings, please let me know. (See the "Here's What I Think Questionnaire" on page 623.)

If you try to contact one of the following organizations and are unable to, because the phone number and/or the address are incorrect, you can:

- *Call the reference room of your local library* and ask if they have a newer listing.
- *Call your local United Way* and ask for the information and referral services department.
- *Contact one of the self-help organizations* listed on page 594. They can either help you locate the group you're looking for, or they can help you start your own self-help group.
- *Call "Lesko's Info-Power" at 1-800 32-LESKO* and ask if one of their many resource books has an up-to-date list of organizations for your particular topic. (Or ask your local library if they have an updated issue.)
- *Call People's Medical Society at 1-800 624-8773 for Dial 800 For Health, or call Pierian Press at 1-800 678-2435 for their Directory of National Helplines: A Guide to Toll-Free Public Service Numbers.* Or ask your library if they have either book. Not all women's health topics are included in their directories, but all numbers are toll-free.

Toll-free 1-800 phone numbers are often busy. If you get a busy signal, you may get through quicker by dialing repeatedly, rather than trying later.

"SASE" in the description means you should send a self-addressed, stamped business-size envelope when you are requesting information.

ABORTION

Committee to Defend Reproductive Rights
25 Taylor Street #704
San Francisco, CA 94102
(415) 441-4434
Focuses on abortion and prenatal care access; provides publications including newsletter, *CDRR NEWS;* and supports legislative reform and direct action. $25/year. SASE for sample copy.

National Abortion Federation
1436 U Street, NW
Washington, DC 20009
1-800 772-9100 (9:30 A.M.–5:30 P.M. Eastern Standard Time) or (202) 667-5881
Provides information about abortion and its availability.

National Abortion Rights Action League (NARAL)
1101 14th Street, NW, 5th Floor
Washington, DC 20005
(202) 408-4600
    Provides information including newsletter, *NARAL News*, and referrals to local affiliates, and works to elect pro-choice officials at all levels of government. $10/year.

Reproductive Freedom Project
American Civil Liberties Union
132 West 43rd Street
New York, NY 10036
(212) 944-9800, Extension 726
    Provides free newsletter, *Reproductive Rights Update*, and litigation on behalf of and public information about reproductive and privacy rights including abortion, contraception, and minors' rights.

ABORTION ALTERNATIVES

Crisis Pregnancy Centers
12959 Jupiter Road #140
Dallas, TX 75238
(214) 343-7283
    Provides pregnancy tests, clothes, prenatal classes, parenting support group, and counseling. All services are free.

National Life Center
686 North Broad Street
Woodbury, NJ 08096
1-800 848-5683
    Provides free pregnancy tests, a place to stay during pregnancy, maternity and baby clothes, and referrals to prenatal care providers through 500 chapters.

Nurturing Network
910 Main Street, Suite 360
P.O. Box 2050
Boise, ID 83701
1-800 866-4MOM
or (208) 344-7200
    Provides counseling, practical support, and referrals nationwide.

Pregnancy Center, Inc.
1327 Dillon Heights Avenue
Baltimore, MD 21228
1-800 492-5530
1-800 521-5530
    Provides information, support, and referrals for abortion alternatives.

(See also "Adoption" and "Single Mothers" in separate entries.)

ABUSE

Battered Women's Directory
Box E-94, Earlham College
Richmond, IN 47374
(317) 966-0858
   Provides more than 2,000 listings of both national and international services and resources for battered women, including an annotated bibliography and more than 100 pages of history, description, and solutions.

Child Help USA Hotline
P.O. Box 630
Hollywood, FL 90028
1-800 4-A-CHILD
or (213) 465-4016
   Provides counseling and referrals for children suffering abuse or adult survivors.

National Clearinghouse on Marital and Date Rape
Women's History Research, Inc.
2325 Oak Street
Berkeley, Ca 94708
(510) 524-1582
   Provides *for a fee* phone consultation, document search and delivery services, date rape packet, speaker's bureau, and volunteer internships.

National Coalition Against Domestic Violence
P.O. Box 18749
Denver, CO 80218
(303) 839-1852
   Provides public education through publications and a speakers' bureau.

National Council on Child Abuse and Family Violence
1-800 222-2000 (9 A.M. – 5 P.M., Monday – Friday, Pacific Standard Time)
   Provides referrals for family violence, child abuse, spouse abuse, and elder abuse.

National Organization for Victim Assistance
1757 Park Road, NW
Washington, DC 20010
(202) 232-6682
   Provides 24-hour crisis counseling and follow-up assistance to crime victims along with publications and national advocacy.

Nine-to-Five Hotline
National Association of Working Women
614 Superior Avenue, NW, Suite 852
Cleveland, OH 44113
1-800 522-0925
or (206) 566-9308
   Provides information for complaints about sexual harassment on the job and other job problems.

Parents United International, Inc.
232 Gish Road
San Jose, CA 95112-4703
(408) 453-7616, Extension 124
　　Provides child sexual abuse treatment; a professional training program; and guided self-help for child victims, siblings, parents, and adults molested as children. SASE.

Sexual Assault Recovery Anonymous Society (SARA)
P.O. Box 16
Surrey, British Columbia V3T 4W4
CANADA
(604) 584-2626
　　Provides mutual aid groups for adult survivors of sexual abuse, SARATEEN groups, and Mothers United for mothers of abused children. (Adult groups are available in the United States, too.)

Voices In Action, Inc.
P.O. Box 148309
Chicago, IL 60614
1-800 786-4238
or (312) 327-1400
　　Helps victims of incest become survivors, and provides workshops to prevent sexual abuse, a national network, and publications including a newsletter, *The Chorus*. SASE.

ACQUIRED IMMUNE DEFICIENCY SYNDROME (AIDS)

AIDS Clinical Trials Information Service (ACTIS)
1-800 874-2572
or (301) 217-0023
　　Provides latest information on HIV/AIDS drugs, treatments, and clinical trials (research studies in which new therapies are tested in humans) for healthcare professionals and the public in English and Spanish. Also provides publications about women and AIDS, a data base of FDA-approved studies, and research updates.

The AIDS Drug Assistance Program (ADAP)
P.O. Box 2052, Empire Station
Albany, NY 12220
1-800 542-2437 (New York only)
　　Pays for AIDS drugs for eligible New York State residents.

The AIDS Drug Assistance Program Plus (ADAP Plus)
P.O. Box 2052, Empire Station
Albany, NY 12220
1-800 542-2437 (New York Only)
　　Pays for primary care and home care for eligible New York State residents with HIV and AIDS.

CDC National AIDS Clearinghouse
P.O. Box 6003
Rockville, MD 20849-6003
1-800 458-5231
1-800 243-7012 (Hearing impaired/TDD)
   Provides information and referrals for HIV and AIDS. Distributes publications including brochures, posters, and videotapes.

CDC National AIDS Hotline
1-800 342-AIDS (24 hours/day, seven days/week)
1-800 342-SIDA (Spanish 8 A.M. – 2 A.M. Eastern Standard Time, seven days/week)
1-800 243-7889 (Hearing impaired/TDD, 10 A.M. – 10 P.M. Eastern Standard Time, seven days/week)
   Provides information and referrals as well as free publications.

Center for Women Policy Studies
2000 P Street, NW, Suite 508
Washington, DC 20036
(202) 872-1770
   Provides information on women and AIDS including fact sheets, video, action kit, policy papers, and annual *Guide to Resources on Women and AIDS*.

Health Information Network
P.O. Box 30762
Seattle, WA 98103
(206) 784-5655 (9 A.M. – 5 P.M., Monday – Friday, Pacific Standard Time)
   Provides speakers' bureau, community resource information, publications, and referral service about AIDS and other sexually transmitted diseases.

Oryx Press
4041 N. Central, Suite 700
Phoenix, AZ 85012-3397
1-800 279-ORYX
or (602) 265-2651
   Publishes *AIDS & Women: A Sourcebook*, an excellent guide to state-by-state resources.

Women's AIDS Network
P.O. Box 426182
San Francisco, CA 94142-6182
(415) 864-4376, Extension 2007
   Provides networking information including brochures and referrals for HIV-infected women and women service providers.

Following are helpful AIDS newsletters. If no subscription price is listed with the publication, contact the newsletter office for rates. Note that the newsletter, *WORLD*, is for women only.

AIDS Treatment News
P.O. Box 411256
San Francisco, CA 94141
1-800 TREAT-1-2
or (415) 255-0588
 Publishes newsletter that is published twice per month. Flexible subscription rates.

Being Alive
People with HIV/AIDS Action Coalition
3626 Sunset Boulevard
Los Angeles, CA 90026
(213) 667-3262
 Provides information and support, dating service, and newsletter in English and Spanish. Flexible subscription rates.

Notes from the Underground
People with AIDS Working for Health, Inc. (PWA Health Group)
150 West 26th Street, Suite 201
New York, NY 10001
(212) 255-0520
 Publishes newsletter with information about experimental or alternative therapies for HIV. $35/6 issues/year for individuals; $75 for businesses; sliding scale for people who can't afford subscription fee.

PI Perspective
347 Dolores Street, Suite 301
San Francisco, CA 94110
(415) 558-8669
 Published quarterly with flexible subscription rates.

Treatment Issues
Gay Men's Health Crisis, Inc. (GMHC)
129 West 20th Street
New York, NY 10011-0022
(202) 807-6664
 Publishes newsletter that provides timely, accurate (from medical journals, clinical trials, and interviews with experts) information about treatments, so that people infected with HIV can make more informed health care decisions. 10 issues/year. Flexible subscription rates.

WORLD
Women Organized to Respond to Life-threatening Diseases
P.O. Box 11535
Oakland, CA 94611
(510) 658-6930
 Provides monthly newsletter by, for, and about women living with HIV. Flexible subscription rates.

ACUPUNCTURE

National Commission for the Certification of Acupuncturists
1424 16th Street, NW, Suite 501
Washington, DC 20036
(202) 232-1404
Provides referrals of certified acupuncturists. Send $3 for list of certified acupuncturists in a particular state.

ADDITIVES, PRESERVATIVES, AND OTHER FOOD CHEMICALS

Aspartame Consumer Safety Network
P.O. Box 780634
Dallas, TX 75378
(214) 352-4268
Provides information, support, and publications including "The Deadly Deception."

Food and Drug Administration
Office of Public Affairs
5600 Fishers Lane, HFE88
Rockville, MD 20857
(301) 443-3170
Provides free pamphlets including *Sweetness Minus Calories = Controversy, More Than You Ever Thought You Would Know About Food Additives*, and *Consumer's Guide to Food Labels*.

National Organization Mobilized to Stop Glutamate (NOMSG)
P.O. Box 367
Santa Fe, NM 87504
1-800 288-0718
Provides information, including a quarterly newsletter, on the food additive monosodium glutamate (MSG) and gives instructions on how to read labels for MSG. SASE.

ADOPTION

Adoptees' Liberty Movement Association (ALMA Society)
P.O. Box 727, Radio City Station
New York, NY 10101-0727
(212) 581-1568 (24-hour answering service)
Provides information and assistance for adopted children who want to find natural parent(s) with international registry for children, parents, and siblings. Groups in 50 states. SASE.

American Adoption Congress
401 East 74th Street
New York, NY 10021
Provides education, search, support on adoption-related matters for adoptees, birth parents, and adoptive parents.

Committee for Single Adoptive Parents, Inc.
P.O. Box 15084
Chevy Chase, MD 20825
　　Provides information on sources of adoptive children and advice to single women and men who are interested in adoption. Publications.

Concerned United Birthparents, Inc. (CUB)
2000 Walker Street
Des Moines, IA 50317
1-800 822-2777
　　Provides mutual support for coping with the ongoing issues of adoption, working for adoption reforms in law and social policy, preventing unnecessary family separations, assisting adoption-separated relatives in searching for family members, and educating the public about adoption issues and realities.

International Soundex Reunion Registry (ISRR)
P.O. Box 2312
Carson City, NV 89702-2312
(702) 882-7755 (9 A.M.–4 P.M. Pacific Standard Time)
　　Provides a confidential mutual consent registry for adults (18 years old) in search of their immediate next of kin by birth.

Interracial Family Circle
P.O. Box 53290
Washington, DC 20009
(703) 719-9887
　　Provides education, social connections, and information for interracial families including adoptive and foster families.

National Adoption Center
1218 Chestnut Street
Philadelphia, PA 19107
1-800 TO-ADOPT
　　Provides referrals and information, specializing in children with special needs.

National Council for Adoption
1930 17th Street, NW
Washington, DC 20009
(202) 328-1200
　　Provides information and advocacy for adoption and maternity services. Referrals to pregnant women for adoption and maternity service and infertile couples for adoption services. SASE.

One Church, One Child
Holy Angels Church
607 East Oakwood Boulevard
Chicago, IL 60653
(312) 624-5375
　　Provides referral service for black children's adoptions primarily through churches. SASE.

OURS, Inc.
3307 Highway 100 North, Suite 203
Minneapolis, MN 55422
(612) 535-4829
Provides information and support for adoptive and prospective adoptive families, including monthly magazine for adoptive families, how-to-adopt information and parenting resource materials for adoptive parents.

REUNIONS Magazine
P.O. Box 11727
Milwaukee, WI 53211-0727
Sells quarterly magazine about planning reunions including those of adoptees and birth families. $24/year.

Triadoption Library, Inc.
P.O. Box 638
Westminster, CA 92684
(714) 892-4098
Provides referrals regarding adoption reform, search/reunion, cooperative adoption. Publications. SASE.

AFRICAN-AMERICAN WOMEN'S HEALTH

Ford Foundation Office of Communications
300 East 43rd Street
New York, NY 10017
Provides free copy of the following booklets: "National Women of Color Organizations" and "Violence Against Women."

Office of Minority Health Resource Center
1-800 248-4344
Provides data base information primarily to health professionals, but also gives organization referrals to consumers.

National Black Women's Health Project
1237 Ralph David Abernathy Boulevard, SW
Atlanta, GA 30310
1-800 ASK-BWHP
or (404) 758-9590
Provides information and support to African-American women and their families about health issues including reproductive rights, teenage pregnancy, and domestic violence.

ALCOHOL

Alcoholics Anonymous (A.A.)
P.O. Box 459, Grand Central Station
New York, NY 10163
Phone number: Look in phone book for local information or write to this address.
Provides fellowship for recovering alcoholic women and men who help each other stay sober and help others recover from alcoholism. Publications.

Al-Anon Family Group Headquarters
P.O. Box 862, Midtown Station
New York, NY 10018
1-800 356-9996
or (212) 245-3151 (New York and Canada)
   Provides information and support for adult children of alcoholics. Worldwide
directory of services and chapters. Newsletter, books, pamphlets.

Coalition on Alcohol and Drug Dependent Women and Their Children
1511 K Street, NW, Suite 926
Washington, DC 20005
   Provides information about alcoholism and drug dependency of women, including
pregnant women, and their families.

National Association of Lesbian and Gay Alcoholic Professionals (NALGAP)
1147 South Alvarado Street
Los Angeles, CA 90006
   Provides quarterly newsletter, bibliography, facilities and services directory, advocacy, support, and workshops.

National Council on Alcoholism and Drug Dependence Hopeline
12 West 21st Street
New York, NY 10010
1-800 NCA-CALL
or (212) 206-6770
   Provides information about alcoholism and teenage drinking, counseling, and local
referrals.

Wisconsin Clearinghouse
315 North Henry Street
Madison, WI 53703-2018
1-800 322-1468
or (608) 263-6884
   Develops and publishes materials about alcohol and other drugs, alternatives to
drug abuse, prevention, mental health, smoking information for youth, families, and
women. Provides free catalog of publications.

Women for Sobriety, Inc.
P.O. Box 618
Quakertown, PA 18951
1-800 333-1606
or (215) 536-8026
   Provides a self-help program for women alcoholics who recognize the need for
self-esteem and self-discovery. Newsletter, publications. SASE.

ALZHEIMER'S DISEASE

Alzheimer's Disease and Related Disorders Association, Inc.
919 North Michigan Avenue, Suite 1000
Chicago, IL 60611-1676
1-800 272-3900 (8:30 A.M. – 5 P.M., seven days/week)
or (312) 335-8882 (Hearing impaired/TDD)
or (312) 335-8700
    Provides information, referrals to local affiliates and services, and publications including a newsletter, *Alzheimer's Disease Newsletter.*

American Health Assistance Foundation
15825 Shady Grove Road, Suite 140
Rockville, MD 20850
1-800 437-2423
    Sponsors research and provide emergency financial help for treatment of people with Alzheimer's disease and their caregivers through the Alzheimer's Family Relief Program.

National Institute on Aging Information Center
2209 Distribution Circle
Silver Spring, MD 20910
(301) 495-3455
    Provides free pamphlet, *Q & A: Alzheimer's Disease.*

ARTIFICIAL INSEMINATION

Donors' Offspring
P.O. Box 37
Sarcoxie, MO 64862
(417) 548-3679
    Provides information and support for women considering donor insemination, offspring of A.I. donors, and their parents. National network of members, newsletter, *Donors' Offspring,* $20/year.

ASPARTAME

(See Additives, Preservatives, and Other Food Chemicals)

BATTERED WOMEN

(See Abuse)

BIOFEEDBACK

Biofeedback Certification Institute of America
10200 West 44th Avenue
Wheat Ridge, CO 80033
(303) 420-2902
    Provides referrals to consumers and certification for biofeedback therapists.

Birth Control

The Alan Guttmacher Institute
111 Fifth Avenue, 11th Floor
New York, New York 10003-1089
(212) 254-5656
　　Provides information about contraception, abortion, and teenage pregnancy, including research, policy studies, and fact sheets.

Association for Voluntary Surgical Contraception
79 Madison Avenue
New York, New York 10016
(212) 561-8090
　　Provides information (including free brochures) about female sterilization, vasectomy, Norplant, and IUDs.

The Couple to Couple League
3621 Glenmore Avenue
P.O. Box 111184
Cincinnati, OH 45211-1184
(513) 661-7612
　　Provides help to couples with the practice of the full sympto-thermal method of natural family planning and child-spacing by breastfeeding. Publications.

Planned Parenthood Federation of America
810 Seventh Avenue
New York, New York 10019
1-800 223-3303
　　Provides publications and referrals to local clinics (or check your phone book for your local office).

Breastfeeding/Lactation Consultants

(See Childbirth and Pregnancy)

Cancer

American Cancer Society
2255 South Oneida
Denver, CO 80224
1-800 227-2345
　　Provides general information about all forms of cancer including publications.

American Institute for Cancer Research
1759 R Street, NW
Washington, DC 20069
1-800 843-8114
or (202) 328-7744 (Washington, DC)
　　Provides registered dietitian to answer personal questions regarding diet, nutrition, and cancer as well as publications.

Breast Surgery Alert
P.O. Box 550642
Dallas, TX 75355-0642
(214) 349-4399
  Sells surgical-alert pendant designed by woman who had mastectomy with brochure regarding arm care following surgery.

Cancer Control Society
2043 North Berendo Street
Los Angeles, CA 90027
(213) 663-7801
  Provides information and physician referrals for nontoxic, nutritional, and nontraditional cancer therapies.

Committee for Freedom of Choice in Cancer Therapy
1180 Walnut Avenue
Chula Vista, CA 91911
(619) 429-8200
  Provides physician referrals and information on metabolic, nutritional, and other alternative therapies for cancer.

Foundation for Advancement in Cancer Therapy (FACT)
P.O. Box 1242, Old Chelsea Station
New York, NY 10113
(212) 741-2790
  Provides information, including the publication *Cancer Forum,* about cancer alternatives, funds research, and campaigns against environmental pollution.

National Alliance of Breast Cancer Organizations
1180 Avenue of the Americas, 2nd Floor
New York, NY 10036
(212) 719-0154
  Provides resource network and publications for people who are interested in breast cancer, including quarterly newsletter, *NABCO News.* $40/year for individuals.

National Cancer Institute Hotline
Rocky Mountain Cancer Information Service
P.O. Box 7021
Colorado Springs, CO 80933
1-800 4-CANCER
1-800 638-6070 (Alaska)
1-800 524-1234 (Oahu, Hawaii and neighbor islands call collect)
or (301) 427-8656 (Maryland)
  Provides information regarding cancer symptoms, treatment, and diagnosis and gives local referrals.

National Coalition for Cancer Survivorship
1010 Wayne Avenue, Suite 300
Silver Spring, MD 20910
(301) 585-2616
Provides local referrals and information about surviving cancer including publications.

The Skin Cancer Foundation
P.O. Box 561
New York, NY 10156
(212) 725-5176
Provides information about skin cancer including newsletter, *Sun and Skin News; The Melanoma Letter*. SASE.

The Susan G. Komen Volunteer and Education Center
111 Park Forest Shopping Center
Dallas, TX 75234
1-800 462-9273 Hotline (8 A.M. – 5 P.M., Monday – Friday, Central Standard Time)
or (214) 247-5513
Provides breast health care and breast cancer information, publications including "Speaking With Your Doctor" series, a drop-in library, and American College of Radiology mammogram referrals.

Y-ME Breast Cancer Support Program
18220 Harwood Avenue
Homewood, IL 60431
1-800 221-2141 (9 A.M. – 5 P.M., Monday – Friday, Central Standard Time)
or (312) 799-8228 (Illinois)
Provides information and support to all women who are concerned about breast cancer and offers publications including a bimonthly newsletter, Y-ME Hot line.

CAREGIVERS

Children of Aging Parents (CAPS)
1609 Woodbourne Road, Suite 302-A
Levittown, PA 19057
(215) 945-6900
Provides support groups for caregivers of the elderly and publications including newsletter and a directory of support groups. $15/year individuals, $25/year professionals or organizations. SASE.

Children's Hospice International
901 North Washington Street, Suite 700
Alexandria, VA 22314
1-800 2-4-CHILD
or (703) 684-0330
Provides information and support for health care professionals, families and the network of organizations within communities that offer hospice care to terminally ill children.

Choice in Aging, Inc.
200 Varick Street
New York, NY 10014
(212) 246-6962
   Provides living wills; will consult with families and individuals regarding their rights to refuse treatment. Professional education workshops.

Helping Ourselves Together (HOT)
8172 Magnolia Avenue
Riverside, CA 92504
(714) 688-5531
   Provides self support groups for anyone caring for a family member with long-term illness and/or disability.

National Hospice Organization
1901 North Moore Street, Suite 901
Arlington, VA 22209
1-800 658-8898
or (703) 234-5900
   Provides support and care for people in the final phase of a terminal disease so that they can live as fully and comfortably as possible and publishes directory of 1,900 hospice programs.

CESAREAN BIRTH

(See Childbirth)

CHILDBIRTH AND PREGNANCY

BIRTH ASSISTANTS

Informed Homebirth/Informed Birth and Parenting (IH/IBP)
P.O. Box 3675
Ann Arbor, MI 48106
(313) 662-6857
   Provides birth-assistant training throughout the United States and Canada with workshops and publications.

National Association of Childbirth Assistants
219 Meridian Avenue
San Jose, CA 95186-2926
(408) 225-9167
   Provides birth-assistant training through workshops and publications.

Pacific Prenatal Education Association
26280 Grant Avenue
Maple Ridge, British Columbia V2X 7E6
CANADA
(604) 462-0457
   Provides birth-assistant training in Canada through workshops and publications.

BIRTH CENTERS

National Association of Childbearing Centers
3123 Gottchall Road
Perkiomenville, PA 18074
(215) 234-8068

Provides information about more than 140 birth centers nationwide. Send $1 for postage and handling—no SASE required.

BIRTH DEFECTS

Alliance of Genetic Support Groups
35 Wisconsin Circle, Suite 440
Chevy Chase, MD 20815
1-800 336-GENE
or (301) 652-5553 (Maryland)

Refers callers to appropriate genetic support groups and provides publications.

Association for Birth Defect Children, Inc.
5400 Diplomat Circle, #270
Orlando, FL 32810
(407) 629-1466

Provides information and support to families of children with birth defects, including a quarterly newsletter; offers birth defects registry; and collects research about birth defects believed to be caused by a parent's exposure to drugs, chemicals, radiation and other environmental agents.

Intensive Caring Unlimited
910 Bent Lane
Philadelphia, PA 19118
(609) 848-1945

Provides information and support for those women who have a high-risk pregnancy; who have experienced a miscarriage, stillbirth, or death of a child; who have a hospitalized child and/or want to breastfeed a hospitalized child; or who have a child with a birth defect or who is developmentally delayed.

March of Dimes Birth Defects Foundation
National Headquarters
1275 Mamaroneck Avenue
White Plains, NY 10605
(914) 428-7100

Provides films, videos, and publications about healthy childbearing, birth defects and their prevention with information sheets on individual birth defects, such as club foot, Tay Sachs, and spina bifida.

National Institute of Environmental Health Sciences
National Institutes of Health
Public Affairs Office
Research Triangle Park, NC 27709
(919) 541-3345
    Provides latest research findings on cancer-causing agents and birth defects.

National Network to Prevent Birth Defects
Box 15309, Southeast Station
Washington, DC 20003
(202) 543-5450
    Supports political action to reduce birth defects and learning disabilities, particularly those from toxins, radiation, and drugs. Occasional newsletter.

Parents Helping Parents (PHP)
The Family Resource Center
535 Race Street, Suite 220
San Jose, CA 95126
1-800 397-9827
or (408) 288-5010
    Provides information and support to those who want to establish family resource centers and to parents of children who have special needs including counseling, support, referrals, and quarterly newsletter, *Special Addition.* $25/year.

(See Down Syndrome entry for other organizations.)

BOOKS, VIDEOS, AND SUPPLIES

Birth and Life Bookstore, Inc.
P.O. Box 70625
Seattle, WA 98107
1-800 736-0631
or (206) 789-4444
    Sells full range of mail-order birth, childcare, and women's health books.

Childbirth Graphics Ltd.
P.O. Box 20540
Rochester, NY 14602-0540
(716) 272-0300
    Sells childbirth education materials, including books, posters, pamphlets, and videos in English and Spanish.

Maternity Center Association
Publications Department
48 East 92nd Street
New York, NY 10128
(212) 369-7300
    Sells books, pamphlets, charts, slides, and videos for expectant parents, parent educators, and health care professionals.

Naturpath Medical & Birthing Supplies
1410 NW 13th Street, Suite 2
Gainesville, FL 32601
1-800 542-4784
or (904) 374-9655
   Sells home birth supplies, books, and baby items.

Spirit-Led Childbirth
Birthing and Parenting Supplies
1001-A East Harmony Road #303
Ft. Collins, CO 80525
(303) 663-6480
   Sells home-birth supplies and books.

WishGarden Herbs
P.O. Box 1304
Boulder, CO 80306
(303) 665-9508
   Sells quality herbal preparations for childbearing and general health.

BREASTFEEDING/LACTATION CONSULTANTS

International Lactation Consultant Association (ILCA)
201 Brown Avenue
Evanston, IL 60202
(708) 260-8874
   Provides professional organization for board-certified lactation consultants and other health professionals interested in breastfeeding. Quarterly publication, *Journal of Human Lactation*, annual conferences, and consumer referrals.

La Leche League International, Inc. (LLL)
P.O. Box 1209
9616 Minneapolis Avenue
Franklin Park, IL 60131-8209
1-800 LA-LECHE (9 A.M. – 3 P.M., Monday – Friday, Central Standard Time)
or (708) 455-7730
   Provides mother-to-mother breastfeeding information worldwide to one million women annually. Publications, including information sheets, newsletters, books for both consumers and health care professionals, and catalog of publications. Also tapes and Braille for the visually impaired regarding pregnancy, childbirth and breastfeeding. Contact for name of nearest LLL counselor.

Nursing Mothers Counsel, Inc.
P.O. Box 50063
Palo Alto, CA 94303
(415) 591-6688
   Provides information and encouragement to women who want to breastfeed and, in some areas, has electric breast pumps for rent. Chapters are located in various cities in California and Colorado as well as in Ft. Wayne, Indiana, and in Atlanta, Georgia. Call for a local number and free pamphlet.

CESAREAN BIRTH

Cesareans/Support, Education and Concern (C/SEC, Inc.)
22 Forest Road
Framingham, MA 01701
(508) 877-8266
   Provides support and information on cesarean childbirth, cesarean prevention, and vaginal birth after cesarean (VBAC).

International Cesarean Awareness Network (ICAN)
P.O. Box 152, University Station
Syracuse, NY 13210
(315) 424-1942
   Provides information about cesarean prevention and vaginal birth after cesarean (VBAC); more than 70 chapters nationwide; book catalog; and quarterly newsletter, *The Clarion.* $25/year.

Public Citizen's Health Research Group
2000 P Street, NW, Room 605
Washington, DC 20036
(202) 833-3000
   Sells publications, including the report "Unnecessary Cesarean Sections: Halting a National Epidemic." $10 for individuals/nonprofits; $20/businesses/hospitals.

Vaginal Birth After Cesarean (VBAC)
10 Great Plain Terrace
Needham, MA 02192
(617) 449-2490
   Provides VBAC information, workshops, and counseling.

CHILDBIRTH EDUCATION

Academy of Certified Birth Educators
2001 East Prairie Circle, Suite I
Olathe, KS 66062
1-800 444-8223
or (913) 782-5116
   Provides certification course for childbirth educators, including curriculum development, relaxation, labor and support techniques, teaching skills, and teen pregnancy.

American Academy of Husband-Coached Childbirth
1-800 423-2397
1-800 42-BIRTH (in California)
   Certifies and trains instructors in Bradley method of childbirth education and provides publications, videos, and referrals to Bradley teachers.

ASPO/Lamaze
1101 Connecticut Avenue, NW, Suite 700
Washington, DC 20036
1-800 368-4404
or (202) 857-1128 (Washington, DC)
Certifies and trains instructors in Lamaze method and provides information for consumers, including referrals to instructors, books about childbirth and family-centered maternity care, and magazines, including *Lamaze Parents* Magazine and *Genesis.* Videos about parenting are available through ASPO instructors.

Birth Works
International Cesarean Awareness Network (ICAN)
P.O. Box 152, University Station
Syracuse, NY 13210
(315) 424-1942
Combines traditional childbirth education classes with prevention of unnecessary cesareans.

Childbirth Without Pain Education Association
20134 Snowden
Detroit, MI 48325
(313) 345-9850 (10 A.M. – 4 P.M., Monday – Thursday)
Offers classes to expectant parents, certifies and trains instructors in the Lamaze method of painless childbirth, and provides publications and public film showings. SASE.

International Childbirth Education Association
P.O. Box 20048
Minneapolis, MN 55420
(612) 854-8660
Supports family-centered maternity care; provides books, pamphlets, and other publications including the *International Journal of Childbirth Education;* workshops; annual conferences. Certifies childbirth educators.

CHILDBIRTH ORGANIZATIONS

American Foundation for Maternal and Child Health
439 East 51st Street
New York, NY 10022
(212) 759-5510
Promotes unmedicated childbirth by sponsoring research and seminars, publishing literature, and lobbying national and state legislators and agencies.

National Association of Parents and Professionals for Safe
Alternatives (NAPSAC)
Rt. 1, Box 646
Marble Hill, MO 63764-9725
(314) 238-2010
Promotes education about all childbirth alternatives with newsletter, books, and other publications including *Directory of Alternative Birth Services.*

Circumcision

National Organization of Circumcision Information Resource
Centers (NO-CIRC)
P.O. Box 2512
San Anselmo, CA 94979-2512
(415) 488-9883

Provides information about avoiding circumcision and publications including a newsletter and pamphlet, *Circumcision Why*.

Peaceful Beginnings
13020 Homestead Court
Anchorage, AK 99516
(907) 345-4813

Provides printed information about avoiding circumcision and other childbirth-related issues.

Drugs and Pregnancy

Food and Drug Administration
5600 Fishers Lane, HFE-88
Rockville, MD 20857
(301) 443-3170

Provides free booklets including *Drugs and Pregnancy* and *The Perplexities of Pregnancy*.

Home Birth

Association for Childbirth at Home, International
116 South Louise Street
Glendale, CA 91250
(213) 667-0839

Provides information and support for home birth, including publications.

Informed Homebirth/Informed Birth & Parenting (IH/IBP)
P.O. Box 3675
Ann Arbor, MI 48106
(313) 662-6857

Trains and certifies childbirth educators and offers classes for couples planning home births; provides referrals to midwives; and offers publications including a newsletter and books; and videos.

Two Attune
Box 12-A
Harborside, ME 04642

Provides information for do-it-yourself, wife/husband home birth. Newsletter, $10/4 issues.

MIDWIFERY

American College of Nurse-Midwives (ACNM)
1522 K Street, NW, Suite 1000
Washington, DC 20005
(202) 289-0171
Provides certification of nurse-midwives; referrals for consumers; publications, including brochures and fact sheets; and a pregnancy calculator — a gestational wheel that estimates a due date.

Apprentice Academics
P.O. Box 788
Claremore, OK 74018-0788
(918) 342-1335
Offers midwifery home study course.

Association of Ontario Midwives
P.O. Box 85
Postal Station C
Toronto, Ontario M6J 3M7
CANADA
(416) 538-4389
Provides referrals for midwives in Ontario.

Association of Radical Midwives
62 Greetby Hill
Ormskirk, Lancashire L39 2DT
ENGLAND
0695-572776
Provides study and support for midwives and mothers, and information on choices in childbirth including quarterly journal, *Midwifery Matters*.

Fellowship of Christian Midwives and Childbirth Educators, International
P.O. Box 642
Parker, CO 80134
Provides information and support for Christian midwives, publications, referral service, childbirth-education certification, and continuing education and degree program for midwives.

Midwifery and the Law
Mothering Magazine
P.O. Box 1690
Santa Fe, NM 87504
1-800 424-3305
or (505) 984-8116
This publication provides current legal status and midwifery contacts in each state. $19.95.

Midwives Alliance of North America (MANA)
P.O. Box 1121
Bristol, VA 24203-2111
(615) 764-5561
 Provides support for all midwives and makes referrals to consumers for midwives in each state.

Seattle Midwifery School
2524 16th Avenue South, #300
Seattle, WA 98144
(206) 322-8834
 Trains direct-entry midwives and offers continuing education, labor support course, and other workshops.

MISCARRIAGE, STILLBIRTH, AND NEWBORN DEATH

A.M.E.N.D.
4324 Berrywick Terrace
St. Louis, MO 63128
(314) 487-7528
 Provides one-to-one contact with parents who lose a baby through miscarriage, stillbirth, or shortly after birth.

The Compassionate Friends
P.O. Box 3696
Oak Brook, IL 60522-3696
(708) 990-0010
 Provides support to parents who have experienced the death of a child. Hundreds of local chapters. Publications, booklist, newsletter.

HOPING
Kaiser Permanente
3288 Moanalua Road
Honolulu, HI 96819
(808) 834-5333, Extension 9903
 Provides a perinatal loss support group for parents, lending library, newsletter, parent-to-parent phone support, and group meetings.

Illowa Guild for Infant Survival
P.O. Box 3586
Davenport, IA 52808
(319) 322-4870
 Provides information and support for families who have lost a child to SIDS (sudden infant death syndrome).

Parents Resolving Infant Death Experiences (PRIDE)
Jersey Shore Medical Center
1945 Route 33
Neptune, NJ 07753
(908) 776-4316

Provides self-help and support groups for parents who have lost an infant for any reason or who have experienced pregnancy loss.

Pregnancy and Infant Loss Center (P.I.L.C.)
1421 East Wayzata Boulevard, Suite 30
Wayzata, MN 55391
(612) 473-9372

Provides referrals to support groups nationwide; publications including literature on pregnancy and infant loss and quarterly newsletter, *Loving Arms;* lending library; educational programs for parents and care providers; and consultation for professional care providers.

Pregnancy and Infant Loss Support, Inc. (SHARE)
St. Joseph Health Center
300 First Capitol Drive
St. Charles, MO 63301-2893
(314) 947-6164

Provides help for parents who have experienced miscarriage, stillbirth or newborn death with local groups; publications including bimonthly newsletter, manual for farewell rituals, book on starting your own SHARE group, and books on children's grief.

Shattered Dreams
21 Potsdam Road #61
Downsview, Ontario M3N IN3
CANADA
(416) 663-7143

Quarterly newsletter offering support, information, sharing and hope for the future to parents experiencing miscarriage. $16/4 issues. $4/sample issue.

The Southern California Pregnancy and Infant Loss Center
5505 East Carson Street, Suite 215
Lakewood, CA 90713
(310) 425-4889

Provides support, resources, information, and education on miscarriage, stillbirth, and infant death; referrals to parent support groups; monthly newsletter; lending library; and subsequent pregnancy support.

MOTHER-HELPERS

National Association of Postpartum Care Services
8910 299th Place, SW
Edmonds, WA 98026
(206) 771-4577

Provides referrals to more than 80 individuals or companies who provide woman-to-woman help after a baby is born. Offers publications, including a quarterly newsletter and cookbook, and national conferences for providers of these services.

MOTHERING ORGANIZATIONS

Healthy Mothers, Healthy Babies
409 12th Street, SW
Washington, DC 20024-2188
(202) 863-2458
   Promotes quality health care and education for mothers and children with national coalition that coordinates activities of member groups.

National Association of Mothers' Centers
336 Fulton Avenue
Hempstead, NY 11550
1-800 645-3828
or (516) 486-6614
   Provides a community program where women meet to explore the experience of becoming and being mothers. Contact them for location of 60 local groups, or how to start a center in your area.

Pacific Postpartum Support Society
#104-1416 Commercial Drive
Vancouver, British Columbia V5L 3K2
CANADA
(604) 255-7999
   Provides treatment program for mothers with postpartum depression and educational materials including the handbook, *Post Partum Depression and Anxiety: A Self-Help Guide for Mothers* for $7.95, plus $2.50 postage and handling (Canada or United States).

Woman's Workshop
P.O. Box 843
Coronado, CA 92118
   Newsletter to help at-home mothers explore outside interests and plan for life after motherhood. $16/4 issues.

MOTHERING PUBLICATIONS

The Birth Gazette
42, The Farm
Summertown, TN 38483
(615) 964-2519
   Publishes quarterly magazine for midwives, physicians, childbirth educators, parents, breastfeeding counselors, health planners, and legislators. $25/year.

Birth Journal
Blackwell Scientific Publications
Three Cambridge Center, Suite 208
Cambridge, MA 02142
(617) 225-0401
   Publishes quarterly journal about birth issues for nurses, consumers, midwives, childbirth educators, and physicians. $20/year, single issues $5.

The Compleat Mother
P.O. Box 399
Mildmay, Ontario N0G 2J0
CANADA
(519) 367-2394
    Publishes quarterly magazine about pregnancy, birth, and breastfeeding. $12/year.
Also sells posters, postcards, and books.

The Doula
P.O. Box 71
Santa Cruz, CA 95063-0071
(408) 464-9488
    Provides women and their families with support, inspiration, and resources to
foster an emotionally satisfying pregnancy and birth and mothering experiences.

Maternal Health News
Box 46563, Station G
Vancouver, British Columbia V6R 4G8
CANADA
    Publishes quarterly magazine about birth issues.

Midwifery Today and Childbirth Education
Box 2672
Eugene, OR 97405
1-800 743-0974
or (503) 344-7438
    Publishes quarterly magazine for midwives, childbirth educators, and others. Offers
books, tapes, and annual conference. $30/year.

Mothering Magazine
P.O. Box 1690
Santa Fe, NM 87504
1-800 424-3308
or (505) 984-8116
    Publishes magazine that celebrates parenting, advocates the needs and rights of the
child, and provides helpful information on which parents can base informed choices.
$22/4 issues per year.

PREMATURE BIRTH

Children in Hospitals, Inc.
31 Wilshire Park
Needham, MA 02192
(617) 482-2915
    Provides information about the need for ample contact between children and
parents when either is hospitalized. Encourages hospitals to adopt flexible visiting and
living-in policies. Offers publications including *1992 Directory of Massachusetts Hospitals*
for $5.

TWINS, TRIPLETS, AND QUADS

Center for Study of Multiple Births
333 East Superior Street, Suite 476
Chicago, IL 60611
(312) 266-9093
    Provides information including publications and books for parents of twins, triplets, and quadruplets.

Double Talk
P.O. Box 412
Amelia, OH 45102
(513) 231-8946
    Provides resource center including a newsletter for parents of twins, triplets, or more.

National Organization of Mothers of Twins Clubs, Inc.
12404 Princess Jeanne NE
Albuquerque, NM 87112-0955
    Offers opportunity for mothers of multiples to share information, concerns, and advice with information sheets, quarterly newsletter, and chapter development kit.

The Triplet Connection
8900 Thornton Road #25
P.O. Box 99571
Stockton, CA 95209
(209) 474-0885
    Provides information including a newsletter to families expecting triplets or more as well as encouragement, an information packet, resources, and networking with parents of other multiples.

Twinline, Services for Multiple Birth Families
P.O. Box 10066
Berkeley, CA 94709
(415) 644-0863 (10 A.M.–4 P.M., Monday–Friday, Pacific Standard Time)
or (415) 644-0861
    Provides services, publications, resource referral, and advocacy for families with twins, triplets, quadruplets, and quintuplets.

Twins Magazine
P.O. Box 12045
Overland Park, KS 66212
(913) 722-1090
    Bimonthly, national magazine offers a wide variety of viewpoints on twins, triplets, and more with research-based child development and family-living guidance. $21/year.

ULTRASOUND

National Institutes of Child Health and Human Development
Office of Research Reporting
Building 31, Room 2A-32
9000 Rockville Pike
Bethesda, MD 20892
(301) 496-5133
    Provides information about ultrasound including booklets and research reports.

CHIROPRACTIC

American Chiropractic Association
1701 Clarendon Boulevard
Arlington, VA 22209
(703) 276-8800
    Represents 20,000 doctors and students of chiropractic and disseminates information to the public and media about the benefits of chiropractic health care. Publications.

CHRONIC FATIGUE SYNDROME

The CFIDS Association, Inc.
P.O. Box 220398
Charlotte, NC 28222-0398
1-800 442-3437
or (900) 988-2343
    Provides referrals to local support groups, information on research and treatments, and publications including *The CFIDS Chronicle*. $25/year.

National Chronic Fatigue Syndrome Association, Inc.
3521 Broadway, Suite 222
Kansas City, MO 64111
(816) 931-4777 (24-hour information line)
    Provides medical journal reprints; quarterly newsletter, *Heart of America News*, brochures, physician packets, and other publications; referrals to at least 400 support groups; and conferences. SASE.

United Federation of CFS/CFIDS/CEBV Organizations
P.O. Box 14603
Tucson, AZ 85732
(602) 298-8627
    Provides clearinghouse information for both health care professionals and the public, as well as referrals to CFS support groups. SASE.

Community Health Care

Information USA, Inc.
P.O. Box E
Kensington, MD 20895
1-800 955-POWER
   Ask for copy of *Free Health Care* which provides 200 federal, state, and local resources for *free* health care.

National Association of Community Health Centers, Inc.
1330 New Hampshire Avenue, NW, #122
Washington, DC 20036
(202) 659-8008
   Contact for the name of your state association to find out the location of one of the 600 clinics providing prevention-oriented medical care near you.

National League for Nursing
350 Hudson Street
New York, NY 10014
(212) 989-9393
   Contact for the name of your state nursing association to find out the location of one of their 300 clinics which provide primary and preventive care, as well as home care to the acutely, chronically, and terminally ill. Staffed by nurses, these clinics are often associated with hospitals, home health agencies, or public health departments.

Visiting Nurse Associations of America
3801 East Florida Avenue, Suite 900
Denver, CO 80210
1-800 426-2547
   Contact for referral to local visiting nurses.

Cosmetic Surgery

American Academy of Cosmetic Surgery
159 East Live Oak Avenue, #204
Arcadia, CA 91006
1-800 221-9808
   Provides information and physician referrals.

American Society for Dermatologic Surgery
930 North Meacham Road
Schaumberg, IL 60173-6016
1-800 441-2737
or (708) 330-9830
   Provides referrals to dermatologic surgeons and information about the cosmetic surgery they perform.

American Society of Plastic and Reconstructive Surgeons
401 North Michigan Avenue
Chicago, IL 60611-4267
1-800 635-0635
   Provides names of board-certified plastic surgeons and for women having breast implant problems, provides information, free phone consultation with plastic surgeon, and — if necessary — one free visit with a plastic surgeon.

Coalition of Silicone Survivors
P.O. Box 129
Broomfield, CO 80038-0129
(303) 469-8242
   Provides information about breast implants and monthly support groups.

Command Trust Network
P.O. Box 17082
Covington, KY 41017
(606) 331-0055
   Provides information, support groups for women who have had problems with breast implants, and referrals to physicians.

Facial Plastic Surgery Information Service, Inc.
1110 Vermont Avenue, NW, Suite 220
Washington, DC 20005
1-800 332-FACE
or (202) 842-4500 (Washington, DC)
   Provides referrals to board-certified plastic surgeons as well as printed information.

FDA Breast Implant Information Line
5600 Fishers Lane, HFE 88
Rockville, MD 20857
1-800 532-4440 (9 A.M.–7 P.M., Monday–Friday, Eastern Standard Time)
or (301) 443-4130 (Maryland)
   Provides free "Update on Silicone Gel–filled Breast Implants," which summarizes FDA's position on implants, explains risks and complications of these implants, and what you can do if you already have an implant.

FDA Problem Reporting Network
5600 Fishers Lane, HFE 88
Rockville, MD 20857
1-800 638-6725
or (301) 638-6725 (call collect in Maryland)
   Call to report problems with implants, but not to get general information. (See listing immediately above for that.)

MedicAlert International Breast Implant Registry
2323 Colorado Avenue, Department 95X
Turlock, CA 95380
1-800 892-9211

Provides system for tracking and notifying women with breast implants and their physicians for advisories on specific implant brands. Contacts doctors first, then notifies each woman directly within two weeks. Also provides publications about breast implants including a newsletter. $25/year, $15/renewal year.

(See also Medical Devices, Implants, and Other Technology in a separate entry.)

DENTAL HEALTH

Environmental Dental Association
1-800 388-8124
or (619) 586-7626
Provides free information packets, research data on mercury fillings, and referrals to more than 700 mercury-free dentists.

National Institute of Dental Research
National Institutes of Health
Building 31, Room 2C35
9000 Rockville Pike
Bethesda, MD 20892
(301) 496-4261
Provides free brochures about tooth decay, oral health, and other dental topics.

DIETHYLSTILBESTROL (DES)

DES Action U.S.A.
1615 Broadway, #510
Oakland, CA 94612
(510) 465-4011
Provides medical and legal referrals, educational information to DES-exposed people and health practitioners, advocacy, support, legislative work, research, and publications including quarterly newsletter. SASE.

DES Cancer Network
P.O. Box 10185
Rochester, NY 14610
(716) 473-6119
Provides information about DES including newsletter, *DCN News*, research advocacy, and person-to-person support.

DISABLED WOMEN

DateABLE
35 Wisconsin Circle, Suite 205
Chevy Chase, MD 20815
(301) 657-DATE
Provides dating service and social club for people with and without physical disabilities and medical illnesses. Newsletter.

Heath Resource Center
One Dupont Circle, Suite 800
Washington, DC 20036
1-800 544-3284
    National clearinghouse that provides information and referrals to local sources as well as publications.

Information Center for Individuals with Disabilities
Fort Point Place
27-43 Wormwood Street
Boston, MA 02210-1606
1-800 462-5015 (Massachusetts only)
or (617) 727-5540
    Provides information, including newsletter, *Disability Issues;* referral; and problem-solving assistance to people (primarily in Massachusetts) who have disabilities, their families, friends, and service providers.

Learning How, Incorporated
P.O. Box 35481
Charlotte, NC 28235
(704) 376-4735
    Provides programs to enable disabled women and men to reach their fullest potential and coordinates chapter development.

National Organization on Disability
910 16th Street, NW
Washington, DC 20006
1-800 248-ABLE
    Provides information, including fact sheets and referrals, regarding disability problems.

The National Shut-In Society, Inc.
P.O. Box 986, Village Station
New York, NY 10014-0986
(212) 255-2596
    Provides cheer and comfort to chronic invalids without regard to race, creed, or color. SASE.

Siblings for Significant Change
United Charities Building
105 East 22nd Street
New York, NY 10010
(212) 420-0776
    Provides peer support for siblings of disabled people, legal direction, access to psychological professionals, social functions. Publications. SASE.

Sibling Information Network
A.J. Pappanikou Center
991 Main Street
East Hartford, CT 06108
(203) 282-7050
Provides information relating to siblings who have a brother or sister with disabilities.

DOWN SYNDROME

Association for Retarded Citizens
2501 Avenue J
Arlington, TX 76006
(817) 640-0204
Provides services to the mentally retarded and their families including education, publication, and advocacy.

National Down Syndrome Congress
1800 Dempster Street
Park Ridge, IL 60068-1146
1-800 232-6372
or (708) 823-7550
Provides political advocacy and clearinghouse for DS information including *Down Syndrome News*, recommended reading lists, and other publications.

National Down Syndrome Society
666 Broadway
New York, NY 10012
1-800 221-4602 Hotline
or (212) 460-9330 (New York)
Provides fact sheets, videos, and other materials and services for parents of children with Down syndrome.

National Institute of Child Health and Human Development
National Institutes of Health
Building 31, Room 2A-32
9000 Rockville Pike
Bethesda, MD 20892
(301) 496-5133
Provides free booklet, *Facts About Down Syndrome for Women over 35*.

(See Birth Defects entry for additional organizations.)

DRUGS

(See Prescription and Over-the-Counter Drugs or see Recreational Drugs)

EATING DISORDERS

American Anorexia/Bulimia Association, Inc.
418 East 76th Street
New York, NY 10021
(212) 734-1114
    Provides information including newsletter and other publications about anorexia and bulimia, support groups, referral network, and speakers bureau.

Anorexia Nervosa and Related Eating Disorders, Inc. (ANRED)
P.O. Box 5102
Eugene, OR 97405
(503) 344-1144
    Provides support and information including free booklet and newsletter, *Anred Alert*. $10/year, 10 issues.

National Anorectic Aid Society
1925 East Dublin-Granville Road
Columbus, OH 43229-35117
(614) 436-1112
    Provides assistance and information packets.

National Association of Anorexia Nervosa and Associated Disorders
P.O. Box 85
Highland Park, IL 60035
(312) 831-3438

National Institute of Child Health and Human Development
National Institutes of Health
9000 Rockville Pike
Building 31, Room 2A-32
Bethesda, MD 20892
(301) 496-5133
    Provides free pamphlet about anorexia.

EMOTIONAL HEALTH

Agoraphobics in Motion
1729 Crooks Road, #101
Royal Oak, MI 48067-1306
(313) 547-0400
    Provides support groups nationwide for the purpose of recovery from agoraphobia and other anxiety disorders.

Depressives Anonymous — Recovery from Depression, Inc.
329 East 62nd Street
New York, NY 10021
    Provides information to the public and training to mental health personnel about depression; local networks; information on starting a local group; publications; newsletter. SASE.

Emotional Health Anonymous
2420 San Gabriel Boulevard
Rosemead, CA 91770
(818) 573-5482

Provides support to persons who are recovering from emotional problems or illnesses. Contact for local group. Publications. SASE.

Emotions Anonymous
P.O. Box 4245
St. Paul, MN 55104
(612) 647-9712

Provides self-help program for people with emotional difficulties.

National Alliance for the Mentally Ill
2101 Wilson Boulevard, Suite 302
Arlington, VA 22201
1-800 950-6264
or (703) 524-7600

Provides information for families of persons with serious mental illness. 1,000 groups nationwide. SASE.

National Association of Psychiatric Survivors
P.O. Box 618
Sioux Falls, SD 57101
(605) 334-4067 (10 A.M.–12 P.M.)

Provides advocacy to promote the rights of mental patients and is specifically opposed to involuntary psychiatric treatment. SASE.

National Foundation for Depressive Illness
P.O. Box 2257
New York, NY 10116
1-800 248-4344
or (212) 268-4260

Provides a recorded message about the symptoms and treatment of depression as well as publications and referrals to both physicians and local support groups.

National Institute of Mental Health
5600 Fishers Lane, Room 15C05
Rockville, MD 20857
(301) 443-4515

Provides free booklets on depression and mental health.

On Our Own, Inc.
5422 Belair Road
Baltimore, MD 21206
(301) 488-4480

Provides advocacy and support for women who have spent time in psychiatric facilities and who are now ex-patients. Publications including newsletter. SASE.

ENDOMETRIOSIS

Endometriosis Alliance of Greater Washington
P.O. Box 11695
Washington, DC 20008-0895
(301) 369-1452
 Provides support groups, public lectures, and newsletter. SASE.

Endometriosis Association
8585 North 76th Place
Milwaukee, WI 53223
1-800 992-3636
or 1-800 426-2END (Canada)
 Provides support and information, including video, book *Overcoming Endometriosis*, and other literature. SASE.

EXERCISE

Melpomene Institute for Women's Health Research
1010 University Avenue
St. Paul, MN 55104
(612) 642-1951
 Provides information about women and exercise, including information about menopause and osteoporosis, original research, and the *Melpomene Journal.* $32/year/3 issues.

President's Council on Physical Fitness and Sports
701 Pennsylvania Avenue, NW, Suite 250
Washington, DC 20004
(202) 272-3421
 Provides free copies of publications about walking, swimming, and other forms of exercise.

Women's Sport Foundation
342 Madison Avenue, #728
New York, NY 10173
1-800 227-3988
or (212) 972-9170 (Alaska, Hawaii, and California)
 Provides educational material about women in sports including exercise guides.

FAT ACCEPTANCE

National Association to Advance Fat Acceptance, Inc. (NAAFA)
P.O. Box 188620
Sacramento, CA 95818
(916) 443-0303
 Provides information and support including the *NAAFA Newsletter;* local chapters; annual convention and regional gatherings; dating service; and special interest groups for feminists, military personnel, lesbians, super-size women, and midsize women.

Radiance
Magazine for Large Women
P.O. Box 30246
Oakland, CA 94604
(510) 482-0680
    Publishes quarterly magazine, $15/year.

FOOD

American Institute for Cancer Research
1759 R Street, NW
Washington, DC 20009
1-800 843-8114
    Call for nutrition questions and to order brochures about diet and cancer prevention.

Beano
AkPharma Inc.
P.O. Box 111
Pleasantville, NJ 08232-0111
1-800 257-8650
    See description of this food enzyme product on page 28.

National Cancer Institute
Office of Cancer Communications
Building 31, Room 10A-24
9000 Rockville Pike
Bethesda, MD 20892
1-800 4-CANCER
1-800 492-6000 (Maryland)
    Offers free 51-page pamphlet, *Diet, Nutrition and Cancer Prevention: A Guide to Food Choices.*

VEGETARIAN

Vegetarian Times
P.O. Box 570
Oak Park, IL 60303
1-800 435-9610
or (708) 848 8120
    Publishes monthly cooking and service magazine featuring articles on health, fitness, the environment, interviews, and other topics as they relate to a vegetarian life-style. $24.95/year for 12 issues.

Food and Drug Administration
5600 Fishers Lane, HFE88
Rockville, MD 20857
(301) 443-3170
    Distributes publications including *The Confusing World of Health Foods.*

Jewish Vegetarians of North America
6938 Reliance Road
Federalsburg, MD 21632
(410) 754-5550
　　Provides publications including quarterly *Jewish Vegetarians Newsletter*. $24/year.

Vegetarian Resource Group
P.O. Box 1463
Baltimore, MD 21203
(410-366-8343)
　　Provides clearinghouse for vegetarian information and publishes 36-page, bi-monthly *Vegetarian Journal*. $20/year.

HEADACHES

(see Migraine Headaches)

HEALTH NEWSLETTERS

Among the dozens of good health newsletters that are available, following are six of the best because they are consumer oriented, well researched, and thorough. Two (indicated with an *) are for women only.

Health Letter
Public Citizen Health Research Group
2000 P Street, NW, Room 605
Washington, DC 20036
(202) 833-3000
　　Provides legislative advocacy and sells books, other publications including a magazine, and a monthly newsletter. $18/year.

HealthFacts Newsletter
Center for Medical Consumers
237 Thompson Street
New York, NY 10012-1090
(212) 674-7105
　　Provides drop-in library and sells other publications, including health resource guides. $21/12 issues per year.

Healthsharing
14 Skey Lane
Toronto, Ontario M6J 354
CANADA
(416) 532-0812
　　Publishes quarterly magazine about women's health issues. $19/USA (individuals), $32/USA (institutions), $15/Canada (individuals), and $28/Canada (institutions).

Network News
National Women's Health Network
1325 G Street, NW
Washington, DC 20005
(202) 347-1140
Provides information and support for women's issues and sells publications, including fact sheets, pamphlets, and bimonthly newsletter about women's health issues. $25/year.

Nutrition Action Healthletter
Center for Science in the Public Interest
1875 Connecticut Avenue, NW, Suite 300
Washington, DC 20009-5728
(202) 332-9110
Provides up-to-date look at nutrition in today's grocery stores and restaurants and sells posters, books, pamphlets, and newsletter. $19.95/10 issues.

People's Medical Society Newsletter
462 Walnut Street
Allentown, PA 18102
1-800 624-8773
or (215) 770-1670
Publishes newsletter and other publications including "Vital Information" packets, books, and other resources. $20/year.

HEART

American Heart Association
7272 Greenville Avenue
Dallas, TX 75231-4596
1-800 AHA-USA1
or (214) 373-6300
Provides local chapters and publications to reduce disability and death from cardiovascular diseases and stroke.

The Coronary Club, Inc.
9500 Euclid Avenue
Cleveland, OH 44195
(216) 444-3690
Provides information and support for people who have had heart attacks including the monthly newsletter, *Heartline.* $20/year.

Mended Hearts
7272 Greenville Avenue
Dallas, TX 75231-4596
(214) 706-1442
Provides help, encouragement, and advice to those who will be having or have had heart surgery.

NHLBI Information Center
P.O. Box 30105
Bethesda, MD 20824-0105
(301) 951-3260
 Provides free copies of publications about cardiovascular risk factors such as cholesterol, high blood pressure, and smoking.

HOME TESTING KITS

Medical Self-Care
5850 Shellmound Avenue
Emoryville, CA 94662-0813
1-800 345-3371
 Call for copy of the catalog which includes kits for ear analysis, bladder infection detection, and blood pressure monitoring.

HOMEOPATHY

Foundation for Homeopathic Education & Research
2124 Kittredge Street
Oakland, CA 94704-1436
(510) 649-8930
 Provides information including a newsletter and books. SASE.

Homeopathic Educational Services
2124 Kittredge Street
Oakland, CA 94704-1436
(510) 649-8930
 Sells homeopathic books, tapes, medicine kits, and software.

National Center for Homeopathy
801 N. Fairfax, Suite 306
Alexandria, VA 22314
(703) 548-7790
 Provides physician referrals and general information packet.

HOSPITAL CARE

U.S. Department of Health and Human Services
Public Health Service
Rockville, MD 20857
1-800 638-0742 (9:30 A.M. – 5:30 P.M., Monday – Friday, Eastern Standard Time)
1-800 492-0359 (Maryland)
 Provides referrals to facilities that have free and/or below cost care. Might be able to provide guidance if your hospital won't give you free medical care even though you're eligible.

HYSTERECTOMY

Hysterectomy Educational Resources and Services (HERS)
422 Bryn Mawr Avenue
Bala Cynwyd, PA 19004
(215) 667-7757

Provides free telephone counseling about alternatives to hysterectomy and coping with the consequences of the surgery. Newsletter, conferences, and physician second-opinion referral list. SASE.

INFERTILITY

The American Fertility Society
1209 Montgomery Highway
Birmingham, AL 35216

Provides information on all aspects of infertility, reproductive endocrinology, conception control, and reproductive biology. Resource lists and publications.

Resolve, Inc.
1310 Broadway
Somerville, MA 02144-1731
(617) 623-0744

Provides infertility support, referrals to doctors and hospitals, nationwide chapters, and publications including newsletter, fact sheets, and books.

INTERSTITIAL CYSTITIS

Interstitial Cystitis and Related Disorders (ICARD)
233 Rohner Avenue
Akron, OH 44319
(216) 644-0838

Provides support and education for women with interstitial cystitis including quarterly newsletter, *ICARD News*. SASE.

Interstitial Cystitis Association
P.O. Box 1533, Madison Square Station
New York, NY 10159
(212) 979-6057

Provides support and education for women with interstitial cystitis including the newsletter, *ICA Update;* video; national and local meetings; and other resources. SASE.

(See also Women Urologists entry)

LASER SURGERY

(See Surgery)

LATINA WOMEN'S HEALTH

Mexican-American Women's National Association
1101 17th Street, NW, Suite 803
Washington, DC 20036
(202) 833-0060
    Provides an advocacy organization for Latina women.

National Conference of Puerto Rican Women, Inc.
5 Thomas Circle, NW
Washington, DC 20005
(202) 387-4716
    Provides training through conferences for Puerto Rican and other Latina women
to enhance their participation in their economic, social, and political lives.

National Institute for Women of Color
1301 20th Street, NW
Washington, DC 20036
(202) 296-2661
    Provides information and support for women of color (Asian-Pacific, African-
American, Latina, Native American, and Alaskan Native) in leadership, reproductive
rights, teenage pregnancy, domestic violence, and families.

National Latina Health Organizations
P.O. Box 7567
1900 Fruitvale Avenue
Oakland, CA 94601
(510) 534-1362
    Provides information, including publications, and support.

U.S. Office of Minority Health Resource Center
P.O. Box 37337
Washington, DC 20013-7337
1-800 444-6472
    Provides data base information primarily for health professionals, but also gives
referrals to organizations for consumers as well.

LESBIAN HEALTH

Lesbian Mothers National Defense Fund
P.O. Box 21567
Seattle, WA 98111
(206) 325-2643
    Provides attorney referral, personal and emotional support, 24-hour answering
service, and alternative conception and adoption information. Quarterly newsletter,
$10/year.

Pacific Women's Resources
1208 East Pine
Seattle, WA 98122
(206) 322-DYKE
Provides groups, workshops, lending library, monthly newspaper, extensive information and referral resources including job and housing files. Drop-in center is open Monday – Friday, 2 – 7 P.M.

LUPUS

American Lupus Society
3914 Del Amo Boulevard, Suite 922
Torrance, CA 90503
1-800 331-1802
or (310) 542-8891
Provides information and support including fact sheets, newsletter *LUPUS Today*, and referrals to physicians and local groups.

Bay Area Lupus Foundation
2635 North First Street, Suite 206
San Jose, CA 95134
1-800 523-3363 (California only)
or (408) 954-8600
Provides information and support including the quarterly *Bay Area Lupus Foundation Newsletter.*

Lupus Foundation of America, Inc.
4 Research Place, Suite 180
Rockville, MD 20850-3226
1-800 558-0121
or (301) 670-9292
Provides information and support including brochures, fact sheets, newsletter articles, and referrals to local groups.

Lupus Research Institute
3 Duke Place
South Norwalk, CT 06854
1-800 82-LUPUS
or (203) 852-0120 (Connecticut)
Provides referrals to lupus centers.

National Arthritis and Musculoskeletal and Skin Diseases Information Clearinghouse
Box AMS
Bethesda, MD 20892
(301) 495-4484
Provides free copy of the kit, "What Black Women Should Know About Lupus."

MAMMOGRAPHY

National Cancer Institute Hot line
Rocky Mountain Cancer Information Service
P.O. Box 7021
Colorado Springs, CO 80933
1-800 4-CANCER
   Call to find out which mammogram facilities in your area (United States only) are accredited by the American College of Radiology.

MEDICAL DEVICES, IMPLANTS, AND OTHER TECHNOLOGY

Device Experience Administration and Monitoring Branch
1390 Piccard Drive, HFZ-343
Rockville, MD 20850
(301) 427-8100
   Provides computer data base on specific medical devices.

Food and Drug Administration
Center for Devices and Radiological Health
5600 Fishers Lane, HFZ-210
Rockville, MD 20857
(301) 443-4190
   Provides information on medical devices and radiologic health products that impact on women's health including mammography, x-rays, contraceptives, dental implants, and contact lenses. Publications in English and Spanish.

Food and Drug Administration
Medical Devices Recall and Notification Office
5600 Fishers Lane
Rockville, MD 20857
(301) 427-1122
   Contact to check status of any medical device.

International Implant Registry
2323 Colorado Avenue
Turlock, CA 95380
1-800 245 1492
   Provides updated information about specific medical implants and tracks patients with implants of any kind, so they can receive notification about recalls and safety alerts

U.S. Congress, Office of Technology Assessment
Publications Order
Washington, DC 20510-8025
(202) 224-8996
   Publishes numerous, thorough reports about medical technology. Contact for publications catalog and prices.

MEDICAL INSURANCE

Health Insurance Association of America
1005 Connecticut Avenue, NW
Washington, DC 20036
1-800 635-1271
   Provides publications and general information about buying insurance, how to evaluate insurance companies and insurance agents, and how to save money.

National Health Information Centers
P.O. Box 1133
Washington, DC 20013-1133
1-800 336-4797 (9 A.M. – 5 P.M., Monday – Friday, Eastern Standard Time)
   Provides pre-recorded messages with referrals to helpful organizations.

National Insurance Consumer Helpline
1025 Connecticut Avenue, NW
Washington, DC 20036
1-800 942-4242 (8 A.M. – 10 P.M., Monday – Friday, Eastern Standard Time)
   Provides consumer tips on insurance and makes referrals for claim problems.

National Insurance Consumer Organization
121 North Payne Street
Alexandria, VA 22314
(703) 549-8050
   Provides information including publications about buying insurance and makes referrals about the handling of specific insurance problems.

Office of Prepaid Health Care
Health Care Financing Administration
Cohen Building, Room 4360
330 Independence Avenue, SW
Washington, DC 20201
(202) 619-3555
   Provides information, legal advice, and investigative resources if you are dissatisfied with your health maintenance organization (HMO) care.

MENOPAUSE

Melpomene Institute for Women's Health Research
1010 University Avenue
St. Paul, MN 55104
(612) 642-1951
   Provides information about women and exercise, including information about menopause and osteoporosis, original research, and the *Melpomene Journal*. $32 for 3 issues/year.

Menopause News
2074 Union Street, Suite 10
San Francisco, CA 94123
(415) 567-2368
   Publishes 6-page, bimonthly newsletter with the latest medical and psychological information, including first-person stories and book reviews. 6 issues/$24.

MidLife Woman
5129 Logan Avenue South
Minneapolis, MN 55419-1019
1-800 88-MIDLIFE
   Publishes 8-page newsletter which discusses menopause, social roles, stress, health, relationships, and sexuality, and provides research updates. Call for free copy. 6 issues/$25.

Older Women's League (OWL)
666 11th Street, NW, Suite 700
Washington, DC 20001
(202) 783-6686
   Provides advocacy about health issues of older women, referrals to local chapters, and newsletter, *The OWL Observer*, 6 issues/year.

MENSTRUAL EXTRACTION

(See Women's Health Centers)

MIDWIFERY

(See Childbirth)

MIGRAINE HEADACHES

National Headache Foundation
5252 North Western Avenue
Chicago, IL 60625
1-800 843-2256
or (312) 878-7715
   Provides publications including fact sheets, booklets, and newsletter.

MINORITY WOMEN

(See Black Women's Health, Latina Women's Health, or Native American Women's Health)

MISCARRIAGE, STILLBIRTH, AND NEWBORN DEATH

(See Childbirth and Pregnancy)

MONOSODIUM GLUTAMATE

(See Additives, Preservatives, and Other Food Chemicals)

NATIVE AMERICAN WOMEN'S HEALTH

Native American Women's Health Education Resource Center
Lake Andes, SD 57356
(605) 487-7072
　　Provides publications on health care issues such as cancer awareness, nutrition, and fetal alcohol syndrome and other resources including a women's shelter.

NUTRASWEET/ASPARTAME

(See Additives, Preservatives, and Other Food Chemicals)

NATUROPATHY

American Association of Naturopathic Physicians
P.O. Box 20386
Seattle, WA 98102
(206) 323-7610
　　Provides referrals to primary-care physicians who have completed four years of naturopathic education and publishes quarterly newsletter, *The Naturopathic Physician*.

NUTRITION

(See Food)

OCCUPATIONAL HEALTH

Massachusetts Coalition for Occupational Safety and Health
555 Amory Street
Boston, MA 02130
(617) 524-6686
　　Provides a health and safety library, videos, many factsheets, and a newsletter, *MassCOSH Health and Safety News*, for the purpose of improving health and safety conditions in the workplace.

Occupational Health Clearinghouse
Technical Information Branch
National Institute for Occupational Safety & Health
4676 Columbia Parkway
Cincinnati, OH 45226-1998
1-800 35-NIOSH
　　Provides information on occupational health hazards.

OSTEOPOROSIS

Food and Drug Administration
Office of Public Affairs
5600 Fishers Lane, HFE88
Rockville, MD 20857
(301) 443-3170
 Provides free publications about osteoporosis.

National Arthritis and Musculoskeletal and Skin Diseases Information Clearinghouse
Box AMS
Bethesda, MD 20892
(301) 468-3235
 Provides osteoporosis information regarding the disease description, diagnosis, treatment, and prevention; patient education, care, and rehabilitation; physical and occupational therapy; diet, exercise, and medication; psychosocial factors; demography, epidemiology, and statistics.

National Osteoporosis Foundation
2100 M Street, NW, Suite 602
Washington, DC 20037
(202) 223-2226
 Provides latest osteoporosis treatment information.

PELVIC INFLAMMATORY DISEASE (PID)

The Canadian Pelvic Inflammatory Disease (PID) Society
P.O. Box 33804, Station D
Vancouver, British Columbia V6J 4L6
CANADA
(604) 684-5704
 Provides counseling; information; referrals; public education, including materials and programs; telephone support networks; and resource materials such as medical research, articles, pamphlets, fact sheets, and videos. Will accept collect calls, even from the United States, if person cannot afford to call.

PREGNANCY

(See Childbirth and Pregnancy)

PREMENSTRUAL SYNDROME (PMS)

Cycles
P.O. Box 524
Sharon, MA 02067
 Provides education, support, and a comprehensive handbook, *Conquering PMS*. Send SASE for table of contents.

PMS Access
P.O. Box 9326
Madison, WI 53715
1-800 222-4767 Hotline
or (608) 833-4767 (Wisconsin)
  Provides free information, books, tapes, and doctor referrals for PMS.

PRESCRIPTION AND OVER-THE-COUNTER DRUGS

Food and Drug Administration
Office of Public Affairs
5600 Fishers Lane, HFE88
Rockville, MD 20857
(301) 443-3170
  Provides free booklets, including *Food and Drug Interactions* and *A Guide to the Proper Use of Tranquilizers.*

Pharmaceutical Manufacturers Association Hotline
1-800 762-4636 (for physicians only)
or (202) 393-5200
  If you have a low income, ask your doctor to call this hotline to find out if a drug you need is available free from a pharmaceutical company.

Pill Addicts Anonymous
P.O. Box 278
Reading, PA 19603
(215) 372-1128 (answering machine)
  Provides self-help groups for those who must get off and stay off prescribed, mood-altering medications. SASE.

World Service Office, Inc.
Narcotics Anonymous
P.O. Box 9999
Van Nuys, CA 91409
(818) 780-3951
  Provides program for addicts to help each other recover. Any addict who has a desire to stop using drugs is eligible for membership and there are no fees. Check local phone book for Narcotics Anonymous.

RECREATIONAL DRUGS

Families Anonymous
P.O. Box 528
Van Nuys, CA 91408
(818) 989-7841
  Provides fellowship for relatives and friends of people involved in the abuse of mind-altering substances or exhibiting related behavioral problems such as runaways, delinquents, underachievers, and so on. Local groups. Publications. Send $2 for information packet.

National Cocaine Hotline
P.O. Box 100
Summit, NJ 07902
1-800 COC-AINE (24 hours/day, seven days/week)
    Refers callers to local cocaine treatment programs.

Wisconsin Clearinghouse
315 North Henry Street
Madison, WI 53703-2018
1-800 322-1468
or (608) 263-6884
    Develops and publishes materials about drugs, alternatives to drug abuse, preven-
tion, and mental health for youth, families, and women. Provides free catalog of
publications.

RESEARCH SERVICES

Boston Women's Health Book Collective
290A Elm Street
Somerville, MA 02144
(617) 625-0271
    Provides more than two dozen pre-assembled information packets from medical
journals and the feminist press on women's health issues. Will also prepare individualized literature search packets. SASE for list of topics as well as description of other
BWHBC projects.

The Health Resource, Inc.
209 Katherine Drive
Conway, AR 72032
(501) 329-5272
    Provides individualized, comprehensive research reports on your medical condi-
tion including treatment options — both conventional and alternative — self-help measures, resource organizations, and specialists. Reports average 50 to 150 pages. Request
brochure.

Planetree Health Resource Center
2040 Webster Street
San Francisco, CA 94115
(415) 923-3680
    Provides free medical library open to the general public including information on
alternative therapies. Sells medical data base information for $25 to $100, depending on
the extent of the search and the scope of your questions.

Your Local Library
    Perhaps will provide a free computer search on a health-related problem and
perhaps will provide up to 20 citations, although usually not the full article. (Not all
libraries provide this service.)

SELF-HELP GROUP CLEARINGHOUSES

California Self-Help Center
UCLA
2327 Franz Hall, 405 Hilgard Avenue
Los Angeles, CA 90024-1563
1-800 222-LINK
or (310) 825-1799
    Provides a statewide resource center to help people find and form self-help groups for a wide variety of personal and emotional health concerns.

Community Care Resources
919 LaFond Avenue
St. Paul, MN 55104
(612) 642-4060
    Provides training, consultation, information, and advocacy to religious congregations, human service programs, government, and mutual-help groups that serve children, families, and older persons. Free mutual-help directory for Minnesotans.

Massachusetts Clearinghouse of Mutual Help Groups
113 Skinner Hall
University of Massachusetts
Amherst, MA 01003
(413) 545-2313
    Provides clearinghouse for all self-help groups currently active within Massachusetts, encourages the formation of these groups, and sponsors conferences.

National Self-Help Clearinghouse
25 West 43rd Street, Room 620
New York, NY 10036
(212) 642-2944
    Provides information and referral services to self-help groups nationwide. SASE.

Self-Help Clearinghouse
St. Clare's Riverside Medical Center
25 Pocono Road
Denville, NJ 07834
(201) 625-9565
    Provides help, including publications, in finding and forming self-help groups and self-help clearinghouses. SASE.

Westchester Self-Help Clearinghouse
456 North Street
White Plains, NY 10605
(914) 949-6301
    Provides information and referral to self-help groups in Westchester County, assistance in starting new groups, and training for self-help group leaders.

SEXUAL ABUSE

(See Abuse)

SEXUAL HARASSMENT

(See Abuse)

SEXUAL HEALTH

Sex Information and Education Council of the U.S. (SIECUS)
130 West 42nd Street, Suite 2500
New York, NY 10036
(212) 819-9770
    Publishes a bimonthly journal, brochures, and other publications related to sexuality research, education, and legislation.

SEXUALLY TRANSMITTED DISEASES (STDs)

Herpes Resource Center
American Social Health Association
P.O. Box 13827
Research Triangle Park, NC 27709
(919) 361-8488 (9 A.M. – 7 P.M., Monday – Friday, Eastern Standard Time)
    Provides education, referrals to support groups, and publications including quarterly journal, *The Helper*. SASE.

National STD Hotline
American Social Health Association
P.O. Box 13827
Research Triangle Park, NC 27709
1-800 227-8922 (8 A.M. – 11 P.M., Monday – Friday, Eastern Standard Time)
    Provides information and referrals regarding STDs.

SINGLE MOTHERS

Women on Their Own
P.O. Box 1026
Willingboro, NJ 08046
(609) 871-1499
    Provides advocacy, networking, loans, workshops, and a newsletter for women raising children on their own (divorced, separated, widowed, single).

(See also Widows in a separate entry)

SKIN HEALTH

Food and Drug Administration
5600 Fishers Lane
Rockville, MD 20857
(301) 443-1240
   Provides information and help if you have a skin problem (burning, itching, or other irritation) due to a cosmetic.

SURGERY

American Society for Laser Medicine and Surgery
425 Pine Ridge Boulevard
Wausau, WI 54401
(715) 845-9283
   Provides referrals to doctors who perform laser surgery.

Laser Surgery Referral Network
P.O. Box 1133
Washington, DC 20013
(202) 429-9091
   Provides referrals to organizations and agencies involved with laser surgery that can then refer you to experts in the field.

Second Surgical Opinion Program
Health Care Financing Administration
330 Independence Avenue, SW
Washington, DC 20201
1-800 638-6833 (8 A.M.–8 P.M., Monday–Friday, Eastern Standard Time)
1-800 492-6603 (Maryland)
   Refers caller to agency in your home state that will give you a list of surgeons in the specialty that you need.

TEMPOROMANDIBULAR JOINT (TMJ) PAIN

Jaw Joints and Allied Musculo-Skeletal Disorders Foundation, Inc. (JJAMD)
140 The Fenway
Boston, MA 02115
(617) 266-2550
or (617) 262-5200
   Provides support to individuals, their families, the public and professionals with support group meetings and newsletter. $20/year. $3/educational booklet (12 pages) with SASE.

TWINS, TRIPLETS, AND QUADS

(See Childbirth and Pregnancy)

ULTRASOUND

(See Childbirth and Pregnancy)

URINARY INCONTINENCE

AHCPR Publication Clearinghouse
U.S. Public Health Service
P.O. Box 8547
Silver Spring, MD 20907-8547
(301) 495-3453
　　Provides free pamphlets about incontinence.

Help for Incontinent People (HIP)
P.O. Box 544
Union, SC 29379
(803) 579-7900
　　Provides information and support to people with incontinence. Publications, newsletter, resource guide. SASE.

The Simon Foundation for Incontinence
P.O. Box 835
Wilmette, IL 60091
1-800 237-4666
or (708 864-3913)
　　Provides information for people with incontinence with videos, lectures, support groups, and publications including the newsletter, *Managing Incontinence*, books, and a reprint series. SASE for information packet.

VARICOSE VEINS

(see Cosmetic Surgery)

VEGETARIAN FOOD

(See Food)

WIDOWS

American Association of Retired Persons (AARP)
Widowed Persons Service
1909 K Street, NW, Suite 570
Washington, DC 20049
(202) 728-4370
　　Provides local, one-to-one outreach by trained volunteers to the newly widowed. Also information, education, referral service, and publications.

Theos Foundation, Inc.
1301 Clark Building, 717 Liberty Avenue
Pittsburgh, PA 15222
(412) 471-7779
    Provides local groups, links individuals for one-to-one support, conducts regional conferences and workshops, publishes material on grief and widowhood, and educates the public on grief.

WOMEN'S HEALTH CENTERS

Oryx Press
4041 North Central, Suite 700
Phoenix, AZ 85012-3397
1-800 279-ORYX
or (602) 265-2651
    Provides *Directory of Women's Health Care Centers.* (Unlike listing below, these facilities are usually located in hospitals.)

Federation of Feminist Women's Health Centers
3401 Folsom Boulevard, Suite A
Sacramento, CA 95816
(916) 737-0260
    Provides referrals to women's health centers and information about menstrual extraction.

WOMEN'S HEALTH RESEARCH

Campaign for Women's Health
666 11th Street, NW, #700
Washington, DC 20001
(202) 783-6686
    Provides a coalition of more than 40 national, state, and grass-roots organizations whose intent is to achieve a U.S. health care system that is responsive to women's needs.

Journal of Women's Health
Mary Ann Liebert Inc., Publishers
1651 Third Avenue
New York, NY 10128
(212) 289-2300
    Published quarterly. $65/year (individual), $120/year (institution).

Melpomene Institute for Women's Health Research
1010 University Avenue
St. Paul, MN 55104
(612) 642-1951
    Provides information about women and exercise, including information about menopause and osteoporosis, original research, and the *Melpomene Journal.* $32/year/3 issues.

WOMEN UROLOGISTS

Jean Fourcroy, M.D.
Women in Urology
6310 Swords Way
Bethesda, MD 20817
(301) 897-5563
  Contact Dr. Fourcroy if you want the name of a woman urologist in your area.
(It is often difficult for women who have bladder problems such as urinary tract
infections or interstitial cystitis to find a woman urologist, since there are so few of
them.)

X-RAYS

Food and Drug Administration
Office of Consumer Affairs
5600 Fishers Lane
Rockville, MD 20857
  Provides free booklets about x-rays.

YEAST INFECTIONS

Acu-Trol, Inc.
2 Willow Road
St. Paul, MN 55127
1-800 594-4675
or (612) 484-2811 (Minnesota)
  Provides information including newsletter, *At Last Newslink*, and product catalog
for treatment of candida yeast infections.

Yeast Consulting Services
P.O. Box 11157
Torrance, CA 90510-1157
(310) 375-1073
  Provides information and a support group to women who have a history of
diagnosed vaginal yeast infections.

RECOMMENDED READING

NOTE TO READER

This list, which includes most of this book's topics, is for those who want more information. The Resource Directory, which starts on page 541, has additional sources of information listed by topic.

Outstanding books and magazine articles are marked with an *. Occasionally, some books are mentioned more than once. One computer program is included. You can find copies of the magazines at libraries and the books at libraries or bookstores. If you want to order a book directly from a publisher, call your library reference room and ask for the address and phone number.

PART I: YOUR PASSAGE TO GOOD HEALTH

CHAPTER 1: YOUR BODY AND ITS SYSTEMS

Clark, John (Ed). *The Human Body. A Comprehensive Guide to the Structures and Functions of the Human Body.* London, England: Marshall Editions Limited, 1989.

Jovanovic, Lois et al. *Hormones. The Woman's Answerbook.* New York, New York: Fawcett Columbine, 1987.

Montagu, Ashley. *The Natural Superiority of Women.* New York, New York: Collier/ MacMillan, 1974.

National Geographic Society. *The Incredible Machine.* Washington, DC: National Geographic Society, 1986.

Reader's Digest. *ABCs of the Human Body.* Pleasantville, New York: The Reader's Digest Association, Inc., 1987.

CHAPTER 2: HOW TO STAY HEALTHY

Earle, Richard et al. *Your Vitality Quotient. The Clinically Proven Program That Can Reduce Your Body Age and Increase Your Zest for Life.* New York, New York: Warner Books, 1989.

Evans, William and Irwin H. Rosenberg. *Biomarkers: The 10 Determinants of Aging You Can Control.* New York, New York: Simon & Schuster, 1991.

Ornstein, Robert and David Sobel. *Healthy Pleasures.* Reading, Massachusetts: Addison-Wesley, 1989.

Pixel Perfect, Inc. *Home Medical Advisor Computer Software.* Merritt Island, Florida: Pixel Perfect, Inc., 1992.

Sagan, Leonard. *The Health of Nations. True Causes of Sickness and Well-Being.* New York, New York: Basic Books, 1987.

Weiner, Michael. *Maximum Immunity.* Boston, Massachusetts: Houghton Mifflin, 1986.

Food

*Balch, James F. and Phyllis A. Balch. *Prescription for Nutritional Healing.* Garden City Park, New York: Avery Publishing Group, 1990.

*Calbon, Cherie and Maureen Keane. *Juicing for Life.* Garden City Park, New York: Avery Publishing Group, 1992.

Carper, Jean. *Total Nutrition Guide.* New York, New York: Bantam, 1987.

*Fuchs, Nan Kathryn. *The Nutrition Detective.* Los Angeles, California: Jeremy P. Tarcher, 1985.

*Gaby, Suzanne K. et al. *Vitamin Intake and Health.* New York, New York: Marcel Dekker, 1991.

Gittleman, Ann L. with J. L. Dotson. *Super Nutrition for Women.* New York, New York: Bantam, 1991.

Hausman, Patricia. *The Right Dose. How to Take Vitamins and Minerals Safely.* Emmaus, Pennsylvania: Rodale Press, 1987.

Hausman, Patricia and Judith B. Hurley. *The Healing Foods.* Emmaus, Pennsylvania: Rodale Press, 1989.

*Hendler, Sheldon S. *The Doctors Vitamin & Mineral Encyclopedia.* New York, New York: Fireside/Simon & Schuster, 1990.

Hirschmann, Jane R. and Carol H. Munter. *Overcoming Overeating. Living Free in a World of Food.* Reading, Massachusetts: Addison-Wesley, 1988.

Jacobson, Michael F. et al. *Safe Food. Eating Wisely in a Risky World.* Los Angeles, California: Living Planet Press, 1991.

Long, Patricia. *The Nutritional Ages of Women.* New York, New York: Bantam, 1987.

Morales, Karla (Ed). "How to Choose a Nutritionist." *People's Medical Society Health Bulletin,* 1991.

The Anti—Breast Cancer, Healthy Heart Diet

Bricklin, Mark and Sharon Claessens. *The Natural Healing Cookbook*. Emmaus, Pennsylvania: Rodale Press, 1981.

Center for Science in the Public Interest. "Face the Fats." *Center for Science in the Public Interest*, 1991.

Dreher, Henry. *Your Defense Against Cancer*. New York, New York: Harper & Row, 1988.

Ornish, Dean. *Dr. Dean Ornish's Program for Reversing Heart Disease*. New York, New York: Random House, 1990.

Prasad, Kedar N. *Vitamins Against Cancer. Fact and Fiction*. Rochester, Vermont: Healing Arts Press, 1989.

Fat Counters

Bellerson, Karen J. *The Complete & Up-to-Date Fat Book*. Garden City Park, New York: Avery Publishing Group, 1991.

Netzer, Corinne T. *The Fat Gram Counter*. New York, New York: Dell, 1992.

The Menopause Diet

*Perry, Susan and K. O'Hanlan. *Natural Menopause*. Reading, Massachusetts: Addison-Wesley, 1992.

*Fuchs, Nan K. *The Nutrition Detective*. Los Angeles, California: Jeremy Tarcher, 1985.

The Pregnancy Diet

Brewer, Gail Sforza. *The Very Important Pregnancy Program*. Emmaus, Pennsylvania: Rodale Press, 1988.

The Vegetarian Diet

Goldbeck, Nikki and David. *Nikki and David Goldbeck's American Whole Foods Cuisine*. New York, New York: New American Library/Penguin, 1983.

Katzen, Mollie. *The Moosewood Cookbook* (revised). Berkeley, California: Ten Speed Press, 1992.

Robertson, Laurel et al. *The New Laurel's Kitchen*. Berkeley, California: Ten Speed Press, 1986.

Thomas, Anna. *The Vegetarian Epicure, Book Two*. New York, New York: Alfred A. Knopf, 1978.

Alcohol

Luks, Allan and Joseph Barbato. *You Are What You Drink. The Authoritative Report on What Alcohol Does to Your Body, Mind, and Longevity*. New York, New York: Villard Books, 1989.

Youcha, Geraldine. *Women And Alcohol*. New York, New York: Crown, 1986.

Tobacco

Delaney, Sue. *Women Smokers Can Quit: A Different Approach*. Evanston, Illinois: Women's Healthcare Press, 1990.

Farquhar, John W. and Gene A. Spiller. *The Last Puff: Ex-smokers Share the Secrets of Their Success*. New York, New York: Norton, 1990.

Ferguson, Tom. *The No-Nag, No-Guilt, Do-It-Your-Own-Way Guide to Quitting Smoking*. New York, New York: Ballantine, 1987.

Exercise

American College of Sports Medicine. *ACSM Fitness Book*. Champaign, Illinois: Leisure Press, 1992.

Fox, James M. et al. *Save Your Knees*. New York, New York: Dell, 1988.

Levine, Suzanne M. *My Feet Are Killing Me!*. New York, New York: Fawcett Crest, 1987.

Melpomene Institute for Women's Health Research Staff. *The Bodywise Woman*. St. Paul, Minnesota: Melpomene Institute for Women's Health Research, 1990.

Pritt, Donald and Morton Walker. *The Complete Foot Book. First Aid for Your Feet*. Garden City Park, New York: Avery Publishing Group, 1992.

Tobias, Maxine and John P. Sullivan. *The Complete Stretching Book*. London, England: Dorling-Kindersley, 1992.

Friends and Family

Pogrebin, Letty Cottin. *Among Friends. Who We Like, Why We Like Them, and What We Do with Them*. New York, New York: McGraw Hill, 1987.

Rubin, Lillian B. *Just Friends. The Role of Friendship in Our Lives*. New York, New York: Harper & Row, 1985.

Ruckert, Janet. *The Four-Footed Therapist*. Berkeley, California: Ten Speed Press, 1988.

Sex

Barbach, Lonnie G. *For Yourself: The Fulfillment of Female Sexuality*. New York, New York: New American Library, 1975.

Edelman, Deborah S. *Sex in the Golden Years: What's Ahead May be Worth Waiting For*. New York, New York: Donald Fine, Inc., 1992.

Kitzinger, Sheila. *Woman's Experience of Sex*. New York, New York: G. P. Putnam, 1983.

Sherfey, Mary Jane. *The Nature & Evolution of Female Sexuality*. New York, New York: Vintage Books, 1973.

Stoppard, Miriam. *The Magic of Sex*. London, England: Dorling-Kindersley, 1992.

Emotions

Jeffers, Susan. *Feel the Fear and Do It Anyway*. New York, New York: Fawcett Columbine, 1987.

Ussher, Jane. *Women's Madness. Misogyny or Mental Illness?* Amherst, Massachusetts: University of Massachusetts Press, 1992.

Walsh, Mary Roth (Ed). *The Psychology of Women: Ongoing Debates*. New Haven, Connecticut: Yale University Press, 1987.

*Werbach, Melvyn R. *Nutritional Influences on Mental Illness*. Tarzana, California: Third Line Press, 1991.

Depression

McGrath, Ellen et al. *Women and Depression. Risk Factors and Treatment Issues*. Washington, DC: American Psychological Association, 1990.

Podell, Ronald. *Contagious Emotions: Staying Well When Your Loved One Is Depressed*. New York, New York: Simon and Schuster, 1992.

Seasonal Affective Disorder (SAD)

Rosenthal, Norman E. *Seasons of the Mind*. New York, New York: Bantam, 1990.

Whybrow, Peter el al. *The Hibernation Response. Why You Feel Fat, Miserable, and Depressed from October Through March — and How You Can Cheer Up Through Those Dark Days of Winter*. New York, New York: Arbor House/William Morrow, 1988.

Worry

Handley, Jane and Robert. *Why Women Worry and How to Stop.* New York, New York: Fawcett Crest, 1990.

Finding a Therapist

Laidlaw, Toni Ann et al. *Healing Voices. Feminist Approaches to Therapy with Women.* San Francisco, California: Jossey-Bass, 1990.

Chronic Pain

Epstein, Gloria J. *Help Yourself to Chronic Pain Relief: The Patient's Point of View.* Seattle, Washington: The Manchester Group, Ltd., 1981.

Fardon, David F. *Stop The Pain!* Los Angeles, California: The Body Press, 1983.

Pitzele, Sefra K. *We Are Not Alone. Learning to Live with Chronic Illness.* New York, New York: Workman Publishing, 1986.

Register, Cheri. *Living with Chronic Illness: Days of Patience and Passion.* New York, New York: Free Press, 1989.

Stress

Barnett, Rosalind C. et al. *Gender & Stress.* New York, New York: Free Press, 1987.

Baruch, Grace et al. *Life Prints. New Patterns of Love & Work for Today's Women.* New York, New York: McGraw-Hill, 1983.

Bliss, Shepherd (Ed). *The New Holistic Health Handbook* New York, New York: Stephen Greene Press/Viking Penguin, 1985.

Katsh, Shelley et al. *The Music Within You. How You Can Enhance Your Creativity, Communication and Confidence Through Music.* New York, New York: Fireside/Simon & Schuster, 1985.

Creativity

Harman, Willis et al. *Higher Creativity. Liberating the Unconscious for Breakthrough Insights.* Los Angeles, California: An Institute of Noetic Sciences Book/Jeremy P. Tarcher, Inc., 1984.

Massage

Feltman, John (Ed). *Hands-On Healing. Massage Remedies for Hundreds of Health Problems.* Emmaus, Pennsylvania: Rodale Press, 1989.

*Goodman, Saul. *The Book of Shiatsu. The Healing Art of Finger Pressure.* Garden City Park, New York: Avery Publishing Group, 1990.

Hofer, Jack. *Mini-Massage. Ten-to-Fifteen-Minute Massage Therapies That Reduce Stress.* New York, New York: Putnam, 1988.1133

Lidell, Lucinda et al. *The Book of Massage. The Complete Step-by-Step Guide to Eastern and Western Techniques.* New York, New York: Fireside/Simon & Schuster, 1984.

Therapeutic Touch

Macrae, Janet. *Therapeutic Touch: A Practical Guide.* New York, New York: Alfred A. Knopf, 1988.

Acupressure

Bauer, Cathryn. *Acupressure for Women.* Freedom, California: The Crossing Press, 1987.

*Gach, Michael Reed. *Acupressure's Potent Points.* New York, New York: Bantam Books, 1990.

Yoga

Monro, Robin. *Yoga for Common Ailments.* New York, New York: Simon & Schuster, 1990.

Meditation

Paulson, Genevieve Lewis. *Meditation and Human Growth.* St. Paul, Minnesota: Llewellyn Publishing, 1994.

Skin Health

Begoun, Paula. *Don't Go to the Cosmetics Counter Without Me.* Seattle, Washington: Beginning Press, 1991.

Brumberg, Elaine. *Take Care of Your Skin.* New York, New York: Harper & Row, 1989.

Dental Health

Engelmann, F. C. *The Iatrogenesis Factor: A Quicksilver Mystery (Mercury Poisoning).* New York, New York: Vantage, 1989.

Morales, Karla (Ed). "How to Choose a Dentist." *People's Medical Society Health Bulletin,* Allentown, Pennsylvania, 1991.

X-Rays

Gofman, John W. and Egan O'Connor. *Radiation-Induced Cancer from Low-Dose Exposure: An Independent Analysis.* San Francisco, California: Committee for Nuclear Responsibility, Inc. Book Division, 1990.

CHAPTER 3: HOW TO GET BETTER HEALTH CARE BY TAKING RESPONSIBILITY FOR WHAT HAPPENS TO YOU

Barsky, Arthur J. *Worried Sick. Our Troubled Quest for Wellness.* Boston, Massachusetts: Little, Brown, 1988.

Boyle, Rodger P. *The Medical Wars. Why the Doctors Disagree.* New York, New York: Morrow: 1983.

Cohn, Victor. *News & Numbers. A Guide to Reporting Statistical Claims and Controversies in Health and Related Fields.* Ames, Iowa: Iowa State University Press, 1989.

Heussner, Jr. and Marla E. Salmon. *Warning: The Media May Be Harmful to Your Health! A Consumer's Guide to Medical News and Advertising.* Kansas City, Missouri: Andrews & McMeel, 1988.

Marion, Robert. *Learning to Play God: The Coming of Age of a Young Doctor.* Reading, Massachusetts: Addison-Wesley, 1991.

Bring a Friend

Howell, Mary C. *Helping Ourselves: Families and the Human Network.* Boston, Massachusetts: Beacon Press, 1975.

Health Detective

Arnot, Robert. *The Best Medicine. How to Choose the Top Doctors, the Top Hospitals, and the Top Treatments.* Reading, Massachusetts: Addison-Wesley Publishing Company, 1992.

Goldstein, Jay A. *Could Your Doctor Be Wrong?* New York, New York: Pharos Books, 1991.

Attitude

Carlson, Richard et al. *Healers on Healing.* Los Angeles, California: Jeremy Tarcher, 1989.

Cousins, Norman. *Head First: The Biology of Hope.* New York, New York: Dutton, 1989.

Cousins, Norman. *The Healing Heart. Antidotes to Panic and Helplessness.* New York, New York: W. W. Norton, 1983.

Cousins, Norman. *Anatomy of an Illness as Perceived by the Patient. Reflections on Healing and Regeneration.* New York, New York: Bantam, 1981.

Hammerschlag, Carl A. *The Dancing Healers. A Doctor's Journey of Healing with Native Americans.* San Francisco, California: Harper & Row, 1988.

Justice, Blair. *Who Gets Sick. How Beliefs, Moods, and Thoughts Affect Your Health.* Los Angeles, California: Jeremy Tarcher, 1988.

Seduction of Medical Technology

Robin, Eugene D. *Matters of Life and Death: Risks vs. Benefits of Medical Care.* San Francisco, California: W. H. Freeman, 1984.

Prescription and Over-the-Counter Drugs

Baker, Charles E., Jr. (Ed). *Physicians' Desk Reference.* Oradell, New Jersey: Medical Economics Company (Revised Annually).

Clayman, Charles B. *The American Medical Association Guide to Prescription and Over-The-Counter Drugs.* New York, New York: Random House, 1988.

Graedon, Joe. *The New People's Pharmacy.* New York, New York: Bantam, 1985.

Griffith, H. Winter. *Complete Guide to Prescription & Non-Prescription Drugs.* Los Angeles, California: The Body Press, 1989.

Morales, Karla (Ed). "How to Choose a Pharmacist." *People's Medical Society Bulletin,* Undated.1138

Wolff, Sidney M. et al. *Worst Pills, Best Pills II.* Washington, DC: Public Citizen Health Research Group, 1993.

Malpractice

De Ville, Kenneth A. *Malpractice in Nineteenth Century America: Origins and Legacy.* New York, New York: New York University Press, 1990.

Medical Insurance

Bloom, Jill. *HMOs. What They Are, How They Work, and Which One Is Best for You.* Los Angeles, California: The Body Press, 1987.

Rooney, Michael A. and People's Medical Society. *Health Insurance. How to Evaluate and Select Health Insurance.* Allentown, Pennsylvania: People's Medical Society, 1985.

Shear, Carolyn and Eliot Shear. *The Health Insurance Claims Kit.* Chicago, Illinois: Dearborn Trade, 1992.

Tracy, Gerry (Ed). "The ABCs of HMOs." *People's Medical Society,* Undated.

CHAPTER 4: HOW TO CHOOSE YOUR HEALTH CARE

Alternative Medicine

Grist, Liz. *A Woman's Guide to Alternative Medicine.* Chicago, Illinois: Contemporary Books, 1988.

*Mills, Simon. *Alternatives in Healing. An Open-Minded Approach to Finding the Best Treatment for Your Health Problems.* London, England: Marshall Editions Limited, 1988.

Olsen, Kristin G. *The Encyclopedia of Alternative Health Care.* New York, New York: Pocket Books, 1989.

Acupuncture

Beinfeld, Harriet and Effrem Korngold. *Between Heaven and Earth: A Guide to Chinese Medicine.* New York, New York: Ballantine, 1991.

Homeopathy

Cummings, Stephen and Dana Ullman. *Everybody's Guide to Homeopathic Medicines.* Los Angeles, California: Jeremy Tarcher, 1984.

Medicinal Herbs

*Castleman, Michael. *The Healing Herbs.* Emmaus, Pennsylvania: Rodale Press, 1991.

Mabey, Richard. *The New Age Herbalist.* New York, New York: Collier Books/Macmillan Publishing Company, 1988.

Mindell, Earl. *Earl Mindell's Herb Bible.* New York, New York: Fireside/Simon & Schuster, 1992.

African-American Women's Health

White, Evelyn C. *The Black Women's Health Book: Speaking for Ourselves.* Seattle, Washington: Seal Press, 1990.

Lesbian Health

Hepburn, Cuca and Bonnie Gutierrez. *Alive & Well. A Lesbian Health Guide.* Freedom, California: The Crossing Press, 1988.

The Hospital Stay

Bogdanich, Walt. *The Great White Lie: How America's Hospitals Betray Our Trust and Endanger Our Lives.* New York, New York: Simon & Schuster, 1991.

Consumers' Checkbook Magazine Editors. *Consumers' Guide to Hospitals, 1992.* Washington, DC: Center for the Study of Services, 1992.

Inlander, Charles B. and Ed Weiner. *Take This Book to the Hospital with You.* Emmaus, Pennsylvania: Rodale Press, 1985.

Your Legal Rights

Annas, George J. *The Rights of Patients.* Carbondale, Illinois: Southern Illinois University Press, 1990.

*Isaacs, Stephen L. and Ava C. Swartz. *The Consumer's Legal Guide to Today's Health Care. Your Medical Rights and How to Assert Them.* New York, New York: Houghton Mifflin Company, 1992.

Common Medical Tests

Eddy, David M. (Ed). *Common Screening Tests.* Philadelphia, Pennsylvania: American College of Physicians, 1991.

Hensel, Bruce. *Smart Medicine. How to Get the Most out of Your Medical Checkup and Stay Healthy.* New York, New York: Putnam, 1989.

Robin, Eugene D. *Matters of Life and Death: Risks vs. Benefits of Medical Care.* New York, New York: W. H. Freeman, 1984.

Sobel, David S. and Tom Ferguson. *The People's Book of Medical Tests.* New York, New York: Summit Books, 1985.

Breast Health

*Love, Susan M. *Dr. Susan Love's Breast Book*. Reading, Massachusetts: Addison-Wesley, 1991.

Mammogram

*Bertell, Rosalie. "Breast Cancer and Mammography." *Mothering* Summer 1992.
*Napoli, Maryann. *Mammography Screening: A Decision-Making Guide*. New York, New York: Center for Medical Consumers, 1990.

Home Testing Kits

Pinckney, Cathey and Edward Pinckney. *Do-It-Yourself Medical Testing*. New York, New York: Facts on File, 1989.

CHAPTER 5: WOMEN IN SPECIAL CIRCUMSTANCES

Caregivers

Banks, Carolyn and Janis Rizzo. *A Loving Voice: A Caregiver's Book of Read-Aloud Stories for the Elderly*. Philadelphia, Pennsylvania: The Charles Press, 1992.

Baussell, R. Barker et al. *How to Evaluate and Select a Nursing Home*. Reading, Massachusetts: Addison-Wesley, 1988.

Friedman, Jo-Ann. *Home Health Care: A Complete Guide for Patients and Their Families*. New York, New York: Ballantine, 1987.

Roberts, D. Jeanne. *Taking Care of Caregivers*. Menlo Park, California: Bull Publishing, 1991.

Silverstone, Barbara and Helen K. Hyman. *You and Your Aging Parent*. New York, New York: Pantheon Books, 1989.

Sommers, Tish and Laurie Shields. *Women Take Care*. Gainesville, Florida: Triad Communications, Inc., 1987.

Strong, Maggie. *Mainstay. For the Well Spouse of the Chronically Ill*. Boston, Massachusetts: Little, Brown, 1988.

Disabled Women

Browne, Susan et al. *With the Power of Each Breath: A Disabled Women's Anthology*. Pittsburgh, Pennsylvania: Cleis Press, 1990.

Price, Reynolds. *Clear Pictures*. New York, New York: Atheneum, 1989.

Rousso, Marilyn et al. *Disabled, Female, and Proud: Stories of 10 Women with Disabilities*. Boston, Massachusetts: Exceptional Parent Press, 1988.

Zola, Irving K. *Missing Pieces: A Chronicle of Living with a Disability*. Philadelphia, Pennsylvania: Temple University Press, 1982.

Abused Women

NiCarty, Ginny. *You Can Be Free: Handbook for Women in Abusive Relationships*. Seattle, Washington: Seal Press, 1986.

Statman, Jan Berliner. *The Battered Woman's Survival Guide. Breaking the Cycle. A Resource Manual for Victims, Relatives, Friends, and Professionals*. Dallas, Texas: Taylor Publishing Company, 1990.

Date Rape

Warshaw, Robin. *I Never Called It Rape: The Ms. Report on Recognizing, Fighting, and Surviving Date and Acquaintance Rape*. New York, New York: Harper & Row, 1988.

Incest

Gil, Eliana. *Outgrowing the Pain: A Book for and about Adults Abused as Children.* New York, New York: Dell, 1983.

Tauris, Carol. "Beware the Incest-Survivor Machine." *The New York Times*, Sunday book review section, January 3, 1993, pages 1, 14, 17.

Sexual Harassment

Bravo, Ellen and Ellen Cassedy. *The 9 to 5 Guide to Combatting Sexual Harassment.* New York, New York: John Wiley & Sons, 1992.

*Petrocelli, William and Barbara K. *Sexual Harassment on the Job: What It Is and How to Stop It.* Berkeley, California: Nolo Press, 1992.

Webb, Susan. *Step Forward: Sexual Harassment in the Workplace.* New York, New York: MasterMedia, 1992.

PART II: THE ALPHABETICAL GUIDE

ABORTION

*Chalker, Rebecca and Carol Downer. *A Woman's Book of Choices: Abortion, Menstrual Extraction, RU-486.* New York, New York: Four Walls Eight Windows, 1992.

Donovan, Patricia. *Our Daughters' Decisions. The Conflict in State Law on Abortion and Other Issues.* New York, New York: The Alan Guttmacher Institute, 1992.

*Gardner, Joy. *A Difficult Decision: A Compassionate Book About Abortion.* Freedom, California: Crossing Press 1986.

*National Women's Health Network. *Abortion Then and Now: Creative Responses to Restricted Access.* Washington, DC: National Women's Health Network, 1989.

Townsend, Rita and Ann Perkins (Eds). *Bitter Fruit: Women's Experiences of Unplanned Pregnancy, Abortion and Adoption.* Claremont, California: Hunter House, 1992.

ACQUIRED IMMUNE DEFICIENCY SYNDROME (AIDS)

The ACT UP/NY Women & AIDS Book Group. *Women, AIDS & Activism.* Boston, Massachusetts: Sound End Press, 1990.

Buckingham, Robert W. *Among Friends. Hospice Care for the Person with AIDS.* Buffalo, New York: Prometheus Books, 1992.

Watstein, Sarah B. and Robert A. Laurich. *AIDS and Women: A Sourcebook.* Phoenix, Arizona: Oryx Press, 1991.

Whitacre, John D. *Confronting Life-Threatening Illness.* Ann Arbor, Michigan: Pierian Press, 1992.

ALZHEIMER'S DISEASE

Carroll, David L. *When Your Loved One Has Alzheimer's. A Caregiver's Guide.* New York, New York: Harper & Row, 1989.

Kippel, Raye Lynne and J. Thomas Hutton. *Caring for the Alzheimer Patient.* Buffalo, New York: Prometheus Books, 1991.

*Mace, Nancy L. and Peter V. Rabins. *The 36-Hour Day—A Family Guide to Caring for Persons with Alzheimer's Disease, Related Dementing Illnesses, and Memory Loss in Later Life*. Baltimore, Maryland: The Johns Hopkins University Press, 1981.

*Weiner, Michael A. *Reducing the Risk of Alzheimer's*. Chelsea, Michigan: Scarborough House, 1989.

Nursing Homes

Lesko, Matthew. *The Great American Gripe Book*. Kensington, Maryland: Information USA, Inc., 1990.

ANEMIA

*Carper, Jean. *Total Nutrition Guide*. New York, New York: Bantam, 1987.

Colbin, Annemarie. *Food and Healing*. New York, New York: Ballantine Books, 1986.

*Fuchs, Nan Kathryn. *The Nutrition Detective*. Los Angeles, California: Jeremy P. Tarcher, 1985.

Hausman, Patricia. *The Right Dose*. Emmaus, Pennsylvania: Rodale Press, 1987.

BIRTH CONTROL

Bullough, Vern L. and Bonnie Bullough. *Contraception. A Guide to Birth Control Methods*. Buffalo, New York: Prometheus Books, 1990.

Chalker, Rebecca. *The Complete Cervical Cap Guide. Everything You Want To Know About this Safe, Effective, No-Mess, Time-Tested Birth Control Option*. New York, New York: Harper & Row, 1987.

Gross, Amy and Dee Ito. *Women Talk about Gynecological Surgery*. New York, New York: HarperPerennial, 1991.

Hatcher, Robert A. et al. *Contraceptive Technology 1990–1992*. New York, New York: Irvington Publishers, 1990.

Winikoff, Beverly and Suzanne Wymelenberg. *The Contraceptive Handbook*. Yonkers, New York: Consumer Reports Books, 1992.

Fertility Awareness

Billings, Evelyn and Ann Westmore. *The Billings Method: Controlling Fertility Without Drugs or Devices*. New York, New York: Ballantine Books, 1980.

Winstein, Meryl. *Your Fertility Signals. Using Them to Achieve or Avoid Pregnancy, Naturally*. St. Louis, Missouri: Smooth Stone Press, 1989.

Menstrual Extraction

Chalker, Rebecca and Carol Downer. *A Woman's Book of Choices: Abortion, Menstrual Extraction, RU 486*. New York, New York. Four Walls, Eight Windows, 1992.

National Women's Health Network. *Abortion Then and Now: Creative Responses to Restricted Access*. Washington, DC: National Women's Health Network, 1989.

BREAST LUMPS

Love, Susan M. *Dr. Susan Love's Breast Book*. Reading, Massachusetts: Addison-Wesley, 1991.

CANCER
All Cancer

Bruning, Nancy. *Coping With Chemotherapy*. New York, New York: Ballantine, 1993.

*Dollinger, Malin et al. *Everyone's Guide to Cancer Therapy. How Cancer is Diagnosed, Treated, and Managed Day to Day*. Kansas City, Missouri: Andrews & McMeel, 1991.

Gerson, Max. *A Cancer Therapy. Results of Fifty Cases. The Cure of Advanced Cancer by Diet Therapy*. Bonita, California: Gerson Institute, 1986.

Lane, I. William and Linda Comac. *Sharks Don't Get Cancer*. Garden City Park, New York: Avery Publishing Group, Inc., 1992.

*Prasad, Kedar N. *Vitamins Against Cancer*. Rochester, Vermont: Healing Arts Press, 1989.

U.S. Congress, Office of Technology Assessment. *Unconventional Cancer Treatments*. Washington, DC: U.S. Government Printing Office, 1990.

Walters, Richard. *Options: The Alternative Cancer Therapy Book*. Garden City Park, New York: Avery Publishing Group, Inc., 1993.

Whitacre, John D. *Confronting Life-Threatening Illness*. Ann Arbor, Michigan: Pierian Press, 1992.

Breast Cancer

Dackman, Linda. *Up Front. Sex and the Post-Mastectomy Woman*. New York, New York: Penguin, 1990.

Gross, Amy and Dee Ito. *Women Talk About Breast Surgery*. New York, New York: HarperPerennial, 1991.

Harris, Linda Brown. *Breast Cancer: A Handbook*. St. Paul, Minnesota: Melpomene Institute for Women's Health Research, 1992.

Kelly, Patricia T. *Understanding Breast Cancer Risk*. Philadelphia, Pennsylvania: Temple University Press, 1991.

*Love, Susan M. *Dr. Susan Love's Breast Book*. Reading, Pennsylvania: Addison-Wesley, 1991.

Wittman, Juliet. *Breast Care Journal: A Century of Petals*. Golden, Colorado: Fulcrum Publishing, 1993.

CARPAL TUNNEL SYNDROME (CTS)

Tannenhaus, Norra. *Relief from Carpal Tunnel Syndrome and Other Repetitive Motion Disorders*. New York, New York: Dell, 1991.

CHILDBIRTH (SEE ALSO "PREGNANCY")
Breastfeeding

Huggins, Kathleen. *The Nursing Mother's Companion*. Boston, Massachusetts: Harvard Common Press, 1990.

La Leche League. *The Womanly Art of Breastfeeding*. New York, New York: New American Library, 1991.

Pryor, Karen and Gale Pryor. *Nursing Your Baby*. New York, New York: Pocket Books, 1991.

Childbirth

*Enkin, Murray, M. Keirse, and I. Chalmers. *A Guide to Effective Care in Pregnancy and Childbirth*. Oxford, England: Oxford University Press, 1990.

Haire, Doris. *The Cultural Warping of Childbirth*. Minneapolis, Minnesota: International Childbirth Education Association, 1972.

Klaus, Marshall, John Kennell, and Phyllis Klaus. *Mothering the Mother. How A Doula Can Help You Have a Shorter, Easier, Healthier Birth*. Reading, Massachusetts: Addison-Wesley, 1992.

Korte, Diana and Roberta Scaer. *A Good Birth, A Safe Birth* (third edition). Boston, Massachusetts: The Harvard Common Press, 1992.

Lieberman, Adrienne B. *Easing Labor Pain. The Complete Guide to a More Comfortable and Rewarding Birth*. Boston, Massachusetts: The Harvard Common Press, 1992.

Odent, Michael. *Birth Reborn*. New York, New York: Pantheon, 1984.

Home Birth

Kitzinger, Sheila. *Homebirth and Other Alternatives to Hospital*. London, England: Dorling-Kindersley, 1991.

Tew, Marjorie. *Safer Childbirth?* London, England: Chapman and Hall, 1990.

Midwifery

Kitzinger, Sheila (Ed). *The Midwife Challenge*. London, England: Pandora Press/HarperCollins, 1991.

Steiger, Carolyn. *Becoming a Midwife*. Portland, Oregon: Hoogan House, 1987.

Newborn Period

Klaus, Marshall H. and Phyllis H. Klaus. *The Amazing Newborn. Making the Most of the First Weeks of Life*. Reading, Massachusetts: Addison-Wesley, 1985.

*Lim, Robin. *After the Baby's Birth. A Woman's Way to Wellness*. Berkeley, California: Celestial Arts, 1991.

Premature Birth

Harrison, Helen. *The Premature Baby Book*. New York, New York: St. Martin's Press, 1983.

CHRONIC FATIGUE SYNDROME

Bolles, Edmund Blair. *Learning to Live with Chronic Fatigue Syndrome*. New York, New York: Dell, 1990.

Feiden, Karyn. *Hope and Help for Chronic Fatigue Syndrome: The Official Book of the CFS/CFIDS Network*. New York, New York: Prentice Hall, 1990.

Fisher, Gregg et al. *Chronic Fatigue Syndrome: A Victim's Guide to Understanding, Treating, and Coping with This Debilitating Illness*. New York, New York: Warner, 1989.

Stoff, Jesse A. and Charles R. Pellegrino. *Chronic Fatigue Syndrome. The Hidden Epidemic*. New York, New York: Random House, 1988.

COSMETIC SURGERY

Berger, Karen and John Bostwick. *A Woman's Decision: Breast Care, Treatment, and Reconstruction*. St. Louis, Missouri: Quality Medical Publishing, 1988.

DIETHYLSTILBESTROL (DES)

Apfel, Roberta J. and Susan M. Fisher. *To Do No Harm. DES and the Dilemma of Modern Medicine.* New Haven, Connecticut: Yale University Press, 1984.

EATING DISORDERS

Brumberg, Joan J. *Fasting Girls.* Cambridge, Massachusetts: Harvard University Press, 1989.

Orbach, Susie. *Hunger Strikes.* New York, New York: W. W. Norton, 1986.

*Werbach, Melvyn R. *Nutritional Influences on Mental Illness.* Tarzana, California: Third Line Press, 1991.

ENDOMETRIOSIS

Ballweg, Mary Lou. *Overcoming Endometriosis.* New York, New York: Congdon & Weed, 1987.

Colbin, Annemarie. *Food and Healing.* New York, New York: Ballantine Books, 1986.

Weinstein, Kate. *Living with Endometriosis. How to Cope with the Physical and Emotional Challenges.* Reading, Massachusetts: Addison-Wesley, 1987.

ESTROGEN REPLACEMENT THERAPY (ERT)

*Cutler, Winnifred B. *Hysterectomy: Before and After.* New York, New York: Harper & Row, 1988.

*U.S. Congress, Office of Technology Assessment. *The Menopause, Hormone Therapy, and Women's Health.* Washington, DC: U.S. Government Printing Office, May 1992.

FATIGUE

Hamner, Daniel and Barbara Burr. *Peak Energy—The High—Oxygen Program for More Energy Now.* New York, New York: Putnam, 1988.

HEART

Anderson, Sharon. *Mitral Valve Prolapse. Benign Syndrome?* Barrie, Ontario, Canada: Wellington House Press, 1990.

Donahue, Peggy Jo. *How to Prevent a Stroke. A Complete Risk-Reduction Program.* Emmaus, Pennsylvania: Rodale Press, 1989.

Folly, Conn and H. F. Pizer. *The Stroke Fact Book.* New York, New York: Bantam, 1985.

Legato, Marianne J. and Carol Colman. *The Female Heart: The Truth About Women and Coronary Artery Disease.* New York, New York: Prentice Hall, 1991.

*Ornish, Dean. *Dr. Dean Ornish's Program for Reversing Heart Disease.* New York, New York: Random House, 1991.

People's Medical Society. *Blood Pressure.* Allentown, Pennsylvania: People's Medical Society, 1992.

People's Medical Society. *Your Heart.* Allentown, Pennsylvania: People's Medical Society, 1992.

Shirk, Evelyn. *After the Stroke. Coping with America's Third Leading Cause of Death.* Buffalo, New York: Prometheus Books, 1991.

HYSTERECTOMY AND OOPHORECTOMY

*Cutler, Winnifred B. *Hysterectomy: Before & After*. New York, New York: Harper & Row, 1988.

Gross, Amy and Dee Ito. *Women Talk About Gynecological Surgery*. New York, New York: HarperPerennial, 1991.

Hufnagel, Vicki. *No More Hysterectomies*. New York, New York: New American Library, 1988.

Payer, Lynn. *How to Avoid a Hysterectomy*. New York, New York: Random House, 1987.

Stokes, Naomi Miller. *The Castrated Woman*. New York, New York: Franklin Watts, 1986.

*Wigfall-Williams, Wanda. *Hysterectomy: Learning the Facts*. New York, New York: Michael Kesend Publishing, 1986.

Wolff, Sidney et al. *Women's Health Alert*. Reading, Massachusetts: Addison-Wesley, 1991.

INFERTILITY

Bellina, Joseph and Josleen Wilson. *You Can Have a Baby*. New York, New York: Crown, 1985.

Behrman, S. J. et al. *Progress in Infertility*, 3rd Edition. Boston, Massachusetts: Little Brown, 1988.

Edwards, Margot (Ed). *A Stairstep Approach to Fertility*. Freedom, California: Crossing Press 1989.

Frank, Diana and Marta Vogel. *The Baby Makers*. New York, New York: Carroll & Grof, 1988.

Harkness, Carla. *The Infertility Book*. San Francisco, California: Volcano Press, 1987.

Menning, Barbara E. *Infertility*. New York, New York: Prentice Hall, 1989.

Schwan, Kassie. *The Infertility Maze*. Chicago, Illinois: Contemporary Books, 1988.

Vancouver Women's Health Collective. *Infertility. Problems Getting Pregnant*. Vancouver, British Columbia: Women's Health Center, 1989.

Adoption

Arms, Suzanne. *Adoption: A Handful of Hope*. Berkeley, California: Celestial Arts, 1990.

Caplan, Lincoln. *An Open Adoption*. New York, New York: Farrar, Straus & Giroux, 1990.

Gilman, Lois. *The Adoption Resource Book*. New York, New York: Harper and Row, 1987.

Lindsay, Jeanne Warren. *Parents, Pregnant Teens, and the Adoption Option*. Buena Park, California: Morning Glory Press, 1989.

Michelman, Stanley B. et al. *The Private Adoption Handbook. A Step-by-Step Guide to the Legal, Emotional, and Practical Demands of Adopting a Baby*. New York, New York: Villard Books, 1988.

National Committee for Adoption. *Adoption Factbook, United States Data, Issues, Regulations and Resources*. Washington, DC: National Center for Adoption, 1989.

Sullivan, Michael with Susan Shulz. *Adopt the Baby You Want*. New York, New York: Simon & Schuster, 1990.

Artificial Insemination

Baran, Annette and Reuben Pannor. *Lethal Secrets. The Shocking Consequences and Unsolved Problems of Artificial Insemination*. New York, New York: Warner, 1989.

Noble, Elizabeth. *Having Your Baby by Donor Insemination.* Boston, Massachusetts: Houghton Mifflin, 1987.

Robinson, Susan and H. F. Pizer. *Having A Baby Without a Man.* New York, New York: Simon & Schuster, 1985.

In Vitro Fertilization

Shar, Geoffrey. *From Infertility to In Vitro.* New York, New York: McGraw-Hill, 1988.

Tilton, Nan and Todd. *Making Miracles: In Vitro Fertilization.* New York, New York: Doubleday, 1985.

Surrogate Motherhood

Kane, Elizabeth. *Birth Story. The Story of America's First Legal Surrogate Mother.* San Diego, California: Harcourt Brace Jovanovich, 1988.

Shalev, Carmel. *Birth Power. The Case for Surrogacy.* New Haven, Connecticut: Yale University Press, 1989.

Whitehead, Mary Beth. *The Truth About the Baby M Case.* New York, New York: St. Martin's Press, 1989.

INTERSTITIAL CYSTITIS

Chalker, Rebecca and Kristine E. Whitmore. *Overcoming Bladder Disorders.* New York, New York: Harper & Row, 1990.

Gillespie, Larrian. *You Don't Have to Live with Cystitis!* New York, New York: Rawson Associates, 1986.

LUPUS

Talman, Donna H. *Heartsearch. Toward Healing Lupus.* Berkeley, California: North Atlantic Books, 1991.

MENOPAUSE

*U.S. Congress, Office of Technology Assessment. *The Menopause, Hormone Therapy, and Women's Health.* Washington, DC: U.S. Government Printing Office, 1992.

Greenwood, Sadja. *Menopause Naturally.* San Francisco, California: Volcano Press, 1992.

*Greer, Germaine. *The Change: Woman, Aging, and the Menopause.* New York, New York: Alfred A. Knopf, 1992.

Ojeda, Linda. *Menopause Without Medicine.* Claremont, California: Hunter House Publishers, 1989.

*Perry, Susan and Katherine O'Hanlan. *Natural Menopause.* Reading, Massachusetts: Addison-Wesley, 1992.

MENSTRUATION

Golub, Sharon. *Periods: From Menarche to Menopause.* Newbury Park, California: Sage Publications, Inc., 1992.

Taylor, Dena. *Red Flower: Rethinking Menstruation.* Freedom, California: Crossing Press, 1988.

Wiler, Stella. *Pain-Free Periods.* Rochester, Vermont: Thorsons Publishing, 1987.

Premenstrual Syndrome (PMS)

Castleman, Michael. *The Healing Herbs. Remedies for over 200 Conditions and Diseases.* Emmaus, Pennsylvania: Rodale, 1991.

Harrison, Michelle. *Self-Help for Premenstrual Syndrome.* New York, New York: Random House, 1985.

Lark, Susan. *Premenstrual Syndrome Self-Help Book.* Los Angeles, California: Forman Publishing, 1984.

*Severino, Sally K. and M. Moline. *Premenstrual Syndrome: A Clinician's Guide.* New York, New York: Guilford Press, 1989.

MIGRAINE HEADACHES

Henneberger, Mary. *Overcoming Migraine: A Comprehensive Guide to Treatment and Prevention by a Survivor.* Barrytown, New York: Station Hill Press, 1991.

Lipton, Richard B. et al. *Migraine: Beating the Odds.* Reading, Massachusetts: Addison-Wesley, 1992.

Mansfield, John. *Migraine: The Drug-Free Solution:* Rochester, Vermont: Thorsons Publishing, 1986.

van der Meer, Antonia. *Relief from Chronic Headache.* New York, New York: Dell, 1990.

OBESITY

Brown, Laura and Esther Rothblum. *Fat Oppression and Psychotherapy.* New York, New York: Haworth Press, 1990.

Ernsberger, Paul and Paul Haskew. "Rethinking Obesity: An Alternative View of its Health Implications." *The Journal of Obesity and Weight Regulation* 6:2 (Summer 1987).

Hirschmann, Jane R. and Carl H. Munter. *Overcoming Overeating.* Reading, Massachusetts: Addison-Wesley, 1988.

Sinaikin, Phillip M. and Judith Sachs. *After the Fast.* New York, New York: Doubleday, 1990.

OSTEOPOROSIS

*Calbon, Cherie and Maureen Keane. *Juicing for Life.* Garden City Park, New York: Avery Publishing Group, 1992.

Fuchs, Nan Kathryn. *The Nutrition Detective.* Los Angeles, California: Jeremy P. Tarcher, 1985.

Hausman, Patricia. *The Right Dose.* Emmaus, Pennsylvania: Rodale Press, 1987.

PELVIC INFLAMMATORY DISEASE (PID)

"Pelvic Inflammatory Disease PID." Vancouver, British Columbia, Canada: The Canadian PID Society, 1987. (See "Pelvic Inflammatory Disease" in the Resource Directory for address.)

PREGNANCY (*SEE ALSO* "CHILDBIRTH")

Baldwin, Rahima and Terra Palmorini. *Pregnant Feelings.* Berkeley, California: Celestial Arts, 1986.

Gardner, Joy. *Healing Yourself During Pregnancy*. Freedom, California: Crossing Press, 1987.

*Jimenez, Sherry. *The Pregnant Woman's Comfort Guide*. Garden City Park, New York: Avery Publishing Group, 1992.

*Stillerman, Elaine. *Mother Massage. A Handbook for Relieving the Discomforts of Pregnancy*. New York, New York: Dell, 1992.

Sussman, John R. and B. Blake Levitt. *Before You Conceive*. New York, New York: Bantam, 1989.

Exercise During Pregnancy

Artal, Raul with G. Subak-Sharpe. *Pregnancy and Exercise*. New York, New York: Delacorte Press, 1992.

*Olkin, Sylvia Klein. *Positive Pregnancy Fitness*. Garden City Park, New York: Avery Publishing Group, 1987.

Prenatal Testing

Blatt, Robin J. R. *Prenatal Tests*. New York, New York: Vintage, 1988.

Holtzman, Neil A. *Proceed with Caution*. Baltimore, Maryland: The Johns Hopkins University Press, 1989.

Rothman, Barbara Katz. *The Tentative Pregnancy*. New York, New York: Viking, 1986.

Down Syndrome

Lott, Ira and Ernest McCoy (Eds). *Down Syndrome: Advances in Medical Care*. New York, New York: Wiley-Liss/John Wiley & Sons, Inc., 1992.

Pregnancy Loss

Borg, Susan and Judith Lasker. *When Pregnancy Fails*. New York, New York: Bantam, 1988.

Creel, Mary-Jane. *A Little Death*. New York, New York: Vantage Press, 1987.

DeFraun, John. *Stillborn — The Invisible Death*. Lexington, Massachusetts: Lexington Books, 1986.

Friedman, Rochelle et al. *Surviving Pregnancy Loss*. Boston, Massachusetts: Little, Brown, 1982.

Panuthos, Claudia and Catherine Romeo. *Ended Beginnings — Healing Childbearing Losses*. South Hadley, Massachusetts: Bergin & Garvey, 1984.

Semchyshyn, Stefan and Carol Colman. *How to Prevent Miscarriage and Other Crises of Pregnancy*. New York, New York: MacMillan Publishing, 1989.

SINGLE MOTHERS

Anderson, Joan. *The Single Mother's Book. A Practical Guide to Managing Your Children, Career, Home, Finances, and Everything Else*. Atlanta Georgia: Peachtree Publishers, 1990.

Merritt, Sharyne. *And Baby Makes Two. Motherhood Without Marriage*. New York, New York: Franklin Watts, 1984.

TEMPOROMANDIBULAR JOINT (TMJ) PAIN

Goldman and McCullough. *TMJ Syndrome*. New York, New York: Congdon & Weed, 1987.

Kaplan, Andrew S. and Gray Williams, Jr. *The TMJ Book.* New York, New York: Pharos Books, 1988.

*van der Meer, Antonia. *Relief from Chronic TMJ Pain.* New York, New York: Dell, 1990.

URINARY INCONTINENCE

*Burgio, Kathryn L. et al. *Staying Dry. A Practical Guide to Bladder Control.* Baltimore, Maryland: The Johns Hopkins University Press, 1989.

Chalker, Rebecca and Kristine E. Whitmore. *Overcoming Bladder Disorders.* New York, New York: Harper & Row, 1990.

Gartley, Cheryle B. *Managing Incontinence.* Ottawa, Illinois: Jameson Books, 1985.

URINARY TRACT INFECTIONS

Gillespie, Larrian. *You Don't Have to Live With Cystitis!* New York, New York: Rawson Associates, 1986.

Schrotenboer, Kathryn. *The Woman Doctor's Guide to Overcoming Cystitis.* New York, New York: New American Library, 1987.

VAGINAL INFECTIONS
Yeast Infections

Burton, Gail. *The Candida Control Cookbook.* New York, New York: New American Library, 1989.

Crook, William G. *The Yeast Connection: A Medical Breakthrough.* New York, New York: Vintage, 1986.

Fuchs, Nan K. *The Nutrition Detective.* Los Angeles, California: Jeremy P. Tarcher, 1985.

Novotny, Pamela Patrick. *What Women Should Know About Chronic Infections and Sexually Transmitted Diseases.* New York, New York: Dell, 1991.

Trowbridge, John P. and Morton Walker. *The Yeast Syndrome.* New York, New York: Bantam, 1989.

VARICOSE VEINS

Navarro, Luis et al. *No More Varicose Veins.* New York, New York: Bantam, 1988.

"HERE'S WHAT I THINK" QUESTIONNAIRE

Dear Reader,

Here's a way you can let me know what you think about this book and make suggestions about future editions. Please answer the following questions and send your opinions to me: Diana Korte, P.O. Box 18873, Boulder, Colorado 80308.

1. What information in this book helped you the most?

2. What information was not helpful?

3. What information was missing?

4. Do you have a favorite book to suggest for Recommended Reading or a helpful group to recommend for the Resource Directory? (If book, give author, title, and publisher. If group, give name, address, zip, and phone.)

_____

_____

_____

5. Anything else you want to tell me?

Optional:

Name _____

Address _____

City/State/Zip _____

Phone _____

HOW TO OBTAIN MY SOURCE NOTES

Unfortunately, due to space constraints, the publisher is unable to include the source notes. Since they should be available to you regardless, please send a postcard to Diana Korte, P.O. Box 18873, Boulder, Colorado, 80308, if you want to buy the complete set of source notes (about 500 manuscript pages) or the abridged version (about 100 pages). Both sets include an alphabetized list of published sources.

My source notes include citations from hundreds of medical journals, magazines, newsletters, newspapers, and books. These notes not only include the sources for information I've used, but the sources for the women's quotes that came from publications as well. Some controversial topics, such as "Cancer and the Pill" and "Non-Medical Reasons for Cesareans," for example, are listed separately within a chapter in these notes.

INDEX

abdomen, 367
  pain and tenderness in, 175, 183, 212, 218, 233, 234, 274, 321
abortion, 127–37, 143, 164, 177, 268
  alternatives to, 132, 134, 545
  as birth control, 168, 462
  birth defects and, 462, 463–65, 468, 472–73, 474–76, 486
  facilities for, 88, 134–35, 137
  history of, 164
  intrauterine instillation, 128, 129
  legal aspects of, 136
  maternal death and, 128
  menstrual extraction, 128
  moral and emotional factors in, 129–33, 136, 468, 475–76
  "morning-after," 121, 128, 218–20
  opposition to, 129–32, 134, 207, 501
  outside pressure for, 133
  possible complications of, 128–29, 135
  prenatal testing and, 462, 463–65, 468, 472–73, 474–76
  resources for, 544–45
  safe, 133–35
  second trimester, 128, 129, 475–76
  sex selection and, 462
  statistics on, 129, 130–31, 136, 315
  teenage, 130, 131, 137
  vacuum aspiration, 127–29, 315
abscesses, 275
abuse, 114, 116–24
  blaming victims of, 118, 123–24
  child, 118, 119–20, 122, 124
  dating and, 118, 120
  getting away from, 118–19
  police and, 118, 119, 121
  psychological factors in, 117–18, 120, 282
  recognition of, 118–20
  resources for, 118, 119, 123, 546–47
  violence and battery in, 53, 116–20, 118, 119–20, 282
  see also incest; rape; sexual harassment
Accutane, 454, 464, 487
acetylcholine, 151
acne, 35, 61, 332, 454, 464

ABOUT THE AUTHOR

DIANA KORTE is an award-winning women's health writer and radio producer. She is the co-author of *A Good Birth, A Safe Birth* and has published articles for The Los Angeles Times Syndicate, and in *Mothering, New Woman,* and *Parade,* among others. Her public radio programs include interview shows and documentaries. She is a frequent lecturer on health issues and has served on local, state, and international health-related boards of directors.